Sven Grawunder

On the Physiology of Voice Production in South-Siberian Throat Singing

Sven Grawunder

On the Physiology of Voice Production in South-Siberian Throat Singing

Analysis of Acoustic and Electrophysiological Evidences

Frank & Timme
Verlag für wissenschaftliche Literatur

ISBN 978-3-86596-172-3

Herstellung durch das atelier eilenberger, Leipzig.
Printed in Germany.
Gedruckt auf säurefreiem, alterungsbeständigem Papier.

www.frank-timme.de

This work I dedicate to all throat singers in South Siberia. They are not only keeping a wonderful singing tradition alive and vital, one that is deeply connected to the local environment and the way of living, and still a true folk art. They also enrich it with new ideas and musical elements and inspire the community of musicians all over the world.

Contents

List of Figures

List of Tables

0.1 Acknowledgements

First of all I need to thank Prof. Volker Gall (Clinics of Johann Wolfgang Goethe University, Frankfurt/Main). He provided me with ideas especially for the development of appropriate methods to be used in the field. I thank my supervisor Prof. Lutz Christian Anders for his helpfulness, agreeing on the acquisition of a laryngograph as a useful tool for the institute and encouraging me greatly during the dissertation process. Also I'm extremely grateful to my second supervisor, Prof. Adrian Simpson, for his support, and for providing me with many useful tips and encouragement to work further on acoustics. Many thanks go to Michael Edgerton for a very inspiring critical discussion, and for providing me with one of the most fascinating manuscripts Edgerton et al. (2003) and for letting me have a look at the endoscopic videos. Surely Ted Levin must be integrated into these thanks, since he provided our contact. I am also obliged to Viktor J. Butanaev, Zoya K. Kyrgys, Mark van Tongeren, and Ludek Brož for kindly making their field recordings available to me for analysis. And I thank Dr. Ernst Röpke and Dr. C. Welzel for their collaboration in obtaining video recordings of fiber endoscopy at the Department for Phoniatrics of Martin Luther University Hospital, Halle, and Jörg Dreyer (engineer at ZAS, Berlin) for his kind assistance and cooperation during the aerodynamic experiment. I am also very thankful to Oliver Ehmer for spending valuable time in adjusting the *Transformer* for my purposes, even though I found another way and never used it. Christoph Walter and Alex King provided me with their help and assistance in filming and video editing. And I wish also to express my gratitude to John Esling, Trân Quan Hai, Viktor J. Butanaev, Zoya Kyrgys, Vjačeslav Kučenov, Sergej Čerkov and Wolfgang Saus for all the inspiring conversations I had with them. I thank my wife Ulli and my daughter Hedi for their tremendous patience while I was not available as partner and papa. Brian and Orin, thank you very much for devoting so much time and for helping me with corrections on the English and for your very valuable comments during the final phase. And I would also like to express my deepest thanks to my colleagues K. David Harrison, Greg D. Anderson and Brian Donahoe for their encouragement and their patience over all the years, and additionally to my German colleagues Ines Bose, Susanne Fuchs and Brigitte Pakendorf for their moral support, back-up and advice in how to write a dissertation without going crazy. And, Josi, Kreatorjane, Franze, Alex, Manuel and Uli, many thanks for your generous help with some tedious numbers and figures. I must also thank my 'chief', Prof. Ulla Hirschfeld, for giving me the great opportunity to work as a graduate at the Institute for Speech Science and Phonetics in Halle, and for being so appreciative of my field expeditions and so helpful and supportive, especially during the final phase of the dissertation. I am grateful to the Volkswagenstiftung for partially covering travel expenses, since parts of the recordings were undertaken in conjunction with the expeditions of an endangered language documentation project situated in the Altai-Sayan-Region (DOBES ASLEP). And last but not least I have to thank my hosts in Kyzyl (Tschoigana, Mergen and Tumen) and all the singers, who have been so nice and friendly to serve as subjects for the field experiments: *Andrej M., Andrej T., Igor, Yuri, Kongar-ool, Kaigal-ool, Anatoli, Sayan, Ajas, Radion, Alim, Stas, Slava, Sergej, Maksim, Oleg, Bady-Dorzhu, Vadim O., Vadim S., Način, Zhenja, Emil, Alexsej, Vadim, Anton, Ajan, Ajan-ool, Sholban, Sedik, Badraa* and *Shanshagaj.*

0.2 Preface

Touring groups of Siberian and Mongolian throat singers and ensembles performing at all festivals no longer cause a sensation nowadays. They can be found in pedestrian zones in bigger metropolises or even in smaller cities in Europe and North America. But their extraordinary vocal techniques continue to evoke the immediate admiration of a large audience, and to hold the attention of researchers all over the world. Since the 1960's (Smith and Stevens, 1967; Smith et al., 1967) a number of attempts have been made to find out what exactly is happening in the singers' throats, how are these strange and sometimes extreme-sounding voice qualities are produced and how this can be explained acoustically (see chapter 1). It is remarkable, too, how variable and alterable throat singing is. Not only are well-known speech and singing styles themselves still in need of further inquiry, and with the recent development of new research methods and techniques, but sophisticated and scientifically well founded theories of throat singing are still lacking. The author's own field expeditions (in 1998, 2000, 2001, and 2002) to Russia and Mongolia encouraged him to apply himself in this dissertation to the experimental study of the characteristics of different voice production types in south-Siberian throat singing. With the exception of a very recent study of Michael Edgerton, Diane Bless and colleagues (2003)[1] most earlier investigations have had to rely only on single subjects (Fuks et al., 1998; Lindestad et al., 2001; Sakakibara et al., 2002c, 2004b). Hence a further goal of this thesis is to provide a large corpus of measured acoustic and electro-physiological data on a number of singers from the field in Hakassia and Tyva. This task largely determined for the choice of methods applied in the field. Additional experiments were undertaken to support and verify predictions based on the acquired experimental field data. Of necessity this thesis still bears traits of a pilot study, due to the relatively unfamiliar subject and the recency of some of the newer methods which have been applied.

[1]At the time of submission of the thesis this manuscript still has not been published, so that its final appearance (including page numbers etc.) could not be taken into account. Nevertheless the author decided to include it into his argumentation because of its outstanding relevance and quality.

0.3 Overview

The organization of the thesis is guided by the main of research on voice. This means instead of other usual structuring where first a chronological review of existing literature would be given, followed by the actual investigations, the author in this work does a subdividing of the different (phonetic) research perspectives (articulation, acoustics, perception) almost right from the outset.

Chapter 1 gives an overview on the context "throat singing in South Siberia" of the subject phenomenon voice production in throat singing. It introduces research questions in the field of physiological phonetics, acoustic phonetics and vocology, which finally lead to the research goals of the thesis.

Chapter 2 focuses on the subject phenomenon and its physiological constituents. Subsequently the few published physical examinations (laryngoscopy, endoscopy etc.) of throat singing (and overtone singing) styles. The author provides some new endoscopic material (applied on himself). Its analysis is added to former discussions on laryngeal settings in throat singing and it leads to preliminary hypotheses about voice production types and vocal tract shape variations in throat singing.

Chapter 3 discusses specifically the research methodology on voice source(s) (glottal source characteristics) and vocal tract characteristics of throat singing applied in the present study. After balancing the needs and possibilities in the field, a filed methodology is suggested and the methods of data acquisition, of data pre-analysis are going to be introduced. Subsequently also the actual data analysis regarding specific parameters are discussed.

Chapter 4 begins with a presentation of the empirical data of the field study: short term analysis of voice parameters. Then questions after correlations of voice source and acoustic phonetics of the vocal tract will be derived and will be led into a preliminary discussion. Subsequently 'smaller' additional experimental settings with one subject are going to be carried out. Within this way a discussion of the enhancement and "articulation" of reinforced harmonics shall be supported with new arguments and hypothesis.

The final **Chapter 5** will bring the results and findings together. It leads into a general discussion and draws further conclusions and questions. It shall also give an outlook on possible continuations in the research of throat singing and overtone singing.

The following **Appendices A and B** encompass a selection of samples of waveform sequences, cascades, and spectrograms, but also the program scripts for the applied automatic data analysis, a glossary of the most used technical terms and the necessary references of involved informants (subjects), recordings and literature.

0.4 Symbols, Abbreviations and Transliteration

The given transliteration of proper nouns and names basically follows conventions in modern Turkology and Slavistics (Comrie, 2001; Johanson, 1998). The relevant characters and transliterations for all native terms used in the text are given in Table 1. In the text they appear in italics.

Cyrillic	[IPA]	Transliteration
ч	tʃ	č
ш	ʃ	š
з	z	z
ж, ,	ʒ, dʒ	ž, dž
	ŋ	ŋ
г,	ɣ	ɣ
х	x	x (or h)
й, я, ю, ё, е	i, j	j, ja, ju, jo, je
	ø*	ö
	ʏ	ü
ы	ɯ	y (or ï)

Table 1: Cyrillic, IPA, and transliteration as used in the text

*For Mongolian the pronunciation of vowels does not match with the representation given in the table. In Mongolian, orthographic <ө> is pronounced [o]. Thus Tuvan <хөөмей> will be *xöömej* and Mongolian <хөөмий> will be *xoomij*.

The individual abbreviations are also introduced at there first appearance in the text. But for better convenience all used abbreviations are given here: For explanation of certain terms please see also the glossary (B.1).

Abbrevations

A	= Republic of Gorno-Altai
AEF	= aryepiglottic folds
AES	= aryepiglottic sphincter
AES-VF	= aryepiglottic-sphincter-vocal-fold (voice)
AQ	= amplitude quotient
CQ	= closed quotient
CiQ	= closing quotient
DEGG	= derived electroglottogram (dLx)
EGG	= electroglottogram (=Lx)
F(V)	= falsetto voice
Gx	= laryngographic signal
H*x*	= Harmonic (e.g. H1 or H12)
H, Ha	= Republic of Hakassia
k	= *kargyraa* (only in filenames)
Lx	= laryngographic signal (EGG)
M	= Mongolia
M(V)	= modal voice
MD	= median
MN	= mean
OQ	= open quotient
OtS	= Overtone Singing
PSD	= spectral power density (power spectral density)
rHs	= reinforced harmonics
RT	= respiration tract
s	= *sygyt* (only in filenames)
SD	= standard deviation
SQ	= speed quotient, skew
Sx	= subglottal voice signal
T	= Republic of Tyva (Tuva)
ThS	= Throat Singing
VF	= vocal folds
VP	= voice production
VPM	= voice (production) mode
VPT	= voice production type
VQ	= voice quality
VT	= vocal tract
VTF	= ventricular folds (false folds)
VTFV	= ventricular fold voice
VTF-VF	= ventricular fold - vocal fold
Vx	= voice (audio) signal
x	= *xöömej* (only in filenames)

Symbols

cps	= cycles per second
dB	= Decibel
Hz	= Hertz
st	= semitones
t	= time
T	=period (cycle)
V	=Volume

Chapter 1

INTRODUCTION

1.1 Subject Context

To treat the two terms, throat singing (ThS) and Overtone Singing (OtS), as synonymous (e.g. Pegg, 2001; Seidner and Wendler, 1997; van Tongeren, 2002) would be justified only if there existed a widely accepted definition that encompassed all the characteristics of both these terms. However, even a classification like: 'singing style which uses emphasized single harmonics (overtones) instead of pitch shifts in order to create melodies', or even simpler "a vocal style in which a single performer produces more than one clearly audible note simultaneously" (Pegg, 2003), would miss already certain integral aspects of both styles. For ThS it is not obligatory to use reinforced harmonics (rHs) (Grawunder, 1999, 2003b; Saus, 2004), yet sometimes there are more than two notes audible. And for OtS, it is not necessarily the case that melodies need to be created. A better approach to a more comprehensive definition would involve an overlapping or intersection, drawing on the fact that OtS and ThS to certain degree share common features, which are mainly the selective modulation of single harmonics which are enhanced against its and the use of a low (non-modal) voice register. And, as will be shown later, both ways of singing use similar articulatory strategies in the oropharynx. In some respects the two genres appear quite similar to each other, even apart from the fact that both are practised in order to make music (almost exclusively in a non-ritual context). But there are major differences. OtS and ThS (1) do not share the same musical principles and concepts ("timbre oriented" versus pitch based) (Ted Levin and Valentina Süzükei, personal communication) (Grawunder, 1999; Kyrgys, 2002; Pegg, 2001), nor (2) do they share the same backgrounds and attitudes. ThS is very tightly bound to folk music and folk art, as opposed to OtS, which is situated in the context of Jazz, Avant-garde Serial and Minimal Music, New Age, and World Music. Previous research (e.g. Dmitriev et al., 1983; Edgerton et al., 2003; Grawunder, 2003b; Neuschaefer-Rube et al., 2001) has pointed to particular specific articulatory and phonatory techniques (strategies) in OtS and ThS. The concrete properties of applied voice production types (VPT), which can auditorily appear as timbre, range (ambitus), and transmitted tension are important in transfer situation, when the technique is being taught. Whereas in OtS VPT seems not to be specific to the concept, VPT (and its timbre) in ThS is essential. For a better understanding of the argumentation and its motivation, it is given here as a rough characterisation of the two different voice genres or ways of singing.

1.2 Throat Singing (ThS)

Throat singing (*Kehlgesang, chant de gorge, горловое пение*) as used here refers to a distinct folk-musical genre in Southern Siberia (or more specifically Southern Central Siberia, see map in figure 1.1). Ethnomusicological research (Aksenov, 1967; Kyrgys, 2002; Pegg, 1992, 2001; Sundui, 2000) shows a distribution restricted to certain areas within the (Republics of the Russian Federation) Rep. Hakassia, Rep. Gorno-Altai, Rep. Tyva[1] and Southern *Kemerovo Oblast* (Šoria), as well as in Western Mongolia. The region in question is located between the Kuznetsk-Basin in the North, the Altai Mountains in the South down to the Mongolian-Chinese-

[1]Tyva is more commonly transliterated as Tuva, which reflects the Russian pronunciation and spelling. Hence also the adjectives, "Tuvan" or "Tuvinian", are derived from Russian "тувинский". A more direct transliteration from the Tuvan would be "Tyva" (Тыва) with the <y> representing a high, unrounded back vowel (<ы> in Cyrillic, [ɯ] in standard IPA, and [ɨ] in turcological convention). Though it would be truer to refer to the people as "Tyva people," which is a direct translation of the Tyvan self-designation "Tyva kizhi," the present work sticks to the more common term "Tuva(n)".

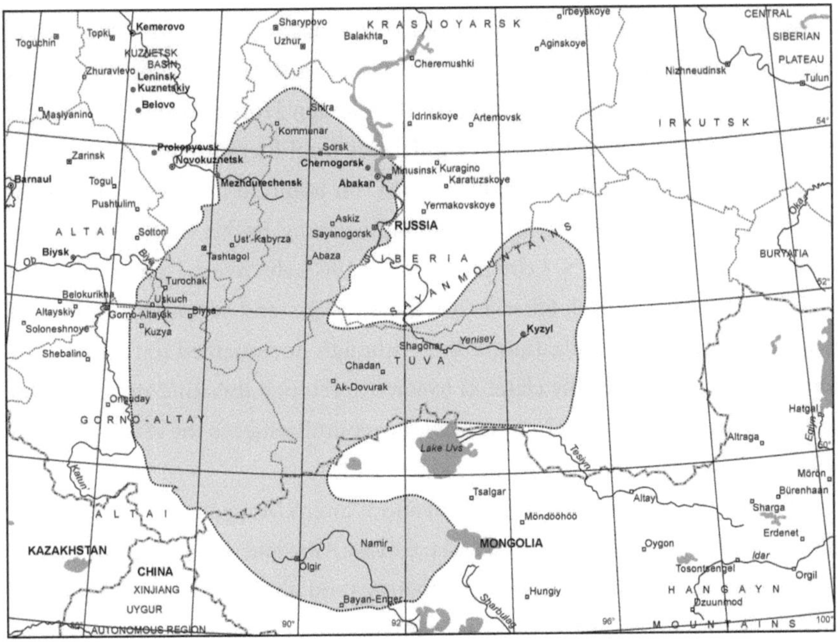

Figure 1.1: South Central Siberia; grey scattered area depicts the approximate area of throat singing as endemic folk art genre

Border, the Sayan Mountains in the East and the steppes of the *Uvs Nuur* Basin in the Southeast.

The marked region in Figure 1.1 shows the area in which it is most likely to find throat singing men. According to records of the *XOOMEJ Research Centre* in Kyzyl there are about 1600 known *xöömejži* ("Throat Singer"), i.e. singers of *xöömej* (Kyrgys, 2002). Even in the Republic of Tyva this would make less than 1% of the population (out of 200,000). According to the author's own research the probable number of singers (*kaiči*) would be about 10-20 in Gorno-Altai and about 20-30 *xajžı* in Hakassia. An approximate number of Mongolian *xöömij* singers (*xöömijč*) might be 150-300 (Wulff, 2001). Throat singing women is subject to a cultural tabu, which is still vivid in the countries listed above. Nevertheless in Tuva and Mongolia there are nowadays also women singing in ensembles, at least in the cities. People (ethnic groups), languages (affiliation to the Turkic language group) and cultural life in the Altai-Sayan-Region all bear the stamps of ancient cultural bonds going back to the Golden Horde (strong Mongolian influence) and show a multitude of similarities (oral literature genres, seminomadic pastural subsistence, kinship system). In addition another region must be included: in the Southern Ural Mountains among Baškir (Baškord) people, the Soviet musicologist L.N. Lebedinskij in the 1930s discovered a musical genre similar to the one in South Siberia. It is called *özljau* and seems to be still vital or in the process of revitalization today. Although documented only with individual singers, who partially claimed to have developed this kind of singing on their own, the timbre and technique used shows similarities to the south-Siberian styles (such as *xöömej* and *sygyt*, see chapter 2.1.1).

Whereas in Central Tuva (Rep. Tyva) and Western Mongolia epic singing and ThS are two separate genres, in Hakassia, Gorno-Altai and Šoria the term *kai/xai* ("ThS") denotes the singing style used mainly (and almost exclusively) for epic singing. The Altai, Hakas and Shor native terms *xai* (*xailaar*), *kai* (*kailaar*) seem related to the Mongolian word *xelex* ("to tell", "to speak") that is used to determine the performance style of story telling, whereas the origin or direction of a possible cultural transfer is hard to determine since epic story telling is a very widespread phenomenon throughout Eurasia, and especially central and middle Asia. The "purpose" of ThS, other than marking the performance of an epic tale and providing self-entertainment and entertainment to others, remains uncertain, but nowadays musical practise tends to show a great detachment from ritual or sacral singing (animistic, shamanistic, burhanist[2], buddhistic). Also the use of ThS for "communicative" purposes, as in Alpine yodeling, can not be described as systemic but only sporadic. Most of the known facts from the first half of the 20th century, like areal distribution and transfer patterns, indicate an association with semi-nomadic pastoralism in the forest steppes and steppes. As one of many other genres of orally transmitted culture in North and Central Asia it has been spread out by and among herdsmen. Those whose profession is that of an epic storyteller (*kaiči* (A), *xajžı* (H), *tooldžu* (T), *tyylč* (M)) partially use the same

[2]prior stadium of a priest oriented monotheistic religion clearly inhering animistic and shamanistic traits

kind of voice production types for 'voice marking' of various characters and for performance enhancement. Besides the gift of musicality, of memory, of narrative performing, and of skillful instrumental playing, the gift of the 'right' voice is and was essential especially to Hakas and Altai epic storytellers (cf. Butanaev, 1998; Pegg, 2001).

Besides very vague Chinese and Mongolian sources from the Middle Ages (cf. Grawunder, 1999; Kyrgys, 1992) and a fairly good description by Manuel Garcia in 1847 (cf. Seidner and Wendler, 1997: 150) about a Baškirean *özljau* singer (Garcia, 1985), there is no record which could clearly be ascribed to throat singing. Surprisingly, other early explorers to these areas, like Philipp Johann von Strahlenberg (1730), Johann Georg Gmelin (1751), Mathias Alexander Castrén and Schiefner (1853), Gerhard Friedrich Müller [about 1760] or Daniel Gottlieb Messerschmidt [1720-1727] do not report on it explicitly in their records. At least, whatever descriptions they did make of singing styles, manner and practises are not unambiguous enough to affirm or recognize a throat or overtone singing style. Hence it remains unclear whether the picture of ThS - as we can observe today - has a history which is centuries old or just a dozen or so decades, reaching back to the mid-19th century, when - according to Kyrgys (2002) and Tatarintsev (1998) - also ethnographs like P.S. Ostrovskih and E.K. Jakovlev described it for the first time.

However myths in Hakassia claim that *xai* (ThS) came from the South, where the *sojon* live (today's *tyva*) (Butanaev, 1998: 281). And nevertheless the Boškordian (Baškirean) musical tradition would provide another reason, since the last Baškir groups are supposed to have moved in the 11th century from South Central Siberia to their new homeland in the West in the Southern Ural mountains (cf. Forsyth, 2000: 25). If this Baškordian singing tradition is a quasi-relict or artefact, it would give a strong argument for a long history of ThS in Siberia.

The first more explicit description, especially on Tuvan ThS, was given by the Soviet ethnomusicologist A. N. Aksenov (1967; 1973). Whereas he speaks of a "double voice solo singing", which has been the established concept among Soviet ethno-musicologists, the American scientists Smith, Stevens and Tomlinson (Smith and Stevens, 1967; Smith et al., 1967), report on Tibetan *mdzo-skad* as just an "unusual mode of chanting". Associations between the two varieties have been made only later Walcott (1974). For an excellent survey of the history of musicological research, historical references and the contemporary state of ThS in Tuva, see Kyrgys (2002).

Only relatively vague reasons can be offered, as e.g. a common history of the Tibetan and Mongolian Empires, the common religion (Buddhism with an animistic background) (incl. exchange of novices) and a similar nomadic subsistence, for also including in ThS a singing technique used in chanting of certain Tibetan monasteries of the Tantra Buddhist *gelugpa* sect. Therefore the monks use a so called *dzo-ke* (*mdzo-skad*) - the bull's voice (*ke*) of a yak-cattle-hybrid (*mdzo/dzo*). Albeit used for a different purpose and in a different musical context (choir), the deep growling voice does sound comparable to the south-Siberian (Tuvan) *kargyraa* and (Altaian) *kai*. For these reasons *dzo-ke* will be treated here as auditorily and therefore supposably "technically" related to the low register styles in Southern Siberia (see chapter 1.3.1 and chapter 2). It will be referred to as Central Asian or simply Tibetan ThS.

South-Siberian ThS, furthermore, must be demarcated from so called throat-games *qattajjaq* (Inuit and Yuit) and *rekutkar* (Ainu) and other special voice techniques, found in Northern and Eastern Siberia and especially those found in the circumpolar regions and sub-arctic regions (*pič eyen* of the Čukči, Even, Evenki, and Koryak) as well as other voice techniques such as *joigan* (Sami) and *oloŋho* (Yakut) (see for discussion Nattiez, 1999). Throat-games (*qattajjaq*) in general seem to feature impulsive, rhythmically structured alternations of short open syllables involving non-periodic non-modal voice (i.e. breath) of different glottal states (breathy, whispered, murmured, open, and closed) and airstreams (ingressive - egressive), with timbre (formant characteristics) serving as a quasi-pitch "anchor" (cf. Charron, 1978). If similarities to Siberian ThS are considered at all, such "melismatic elements" in the vocal techniques of Tuvan folk singing and especially Mongolian *urtin-duu* singing could count as such a similarity (Nagakawa, 1980).

Other, more similar low-register VPTs are found in special voice techniques used in Bahrain, in Corsica and finally among Xhosa women in South Africa. The latter (named *umŋqokolo*)[3] comes closest to the voice quality, timbre and ambitus of certain south-Siberian ThS techniques (Dargie, 1991, 1993; Grawunder, 1999; van Tongeren, 2002; Zemp and Trân, 1991). Unfortunately only very little is known about the status, distribution, elaborateness, usage, origin, transfer and performance practice of *umŋqokolo* (or *umxhube*).

1.3 Overtone Singing (OtS)

Unlike the history of ThS in the Sayan-Altai-Region, the origins of modern OtS are well documented. The starting point is defined by Karl Heinz Stockhausen's vocal concerto "Stimmung" in 1960. Stockhausen, a student of acoustics with Meyer-Eppler in Bonn, used for his composition overtones inherent in the vowel by pitching the voices very high, so that formants and overtones overlay and these ranges become prominent.

During that period other composers like Philip Glass, Luigi Nono, John Cage, Arnold Dreyblatt, Terry Riley and Steve Reich also started to experiment with harmonic components in musical sounds (cf. Edgerton, 2005; Laurion, 1996). Within the avant-garde musical scene OtS was part of other exploratory phases of so-called Minimal Music or Serial Music. It was probably also at that time (late 1970s), however, that the first records of folk music from Mongolia (recording of Robert Hammayon), Tuva ([A1, A2]) and Tibet became available. These recordings may well have influenced composers and performers, who were already independently creating and discovering their own vocal styles. David Hykes is considered to be the founder of the first Overtone Singing choir - the "Harmonic Choir"- in the US in 1975. In Germany the flautist Michael Vetter, who had been among the singers performing in Stockhausen's Stimmung, developed his own overtone singing style ([A53]), inspired by Neo-Buddhistic, New Age, and Avant-garde Music concepts. His students, e.g. Michael Bollmann and Michael Reimann in Germany ([A54, F9]), and others, like Rollin Rachele in the UK, fol-

[3]The closest to be found in the Xhosa dictionary by McLaren (1936: 107r) is *ngqokola* "growl, bellow, (of boys imitating a bull)". The prefix *um-* works as classificator in terms of "human being", and *-a* ending to *-o* ending change is a morphological change in transforming a verb into a substantive. As result *umngqokolo* could be translated as "the bellower, the growler" or "the imitator of the bull's voice".

lowed in the 1980s and began to propagate their own understanding of Harmonic Singing (Bollmann, 1999; Laurion, 1996). Recent influences from south-Siberian ThS and other musical genres (Free Jazz, Traditional Music, and European Folk Music) have enriched the spectrum of OtS. Nevertheless it is a persistent "urban myth", which is believed by many overtone singers themselves and which has even entered the scientific literature (Gundermann, 1994; Klingholz, 1993), that OtS derives directly from Siberian and Central Asian (Tibetan) roots. OtSingers like Saus (2004) and Laurion (1996) have tried to rectify this, emphasizing the autonomy of OtS as its own distinct genre in Western culture. Besides a crossover from improvisational vocal music to world-music, such OtSingers see their traditional ties as being more with medieval Gregorian and Hellenistic singing (see `www.oberton.org`).

Considering the musical scene as a whole, OtS seems as yet to have established little more than a marginal "niche existence". This is perhaps caused by the conceptual unclassifiability or "homelessness"of the voice technique, as it can also be seen in other musical sub-domains that are defined in terms of a single instrument (bagpipe, harmonica; yodelling etc.). Nevertheless the OtS scene itself is still prospering and growing (see e.g. van Tongeren, 2002: 165ff), as increasing numbers of concerts, workshops, websites, and festivals testify.

Indeed, it is not surprising to observe that the Mongolian ThSinger Tserendava performs Western opera melodies and the Swiss performer C. Zehnder sings folk-music-inspired songs using OtS and yodelling techniques ([F11]). Such musical crossbreeding is surely happening all the time and clashes with the concept of "stylistic purity" even less than the routine transfer and adaptation of tunes and melodies (cf. Lomax, 1968: 13).

1.4 Theoretical Context Of Voice Description

1.4.1 Perspectives, Layers and Definitions

In principle it would seem obvious that acoustics, aerodynamics, articulation and perception should be kept apart as different aspects of a phonetic description. In practise, however, this would either mean already having a clear, pre-existing conception of all these terms, an existing concept of all kinds, which is certainly not the case, or it would force us to leave explicit gaps. But even in the more familiar, simpler, two-dimensional realm of perception and acoustics as applied to voice production a clear and unambiguous taxonomy and terminology has still not been developed. Thus, after decades of research it often remains uncertain whether a researcher has described a new phenomenon or just made up a new term. This is especially true for cases of nonmodal phonation (Gerratt and Kreiman, 2001), which have been called diplophonia (Ludlow et al., 1983), diplophonic double pulsing (Klatt and Klatt, 1990), harmonic doubling (Keating, 1980), creak (Laver, 1980), period doubling bifurcation (Svec et al., 1996), pulse register phonation (Hollien, 1974) or vocal fry (Hollien and Michel, 1968). These must be addressed in the context of voice in ThS (and cover only a subset of the occurring phenomena).

A different problem inheres in the term voice quality (VQ) measurement. As Kreiman and Gerratt (1998) put it,

> "voice quality is an interaction between an acoustic voice stimulus and a listener; the acoustic signal itself does not possess vocal quality, it evokes it in the listener. For this reason, acoustic measures are meaningful primarily to the extent that they correspond to what listeners hear" (159).

Since VQ is a perceptual category, it cannot be directly or straightforwardly "measured" at all, only indirectly via the reaction of the listener. Therefore it needs to be emphasized that between evaluated voice quality and acoustic, aerodynamic and articulatory parameters only statistical correlations can be made. Most correspondences which have been made for ThS are based only on assumptions and tentative conclusions.

The various descriptive layers naturally demand a clear taxonomy when going from very detailed to macroscopic views. The taxonomy which follows and which is used in this thesis has been partially adapted and derived from practice in phonetics Crystal (1992); Laver (1980, 2002) as well as from common terminology in vocology (voice research) Titze (1994b) and (ethno-)musicology Sadie (2001); Nettle (2005). Terms that will be dealt with in this context are genre, style, substyle, technique, modus, type, mechanism, (articulatory) strategy, function, principle, concept, pattern, characteristic, and parameter. Most of these will be discussed and defined in this section:

Genre The term genre is defined as a particular style or category of works of art, especially a type of literary work characterized by a particular form, style or purpose. Specifically in music, as a type of music (or singing), a genre would be specifiable in terms of technique, rhythm, melisma, geographical provenience, and application (purpose).

Style as a term denoting "manner, mode of expression, type of presentation" is a complex classification concept which can be based on technique (mechanism, strategy), genre exclusivity (the exclusive use within a genre, what could be defined by text), or musical patterns such as ambitus, beat, meter, rhythmic ornamentation and phrasing. Certainly a style would be defined by a specific VQ which must be acquired as a technique what may vary or not.

Technique Voice technique or singing technique encompasses both phonatory as articulatory strategies to formulate, shape, and embellish both melismatic as static elements of a style. It would include such essentials as breath support, voice production, resonance adjustment (formant shifting, voice onset), and other resonance strategies for voice coloring (velar opening, larynx height, epiglottis position). Voice technique or singing technique can be a very broad and unspecific concept, since the terms also incorporate also the actual interpretation of style.

Mode (Modus) and **Type (Typus)** Mode (modus) involves the way (and manner) a process is carried out (e.g. the way a vocal fold oscillates), whereas the term type (typus) would determine the kind and variety of an entity or category. Both terms occur under a variety of circumstances (e.g. voice production type, phonation mode, articulation type).

Mechanism The term involves the interaction of moving parts, meaning also the transmission of forces between the articulating bodyparts.

Strategy This term is most used in connection with articulatory gestures and their specific performance. Multiple appearance in order to conceive a certain (auditory) phonetic goal. This may be in depend on the context (speech or singing), categorized, grammaticalized or canonized already

Function Function is usually understood here as compound of naturally provided degrees of freedom of a given subsystem in respect to its superordinated environment. Efficiency pathological modal-harmless (aerodynamics) Physiological Patterns is Singing and Speech

Basic concept vs. Basic principle. A good example basic principle is the fact that, in most of the styles in OtS and ThS, various techniques are employed that use a shifting of formants onto harmonics in order to enhance (or reinforce) the harmonics and ultimately to create melodies. This again reveals differences in the basic concepts in ThS and OtS (see above). Especially the *xakas*, *shor* and *altai* epic singers make very little use of reinforced harmonics (rHs) in *xai/kai* to create melodies, which depend more on the specific timbre and pitch. As van Tongeren (1994) points out, there are also styles in Tuvan ThS (e.g. *tespeŋ xöömej*) in which reinforced harmonics do not appear or not necessarily need to appear (see also Kyrgys, 2002).

1.4.2 Principles of Phonation

Biosystem Voice. Since voice in both singing and speech is one of the most complex human processes, a description of the characteristics of voice production and its usage must take into account a bundle of interlocking and interacting cause-and-effect circles. Thus voice and its physically recordable signal necessarily reflect emotional state, congenital and physical background, habitual modulations and settings.

The scheme (Figure 1.2) follows Titze (1994b: 5) and shows the bundle of factors influencing the biomechanical system of 'voice' or voice production respectively. Other interdependencies, especially between external factors, like acoustic environment and auditory feedback, or emotional state and breathing, are not shown in the figure but of course need to be considered too. In this study the relation between the cultural specific accommodated factors (the box in the upper left corner of Figure 1.2) and the voice production with its acoustic correlates has been focused.

Phonation Within the phonetic sciences the term phonation is used "to refer to

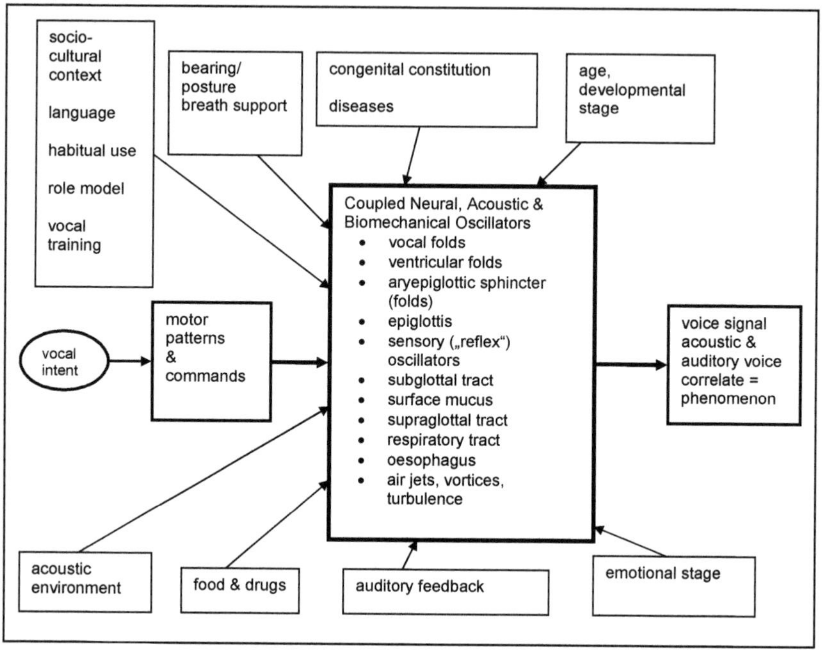

Figure 1.2: Components of voice production

any vocal activity in the LARYNX whose role is one neither of INITIATION nor of ARTICULATION" (Crystal, 1992)

Voice Production (VP) VP is generally described in terms of the myoelastic-aerodynamic theory of vocal fold vibration (van den Berg, 1958), wherein the vibration of vocal folds is induced by a complex combination of aerodynamic, muscular and elastic forces in the larynx. Under a combination of suitable pre-conditions - low glottal resistance, relatively small glottal width, high airflow and high transglottal pressure (difference between sub- and supraglottal pressure) - a single cycle of vocal fold vibration would be produced as follows: Subglottal pressure rises after the vocal folds have been adducted. As soon as the subglottal pressure becomes greater than the medial compression of the vocal folds, they are blown apart and a puff of air escapes into supraglottal space. Given a narrow glottis the airflow (air velocity) increases, and due to the Bernoulli Effect the (intraglottal) pressure decreases in the *rima glottidis*. Subglottal air pressure has also decreased and through combined agency of the Bernouilli Effect and vocal fold elasticity the two folds are sucked together (cf. Schutte, 1980; Hirose, 1997). Modifications to this theory have been proposed, however on the one hand the importance of the Bernouilli Effect has been challenged, and on the other hand airflow has been suggested as factor fostering a flow-induced oscillation as self-sustained mode (Titze, 1980, 1994a). In this respect also subglottal resonance pressure waves have been discussed by Schutte and Miller (1988). An explanation for loud voices on the basis of compressed air bubbles has also recently been suggested by Misun and Prikryl (2002, 2003). The most important event for the speech signal is the abrupt closing of the glottis (see Figure 3.5). This results in a sharp dip in the phonation (air flow) signal, which is responsible for the presence of frequencies up to several kHz in voice(d) signals (Vary et al., 1998: 11).

Phonation Mode vs. Phonation Type The concept of mode needs to be discussed especially in connection with such terms as phonation mode, voice mode and the like. The term Voice Mode was coined by Colton and Estill (1981) in order to refer to different voice (timbre) qualities of emotional expression. The term phonation mode has been applied to such mechanisms as ventricular fold-vocal fold oscillations (Fuks et al., 1998; Kob, 2002), i.e. a non-homorganic non-modal phonatory activity. Given that mode (modus) reflects the way and manner of a process is carried out, the usage of this term has, with regard to a change of the basis for this process, to be rejected. Here it is proposed to use phonation mode either only for varieties of the same VPT that applies different modes of vibrational states and patterns, or in the sense of acoustical or auditory properties. Similarly the term larynx mode was used by Stevens (1977) to refer to "different mechanical action…" but "…in the vocal cords". Since the term phonation mode remains unspecific as to whether it reflects articulatory, acoustic or auditory categories, it will be here preferentially applied in the context of auditory classification, or perception.

Therefore it is proposed to apply voice production type (VPT) to such types of the mechanism of phonation, where different sources or oscillators (vocal folds, ventricular folds, oesophagus, aryepiglottic folds, epiglottis) are used. Phonation type as far as possible should be preferred in the context of auditory categories especially within the linguistic description of phonetic (phonological) entities (Laver, 2002). By analogy, articulation type would then characterize (perceptually) distinguishable articulatory categories (types of articulatory movements).

The term phonation mode will continue to be used for such auditorily evaluated phenomena as tensed, breathy, harsh (Fuks et al., 1998: cf.), whether they are linguistically relevant or not.

Modal vs. Nonmodal Phonation Since the term modal voice originated in the study of vocal registers in singing, it should contrast only with falsetto, whistle and pulse (fry). In a broader phonetic context modal phonation would represent the neutral "unmarked" case and be treated as a phonation type (cf. Laver, 1980: 95) As pointed out above there are several confounded categories of nonmodal phonation. Basically the following classes may be suggested:

MODUS	SUPERPERIODIC PHONATION	BIPHONATION	NONPERIODIC PHONATION
IMPRESSIONISTIC DESCRIPTION	two or more audible coupled pitches	two independent audible pitches	deterministic chaos, noise-like
ALTERNATIVE NAME	subharmonic or period double phonation	diplophonia	creak, fry, breathy

Table 1.1: Classes of nonmodal phonation modes

1.4.3 Voice Production – Source and Vocal Tract

One of the most basic models in the acoustic theory of Voice (Speech) Production is the source filter concept (Fant, 1970), which is a linear theory involving the glottis as source and the vocal tract as a concatenated filter. The laryngeal source spectrum, U(f), is filtered by the vocal tract transfer function, T(f) and the radiation characteristic, R(f), to yield the output spectrum, P(f) Kent and Read (1992).

$$P(f) = U(f)T(f)R(f) \tag{1.1}$$

The equation (1.1) depicts the vocal tract transfer function; P(f) is a coproduct of U(f), T (f) and R(f) where f = frequency. The (ideal) source spectrum would show the amplitude of all harmonics decreasing by around -12dB per octave for a normal vocal quality. This would mean that the harmonics amplitude falls off constantly with increasing frequency, so that for every doubling of frequency the amplitude drops by 12 dB. Source harmonics which fall at or near the peaks of the transfer function of a given vowel (vocal quality) would be amplified by the filter, whereas those which do not come near the peaks and are attenuated. The resulting filter output (oral airflow) consequently has a spectrum that reflects the filter rather than the relatively evenly falling source spectrum. Finally the radiated sound pressure at the lips has a spectrum tilted by approximately +6dB per octave in comparison to the spectral slope of the oral airflow. This radiation effect is due to the acoustic coupling from the mouth to the atmosphere, and it acts like high-pass filter. In reality the source varies dynamically and constantly, reflecting the configuration of the glottis, the degree and type of laryngeal tension, the respiratory effort and the aerodynamic turbulence created by any supraglottal constriction (cf. Kent and Read, 1992; Ní Chasaide and Gobl, 1997).

1.4.4 Voice Quality (VQ)

Basic "Commonly Occurring" Voice Qualities The terms voice quality (VQ) (Laver, 1980), phonatory quality (Gobl and Chasaide, 2003) and vocal quality (Titze, 1994a) have been used synonymously for both singing and speech voice. However, meaning and associated organic and acoustic correspondences of the applied categorical 'parameters' are heavily dependent on the theoretical framework in which they are applied. Thus modal, creaky, whispery, breathy and falsetto appear as phonation types which are partially constrained relative to each other (Laver, 2002: 174). Voice quality labels also appear as parameters in the description and evaluation of voice in singing styles or singing techniques: more generally (and from an auditory perspective) there are voice quality labels which come along with auditory parameters of pitch, timbre, ambit, and noisiness, but also articulatory based ones such as tension, reinforcement, constriction or specific articulatory settings. In part such labels are exclusively used for pathological voice description, meaning that their use already indicates the exceeding of a certain 'psychophonetic' threshold (hoarse, throaty).

Voice Source Variation Frequently used and fairly established (label) categories of voice quality or phonatory quality are given in the following table (1.2). Especially in the discussion of pathologic vocal qualities these terms (roughness/breathiness/hoarseness) had been proven and correlated with acoustical parameters (Anders, 1997; Michaelis, 1999). In singing voice research, however, modal voice is usually regarded as modal register vs. falsetto (loft) vs. vocal fry (sometimes pulse, or even *strohbass*) vs. whistle register. A distinction would also be made between glottalized voice, creaky voice, and pulsed phonation (Titze, 1994b).

Non-Source (supraglottal) Variation Laver (1999) uses for the "phonetic evaluation of voice quality" of speech a selection of categories referring to multiple persisting articulatory settings which are applicable to scalar degrees: pharynx width, lingual root position, lip protrusion, lip rounding, jaw opening, larynx height. Another (more idiosyncratic) terminology (cf. Fischer, 1998; Garcia, 1985) had been established before in the context of research and teaching of the singing voice, which is associated with vocal tract adjustments: epilaryngeal narrowing (diameter and length adjustment of the ventricle and rima ventricularis) with a ring quality, velar coupling with honk and twang, pharyngeal widening with sob or cry (Colton and Estill, 1981) and effective VT lengthening with a covered sound and a muffled quality (cf. Seidner and Wendler, 1997; Titze, 1992).

Covered Voice"A darkened quality obtained by rounding and protruding the lips or by lowering the larynx. The term is likely to stem from covering (fully or partially) the mouth of a brass instrument to obtain a muffled sound; acoustically, all formants are usually lowered and a stronger fundamental is obtained" (Titze, 1994b). Resonant (ringing) Voice is described as having "a voice quality that rings on, 'carries' well; acoustically, ample formant energy is excited" (Titze, 1994b).

Twang (Twangy Voice): A sharp, bright quality, as produced by a plucked string. Twang is often attributed to nasality, but it is probably more laryngeally-based. It is often part of a dialect or singing style. (cf. discussion in Titze, 2001)

Ringing (Resonant) Voice To the contrary is a ringing (resonant) voice: defined by "a brightened quality, apparently obtained by enhanced epilaryngeal resonance, which produces a strong spectral peak around 2500-3500 Hz. In effect, there is a clustering of the formants F3, F4 and F5; the combined resonances are often called the "singer's formant" (Titze, 1994b).

MODAL	normal neutral 'non'-derived "the voice is perceived to be continuous (non-pulsed) and relatively rich in timbre; acoustically, the spectral slope of the glottal source (volume velocity)waveform is on the order of 12-15 dB/octave" (Titze, 1994b)
BREATHINESS	"Impression of turbulence noise and audible escape of air through the glottis due to insufficient closure; vocal folds are vibrating, but somewhat abducted" (Kreiman & Gerratt, 1999: 77) "Breathy Voice: Containing the sound of breathing (expiration) during phonation; acoustically, breathy voice, like falsetto, has most of its energy in the fundamental, but a significant component of noise is present due to turbulence in the glottis. In hyperfunctional breathiness, air leakage may occur in various places along the glottis, whereas in normal voice, air leakage is usually at the vocal processes." (Titze, 1994b)
HARSHNESS/ ROUGHNESS	"Harsh quality is characterized by noisy, rasping, unmusical tone" (Kreiman & Gerratt, 1999: 77) Rough Voice: "An uneven, bumpy quality that appears to be unsteady in the short-term, but stationary in the long-term; acoustically, the waveform is often aperiodic, with the modes of vibration lacking synchrony, but voices with subharmonics can also be perceived as rough." (Titze, 1994b)
HOARSENESS	the combination of rough voice and breathy voice
PRESSEDNESS	(tightness, narrowness) reflects the (mainly) laryngeal constriction Pressed Voice: Phonation in which the vocal processes of the arytenoid cartilages are pressed together, resulting in a constricted glottis with relatively low airflow; there is also medial compression of the vocal fold tissue; acoustically, the fundamental is weakened relative to the overtones." (Titze, 1994b)
THROATINESS	reflects dislocation, misplacement of articulatory patterns especially in the lower pharyngeal area; alternatively "strangled voice" (Laukkanen, Sundberg, & Björkner, 2004)
TENSEDNESS	reflects the associated tenseness in phonation; strained voice, stiff voice

Table 1.2: Pathological vocal qualities and the usually assumed perpectual correlations

1.5 Research Goals

To circumscribe the scope of the inquiry and avoid a completely general discussion of variation in human voice, this thesis sets out to examine only the variation in a described definite context: ThS in the Altai-Sayan region. Accordingly the subject matter is expected to be reasonably homogeneous, given that a particular predefined, culturally conditioned background to the voice usage can be assumed. Rather than looking only at single subjects this study will look at groups of singers in order to describe those groups.

Even though they might turn out to be of the same acoustic or articulatory nature, the other known examples from Europe (Sardia)([65]), Bahrain ([A67]), South Africa (Dargie, 1991, 1993) and Rajasthan (Trân, 1991) will not be considered. Given the very sparse sources for these phenomena, they might easily represent only rare and unique cases, which have arisen spontaneously rather than being transferred[4].

In rough terms, the main aims of this thesis are:

1. discussion of possible VPT used in ThS
    (a) bringing together all the anatomical structures that are known to be involved
    (b) suggesting possible physiological mechanisms
2. developing an adequate noninvasive method for field research on ThS and applying it to research questions on acoustic and electrophysiological properties of different styles
    (a) providing a broader data collection of relevant voice-source measurements
    (b) analysis of source characteristics on the basis of acoustic and other data in order to reveal significant distinctive features for group and style differentiation

[4]Such an isolated example can be found in the singing of an American Country & Western Singer of the 1930s (Arthur Miles)

   (c) presenting hypotheses on voice source (variation) in ThS
   (d) presenting hypotheses on vocal tract function in ThS

3. proposal and introduction of a number of additional experiments for further research into voice source acoustics and acoustic phonetics of ThS
4. discussion of how to extend the implementations of the results to more general research on voice (in speech, singing)

Chapter 2

SUBJECT

2.1 Physiological and Acoustical Correlates of Phonatory Qualities in Throat Singing

2.1.1 Styles in South-Siberian Throat Singing – Ethnomusicological vs. Phonetic Perspective

As noted, voice production types may appear in the context of a specific technique which is defined by a certain style (and sometimes genre, as e.g. epic singing). Besides speculations about a possible ancient age of ThS in South Siberia (cf. Tatarintsev, 1998) one of the other main questions in ethnomusicological research in Tyva is: How many styles are there in ThS? And also: What are the basic styles? What is the basic concept which covers all style definitions, rather than what is the basic principle in all ThS varieties (styles). This is an ongoing debate among singers and singing teachers. For Tyva Sundui (2000) brings into the discussion a perspective which reflects singers' opinions and their perceptions regarding voice generation or production. The singers' notions in her study would support a hypothesis of just two production types in Tuvan ThS, with the styles *sygyt* and *xöömej* on one side and *kargyraa* on the other. And in fact, while ignoring the different techniques and modulations of rHs, it is also possible to arrange the ThS styles throughout Southern Siberia in a classification of just two registers (see table 2.1), indicating, this would be a very simple (or rather simplified) division by source quality (VPT), which also demarcates ranges of fundamental tones. Within the registers a further distinction could then be made between different modes of enhanced harmonics singing, caused by different articulatory strategies.

ThS in	Tyva (xöömej)	Mongolia (xoomij)	Bashkir (özlyau)	Hakas (xai)	Altai (kai)	Shor (kai)	Tibet (yang)
middle register	*sygyt* *xöömej*	*xoomij*	*özljau*	*syyyrtyp* *külenge* *xai*	*sybysky* *kiomioi*	*kai*	*dzo-ke*
low register	*kargyraa*	*xarxiraa*		*xai*	*kai,* *karkiraa*		*dzo-ke*

Table 2.1: Division of south Siberian throat singing into two "registers"; style names (cells) correspond either in register (rows) or area (columns)

Of course is this a perspective which is not oriented to a general ethnomusicological view. The latter type of approach would indicate a Tuvan system of at least 3 or 5 basic styles and a considerable number of auxiliary styles, para- and substyles, according to native terminology. Another recently applied approach is to derive all styles from the single feature: *xörekteer*. This Tuvan term is a derived verb from the root *xörek* ("chest"), so it would mean roughly 'to chest'. It is already used in Tuvan in the meaning "to raise sbs. voice, to shout" . This concept "to sing with the chest" (alternatively: "to sing with a chesty tone or voice") seeks to provide a common basis for all (Tuvan) throat singing styles. But this approach seems also to be reflected by the native conceptualization of ThS in Tyva (cf. Kyrgys, 2002: 79). Also the word *xöömej* and its suggested etymology ['throat, larynx, lower pharynx' (cf. Tatarintsev, 1998)] would support the basic concept (see above). But how homogeneous are ThS styles even within a single region (e.g. in Tyva or Hakassia)?

The terminological and conceptional distinction of styles in Tyva and Mongolia is actually more complex. **Tuvan styles** are partially named according to sound description: *sygyt* ("whistle"), *kargyraa* ("to caw, to croak"), *birlaŋnaadyr* ("to glimmer"), *borbaŋnaadyr* ("to wallow, to roll"), *čylandyk* ("cricket" a birds name), *kaŋzyp* ("to sob"). Only *xörekteer* ("to chest"), *dumčuktaar* ("to nose"), tespeŋ("pressed") and *ezeŋgileer* ("to stirrup" from *ezeŋgi*, "stirrup") reflect the manner of production. Tuvan style labels are often onomatopoetic and are sometimes named after a person, i.e. a performer who has become well known for his individual way of singing (*Gombu, Gennadi Tumat, Oidupa*). **Mongolian style** names, as commonly presented (Pegg, 1992; Trân, 1991) reveal a different system. Their names evoke the image of a certain resonator or better the body (surface) sensation (IN Odsuren Badraa)[1] and its imagined origin: *tagnain xoomij* (*palatal xoomij*), *bagalzuuryn xoomij* (*labial xoomij*), *xevlin xoomij (belly xoomij)*, *xamryn xoomij (nose xoomij)*, *cedžnij xoomij (chest xoomij)* and *xarxiraa (croak)*. The style *xarxiraa* whose name corresponds in appearance to Tuvan *kargyraa* is sometimes even treated as separate from *xoomij*, and it can receive the same kinds of attributes as *xoomij*. Focussing now only on Mongolian and Tuvan ThS styles, since these seem to be the most diversified in Southern Siberia, another (more articulatory) perspective can be applied.

The grouping in table 2.2 is still very rough and is led again by a register distinction. The middle register is undoubtedly detached from low register and differs clearly in pitch, timbre and phonation mechanism type. Therefore these two registers are determined as phonation modes (PM1 and PM2). But a third high register is also sometimes used, e.g. in Hakas, Tuvan and Mongolian folk singing. This encompasses other ornamental techniques which use a tensed head or falsetto voice and very short and fast register downshifts between falsetto and modal register (Hasumi, 1980; Pegg, 2001). From mapping of *xöömej* in Tuva it becomes also obvious that combinations on the basis of different characteristics are 'allowed', e.g. *xöömej kargyraazy* or *borbaŋnaadyr*.

Aksenov (1967) and (van Tongeren, 1994: 24) have given musical ranges of the fundamentals and harmonics used in the different styles (Table 2.3). However, it remains unclear, if these findings hold true for a large group of singers, how this pitch preference could be explained.

"(S)ongs without text" is one of the earlier labels and characterizations used by the first investigators of ThS Jakovlev, Ostrovskix, and Grumm-Grzhimailo (cf. Tatarintsev, 1998)(cf. Vajnštejn, 1988). This may reflect an overall auditory

[1]personal comunication (Ulan-Bator, June 2002)

impression, since long improvisational vocal passages seem to be a basic feature of the genre in Inner Asia, rather than "plain" sung text. This tendency may have begun to change in recent times in Tuva (and Mongolia?), however, at least for some performance practice. Song texts and melodies (or tunes) would then have been mostly adapted from traditional or popular folk songs. Those text passages could either be performed exclusively by means of a ThS 'register' or alternated by such passages without words as a kind of phrasing. Presumably in Altai, Shoria

QUASI register	PM	TUVAN XÖÖMEJ		MONGOLIAN XOOMIJ
high falsetto register	1	*epic tale singing* *certain songs* *(praise, lament)*	*fairy tale singing*	*long songs, laments, praise songs, türlegt, xevlin xoomij*
middle register	1	*sygyt* *xöömej* *tespeŋ*	*kaŋzyp* *borbaŋnaadyr* *ezeŋgileer*	*tšedžiin xoomij, tagnain xoomij, uruulyn xoomij*
low register	2	*čylandyk* *(sygyt kargyraazy)* *borbaŋnaadyr* *(borbaŋ kargyraazy)* *ezeŋgileer* *(ezeŋgi kargyraazy)* *dag-kargyraa*	*xöömej-kargyraa* *tespeŋ* *xovu-kargyraa*	*xailax** *xarxiraa*

Table 2.2: Tuvan and Mongolian basic ThS and folk singing styles sorted by singing registers and corresponding phonation mode (PM); numbers in the PM column refer to single cycle and double cycle modes (see chapter 2); * It stays unclear whether this singing style of the epic tale performance does actually belong to low register voices or there are just some recordings (e.g. B.2.1 rec: 34), which are reminiscent of them.

	xöömej	*sygyt*	*kargyraa*	*borbaŋnadyr*	*ezeŋgileer*
PITCH OF THE FUNDAMENTALS	c-f	d-g	C-E	F G	c C
HARMONICS OR PARTIALS USED	6, 8, 9, 10 12	6, 7, 8, 9, 12, 13, 14	7, 8, 9, 10, 11, 12	6, 7, 8, 9, 10, 12	7, 8, 9, 10, 12, 13

Table 2.3: Perceived musical ranges of fundamental pitch regarding several Tuvan ThS styles

and Hakassia *xai/kai* has only been recently (in the last 50 years) adapted stylistic features as known from *xöömej*, *xoomij* and *özljau*, namely (Grawunder, 1999; van Tongeren, 2002). So e.g. the styles *sygyt* (T), *sygyrtyp* (H, A), or *sikit* (A) appear not only from their name ("whistle, whistling") very similar. This is an ongoing process of mutual influence among the singers, and it is especially maintained since nowadays revitalization of traditional music, including re-creation of traditions and self-identity finding processes are also supported also by the audience.

Table 2.6, as a kind of continuation of Table 2.2, introduces a classification regarding the timbre and harmonic appearance of south-Siberian ThS styles which reflect not register or phonation mode/type but (musical) articulation of reinforced harmonics and formants. This order would lead us to the different main strategies in articulating enhanced harmonics (see section 2.4.2). The French ethnomusicologist Trân Quan Hai had introduced the terms of one-cavity technique and two-cavity technique as a basic principle in the description of his method of overtone singing, implying there from an analogy with the techniques used in all styles of ThS. Following his mapping, such styles as *kargyraa, xarxiraa xoomij, borbaŋnaadyr* and ("deep") *xöömej* would be classified as one-cavity styles because the singer would use only one (oral) cavity while producing overtones. Others styles like *sygyt, tšedžnii xoomij* or *sybysky* would be called two-cavity technique because here the oral cavity is devided by tongue into two separate cavities Trân and Guillou (1980); Trân (1991).

An essential principle in explaining the types in Table 2.4 is the demarcation of VPT, which is based on the introspection of singers (see Sundui, 2000; Fuks et al., 1998; Grawunder, 1999; Kyrgys, 2002; van Tongeren, 1994). Note that Kyrgys and van Tongeren do not agree on the assumption of *xöömej* and *sygyt* produced by the same VPT, although Kyrgys' model (Kyrgys, 2002: 82) assumes *xörekteer* as origin or base of all other styles (incl. *sygyt, xöömej* and *kargyraa*, with substyles). So far Table 2.4 is based on the VPTs that are used in ThS (espec. Tuvan), though it does not reflect the quantitative extent of the various VPT usages, i.e. especially type 2 might occur only rarely. But presumably the table does not reflect totally isolated or deviant phenomena. The focus in this work

	1	2	3	4	5
PHONATION TYPE/ VOICE PRODUCTION TYPE	kargyraa 1	kargyraa 2	kargyraa 3	xöömej/ xörekteer (sygyt) xoomij	xörekteer /xöömej
VQ DESCRIPTION	fry, "raspy"	growling, rough	soft pulse	tensed, pressed	tensed, stiff
EXAMPLE	kargyraa [GT]	kargyraa [TK], umŋqokolo [NM]	kargyraa [DB, SI]	xoomij [TG]	xöömej [KX]

Table 2.4: Rough categorization of "voice modes"(phonation modes) used in Tuvan ThS based on auditory observations and informant's introspectives

will be not on any theoretical ethnomusicological question in terms of style differentiation or systematization, but on the investigation of VPTs as actually used in ThS. Ideally this would involve a differentiation which is based just on acoustic and (easily obtainable) electrophysiological data rather than on semi-invasive imaging procedures.

Following Grawunder (1999, 2003a,b) this non-invasive methodology has been shown to be feasible in the framework of other descriptions of differences in vocal style (Stone et al., 2003). It is suggested that group style behaviour be correlated with voice source selected and with other parameters. In previous research vocal quality of ThS has already been evaluated by others, so that the tentative compilation of attributes given in Table 2.6 is possible.

The middle register in ThS is often associated with "stiff", "tensed", "pressed", or "strained" voice (Klingholz, 1993; Sakakibara et al., 2003; Trân, 1991). Interestingly, in Tuvan ThS the style *tespeŋ* ("pressed") would be according to its label the only style of this kind, which would rule out an absence of such a category in the native concept of *xörekteer* (which means in fact "to chest", see above). Tuvan singers also evaluate Mongolian ThS as more pressed and tensed than their own ThS phonation. The lower register has been described as "rough, raspy, growling" voice (Fuks et al., 1998; Lindestad et al., 2001; Sakakibara et al., 2002b; Trân, 1991).

To a trained ear, meaning experienced listeners (singers, musicologists, etc.)

of ThS in South Siberia, there is usually no problem at all in distinguishing between ThS recordings from different regions. It is questionable if the same could be proven also for context-free samples of e.g. sustained vowels or other stable passages. Nevertheless, it is one of the aims of the present work to ultimately provide some arguments for a differentiation based on acoustic and other experimentally measurable properties of VQs. This work is explicitly not intended to provide an analysis of any musical structure present in ThS (see for these Aksenov, 1967, 1973; Kyrgys, 2002; Levin and Edgerton, 1999; Sundui, 2000; Süzükei, 1993; van Tongeren, 1994), though some musical features (e.g. formant structure and rHs) may impinge on the analysis.

Since those qualities (see Table 2.5) reflect a certain assignment in the field of pathology-linked terminology for phonation types (diagnostics), the question arises as to whether those modes voice pathology belong here, meaning that a certain "hazard" is coupled with the extensive use of such techniques. On what bases are they differentiated? Is there a certain threshold? ... of what parameters? Are they differentiable at all? At this point it needs to be made clear that this work does not aim to provide evidence for a potential impact of use or abuse of certain voice techniques in ThS. Rather it aims to contribute to the description of variance and extreme ranges the human voice can be used in. The ThS voices are of course characterized as "extra-normal" (cf. Edgerton, 2005), but according to my experience ThS performers strive in the same way for perfection in terms of voice brilliance, transparency and economy of effort (breathing, support and tension) as singers in other genres do.

AUTHOR	SUBJECT/OBJECT	VOICE QUALITY ATTRIBUTES GIVEN BY THE AUTHORS
Adachi (Adachi & Yamada, 1999)	"xöömij" (M)	pressed
Trân (Zemp & Trân, 1991)	xoomij (Mongolia)	tensed, stiff
Gunji (Gunji, 1980)	xoomij (M)	tensed
Lindestad (Lindestad et al., 2001)	modal (bass range)	sonorous and slightly hyperfunctional/pressed
Sakakibara (Sakakibara et al., 2003)	xöömej (Tuva)	pressed
Smith (H. Smith& Stevens, 1967; H. Smith et al., 1967)	dzo-ke (Tibet)	sonorous, pulsing
Esling (Esling, 2002a)	dzo-ke (Tibet)	resembling tense/harsh/ low-tone register in Bai
Lindestad (Lindestad et al., 2001)	low register (Mongolian "kargyraa")	extremely low pitched, high intensity, sonority, slight press
Tsai (Tsai, 2003)	kargyraa (xarxiraa)	pulse like
Sakakibara	"kargyraa" (Mongolia)	growl voice
Deutsch (Deutsch & Fördermayr, 1992)	sygyt (Tuva)	[tensed]
Grawunder (1999)	xöömej (Tuva)	[throaty, tensed]
Klingholz (Klingholz, 1993)	overtone singing	[stiff voice, tensed]
Van Tongeren (2002: 64-65)	xovu-kargyraa xöömej sygyt (Tuva)	 constrained pressed, tight
Anlauten, Harvilahti (Aulanko & Harvilahti, 1999)	kai	"even creaky laryngeal VQ"
Walcott (Walcott, 1974)	xoomij (Mongolia)	nasal character above melodic range
Ellingson (1970: 70)	dzo-ke (Tibet)	vocal fry-like, inspiratory like
Fuks (Fuks et al., 1998)	kargyraa (Mongolia)	pulse register -like
Fuks (Fuks et al., 1998;	voice growl	growling
Sakakibara, Fuks, Imagawa, & Tayama, 2004b	voice growl	growling

Table 2.5: VQ attributed to ThS styles from different authors within the scientific literature; the table resembles most known publications of 'phonetic' research on throat singing

Class	Atype	Generalized auditory description	Tyva	Mongolia	Hakassia, Altai	others
A	1	ThS with a high whistling overtone as melodical "leader", very prominent	*sygyt, čylandyk (sygy-tyŋ kar-gyraazy), borbaŋ-naadyr*	*tagnain xoomij, xarxiraa*	*xai, kai (sygyrtyp, sikit)*	*özljau 1*
B	2	ThS with a mid high whistling tone, less prominent than A (vowel quality hardly to perceive)	*xöömej, ezeŋgileer, borbaŋ-naadyr, xöömej kargy-raazy*	*xarxiraa*	*xai, kai (kölenge)*	*özljau 2*
C	3	ThS with a (clearly) per-ceivable vowel quality	*xöömej, kargyraa*	*xarxiraa*	*xai, kai*	*dzo-ke*
D	4	Humming (A) and Hum-ming (B) with (nearly) closed mouth	*dumčuk-taar, xaajing xöömej/ kargyraa*	*xamryn xarxiraa*	*unspecified*	

Table 2.6: Tentative and rough classification by auditory description of vowel and voice quality; second column gives articulation types (Atype) in anticipation of chapter 2.4.1, according to observable articulation strategies

2.1.2 Physiological Phonetics of Throat Singing

The differentiation of OtS and ThS suggested by Grawunder (1999, 2003a) is based on the hypothesis of certain cardinal anatomical features which are exclusive to (or at least highly characteristic of) OtS and ThS; these would be primarily the ventricular folds (VTF) and the (upper) aryepiglottic sphincter (AES) as articulator and source. The behaviour of these anatomical features has been observed in previous research (Edgerton et al., 2003; Esling, 2002b) (see chapter 2.3.1.5). Additionally an assumption was made in the author's earlier work about the usage of the aryepiglottal folds as an alternative voice source for ThS styles belonging to the suggested phonation mode 2 (see chapter 2.5.3) (Grawunder, 2003a,b). The involvement of these structures may also provide justification for the term throat singing at least from a physiological perspective. The exact biomechanisms (tissues, forces and neural control) at work in the suggested laryngeal configuration are still a matter of controversy (Kotby et al., 1991; Kruse, 1981; Reidenbach, 1998b; Rethi, 1952). It is for instance not that apparent which specific muscular and neural structures are involved in the upper sphincter. Nor is it clear to what degree which structures are involved since multiple mechanisms may intertwine spatiotemporally as seen in voice registers?

From the standpoint of (physiological) phonetics and vocology a central question is: What makes the difference to other (known) voice production types and articulatory uses of these supraglottal structures? In particular, what makes the difference between *dysphonia plica ventricularum* ["Taschenbandstimme"] a la Panconcelli-Calzia (1953), Kruse (1981) and van Buuren (1983)? How could this be brought into relationship with creaky voice, pulse register phonation or vocal fry, since there too an involvement of supraglottal structures has been suggested (Blomgren et al., 1998; Henton and Bladon, 1988)? How is such a singing 'device' comparable to similar linguistically relevant configurations? And with regard to the tensed (/pressed) phonation mode 1, how could the difference to hyperfunctional or spasmodic pressed voice in non-pathological terms be described? How generally used and widespread is such a supralaryngeal setting in normal voice use (speech and singing)?

2.1.3 Voice Sources in Throat Singing

Chernov, Maslov and Dimitriev were to do the first physiological research on Tuvan ThS (see chapter 2.3.1.1) especially the styles (*sygyt, xöömej*) featuring a prominent whistling sound. They described ThS as "double voice singing" (Chernov and Maslov, 1987) and argued that only a whistle-like device could generate such prominent sound. The possibility of an interaction of harmonic scale and superimposed melodic tone was completely ignored. On the other hand several observations have been made on spectral slopes in ThS regarding a strong high ostinato acting "independently" from the melodic overtones, which needs to be explained. Based on the observations (given in 2.1.1) and on preliminary research Edgerton et al. (2003); Fuks et al. (1998); Grawunder (2003a); Lindestad et al. (2001) it is plausible to associate the suggested phonation modes with patterns of the different signals reflecting the source (glottal flow, EGG). At the moment, however, it remains questionable if any of the available oscillation models (body cover model, multimass model, air bubble model) or voice source models (LF-Model, KLSYN88, see also chapter 3.3.2.5) could also be applied to the vibrating VTFs, AEFs, since - as will also be shown later - it is not always clear to what extent the VTFs and AEFs are involved and which vibratory pattern they follow. Therefore it may be appropriate to discuss alternative models as suggested by Fuks et al. (1998), Tsai (2003) and Sakakibara et al. (2002a, 2003). The voice function of as acoustic and aerodynamic voice sources as such also needs to be looked at in order to explain such characteristics as spectral slope and also the classification of the different voice types under certain voice qualities. Other special phenomena like voice onset and offset (harsh glottal stop or pressed glottal release) can be expected to reveal predictions about specific transglottal pressure adjustments in ThS.

2.1.4 Vocal Tract in Throat Singing

Rejecting a "double source generator" as the explanation for sound production of the whistling melodic tone occurring in certain ThS styles, it still remains an open question how this enormous enhancement or reinforcement in the spectrum works Edgerton et al. (2003). Of course the term reinforcement brings VT properties and their function in Source-Filter-Theory into the argumentation. A preliminary comparison of examples from ThS with those of OtS Grawunder (2003a) leads to the assumption, that the effective enhancement of a single harmonic for both singing types in good singers may be not very different. Nevertheless it has to be enquired how the reinforcement of harmonics and the specific timbre changes and stylistic features specifically in ThS are obtained. It was suggested by Bloothooft et al. (1992) and Klingholz (1992) that not (only?) voice source but the interacting VT has to be responsible. So, Klingholz argued for an increased stiffness of the VT walls. Regardless the impropriety of this theory, consequently the amplitudes of partial tones (harmonics) to be looked at in their relation to formants and bandwidths. The "effort" of reinforced harmonic shifts or better formant shifts in the relation of articulatory movements and resulting time-frequency alterations. Because of the various constrictions, including the constriction close to the larynx, stronger feedback effects can reasonably be expected. It would thus not be very surprising to observe coupling effects between the resonators. Especially the described ostinatos and the ringing quality that have been described may be linked in that way (see chapter 2.4.2). Additional testing of tuning effects caused by selective lip rounding reveal a specific radiation function. But the source is also closely coupled to the whole respiration tract, which would be expected to have an effect on the first formant. A further question involves the nasal coupling and its tuning effect for certain several ThS styles, namely *xamryn xoomij* (M), *dumčuktaar* (T), and *ezeŋgileer* (T). A search for 'places' of enhancement, i.e. looking at associated articulatory modes and the corresponding resonators (R1, R2, R3, R4, R5), would also require an appropriate procedure for VT-movement tracing and VT measurement (MRI, EMMA, ultrasound etc.) but is certainly remaining for further research.

2.2 Specific Anatomy of Certain Laryngeal Structures

The following four sections discuss the anatomic structures of the lower vocal tract, specifically those of the larynx entrance.

2.2.1 Basic Functional Anatomy of the Larynx

A basic function of the larynx clearly inheres in the closure of the airways (trachea) and so in preventing possible inhalation of foreign objects. The organization of laryngeal musculature could be described as a system of three sphincters (cf. e.g. Rohmert, 1991: 17):
(1) the sphincter internus, composed of the intrinsic larynx muscles: *m. vocalis* (VOC), *m. thyreoarytenoideus* (TA), *m. cricoarytenoideus lateralis* (LCA), *m. interarytenoideus* (IA) (*mm. arytenoideus transversus* and *obliquus*) and *m. cricoarytenoideus posterior* (PCA),
(2) the sphincter externus, composed of the *m. cricothyreoideus* (CT) and *m. constrictor pharyngis inferior* (only this sphincter also encloses the pharynx),
(3) and the upper sphincter, formed by the epiglottis (EP), aryepiglottic folds (AEF) and ventricular folds (VTF). The upper sphincter would include the *m. aryepiglotticus* (prolonged fibers of *m. arytenoideus obliquus*), *m. ventricularis* and *m. thyroepiglotticus* (as the vertical part of TA), which are still part of the intrinsic laryngeal muscle system since they are (supposed to be) controlled by the inferior larynx nerve (*n. recurrens*, RLN). In general it seems widely accepted that the RLN innervates the intrinsic laryngeal muscles while the external branch of the superior laryngeal nerve (SLN) innervates the cricothyroid muscle. Kruse (1991) describes a secondary laryngeal function: vocal folds (VF) and ventricular folds (VTF) here make up a double valve system, which stabilizes the thorax in cases of outward (distal) movements of the limbs. This stabilizing function should be considered as one of the triggering factors of the upper sphincter constriction. Basic features of laryngeal adjustments (Hirose, 1997) for the different phonetic conditions are (1) abduction vs. adduction of the vocal folds, (2) constriction of the supraglottal structures, (3) adjustments of the length, stiffness and thickness of the vocal folds, (4) elevation and lowering of the entire larynx. As a result, al-

terations in pitch, loudness, penetration power, timbre, noisiness and phonatory quality are observed. The laryngeal framework is made up of five basic cartilages: epiglottis, thyroid, cricoid and two arytenoid cartilages, connected by a cricothyroid joint and two cricoarytenoid joints. Movements of the cricothyroid joint (rotation influencing the length of the VFs) are controlled mainly by CT and the cricoarytenoid joints (abduction, adduction) are mainly controlled by the intrinsic laryngeal muscles (PCA, TA, IA, LCA). Hence PCA is the only abductor, and so the default tendency in larynx configuration is adduction (by TA, IA, LCA). Elongation of the VFs is achieved by contraction of CT, and LCA causes a vertical inward turning of the arytenoids for the phonatory "whisper configuration". VOC as medial part of TA contributes to the effective mass and stiffness of the VFs. The entire larynx is suspended in a framework of extrinsic larynx muscle and ligaments, of which suprahyoid and infrahyoid as well as the pharyngopalatal muscles are primarily involved. As pointed out above, non-modal phonation is considered to be induced especially by vertical larynx movement and supralaryngeal constriction. Hence the mechanisms involved and the underlying anatomical structures need to be examined.

2.2.2 Ventricular Fold (*plica ventricularis*) and Ventricular Voice (VTFV)

Histoanatomy Ventricular fold (false vocal fold) anatomy and histo-anatomy have been investigated only very sparsely and marginally. One very inconsistently described aspect of the anatomy of the laryngeal ventricle is the muscle morphology, such as the proportion of muscular tissue especially in the medial part of the vestibular or ventricular or false folds (see table 2.7). Thus Kotby et al. (1991) found in 16 specimens a "superior thyrorytenoid muscle", which consisted of round or oval bundles "...coursing from near the upper border of the inner surface of the thyroid lamina to the muscular process of the arytenoid cartilage and lying lateral to the fibres of the thyroepiglotticus and thyroarytenoideus..." (398).

In her examination of plastinated serial sections of 32 adult larynges Reidenbach (1998b) succeeded in finding three different layers distinct from the thy-

Zemlin, 1984 (after Kotby et al., 1991)	Kotby (Kotby et al., 1991)	Kruse (Kruse, Kleinsasser, & Schönhärl, 1975) supported by Mielke and Tonndorf	Schiel, Olthoff, Kruse (2003)	Reidenbach (1998b)
in 6 out of 15 unilateral in 6 out of 15 bilateral	16 out of 20 subjects	isolated fibres "almost alsways"	8 out of 10 subjects	32 out of 32 subjects

Table 2.7: Proportion of findings of muscular tissue in the ventricular folds per investigated subjects

roarytenoid muscle. First, there is a posterolateral muscle layer (PLM) that courses in a sagittal direction and as a separate fibre parallel to the free margin of the VTF. Then, "towards the anterior half or third of the vestibular fold, the PLM split into an anterolateral (ALM) and anteromedial muscle layer (AMM)... " Whereas the anteromedial muscle layer appeared to be more variable, the structures of the anterolateral muscle layer and the posterolateral muscle system (PLM) remained fairly constant. So, it seems that Kotby's superior TA corresponds to Reidenbach's PLM. Schiel et al. (2003) made a complementary examination of 10 larynges and described *m. ventricularis* also as coursing isolated from the fibres of LTA within the tissue of the VTF parallel to its free margin towards the medial axis of the vertical part of the *sinus morgagni.* By contrast, LTA fibres would course in the septum of the ventricle laterally to the VTF.

Medial "Supraglottic" Compression - Approximation of the Ventricular Folds. Kruse (1981) suggested a different explanation and concept from that of Rethi (1952). Since Rethi had derived the function of *m. aryepiglotticus* (as part of *m. obliquus*) as the laryngeal component of the stylopharyngeal system, this ought to serve as the main function in the mechanism of the ventricular voice. Even though there are fibres (*m. stylopharyngeus, m. palatopharyngeus* vs. *m. aryepiglotticus*) drawing in opposite directions and joining each other, nonetheless a common innervation could not be proven. In clinical voice treatment it is

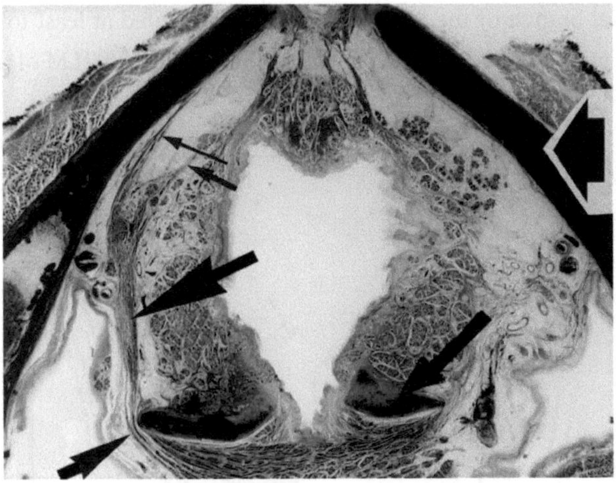

Figure 2.1: Horizontal section at the level of the VTFs (after Reidenbach, 1998b): "Left side: the posterolateral muscular system (PLM) of the vestibular fold [large arrow] splits into an anterolateral (thin long arrow) and a weak anteromedial portion (thin short arrow). Lateral muscle fibers of the PLM may extend beyond the lateral margin of the arytenoids cartilage [small thick arrows]."

a well-known fact, that medial compression of the VTFs (e.g. as a compensatory function) is not impaired after RLN paralysis. It is assumed that this movement is controlled by the internal branch of the SLN. This finding has been sofar supported by a number of authors (Reidenbach, 1998b; Sanders and Mu, 1998; Schiel et al., 2003). Hence Kruse suggested the agency of *m. ventricularis* as an alternative mechanism of VTF medial compression. According to Reidenbach's findings a contraction of the PLM and ALM probably forces the entire tissue mass of the vestibular fold towards the midline, i.e., acts in an adductor manner. "This effect may be enhanced by the action of the weaker AMM. If the AMM is pushed into a horizontal orientation by the periepiglottic adipose tissue, its muscle fibers may exert an additional downward pressure onto the vestibular folds" (Reidenbach, 1998b). It can so also be assumed that the AMM demonstrated by Reidenbach probably corresponds to the ventricular muscle described by Kruse et al. (1975); Kruse (1981). Kruse's *m. ventricularis* was also shown to extend medially to the laryngeal ventricle in an oblique orientation. Additionally, a "motor component of the internal branch of the SLN has been demonstrated at least to supply the transverse arytenoid muscle, which may be connected to the PLM of the vestibular fold"(Reidenbach, 1998b).

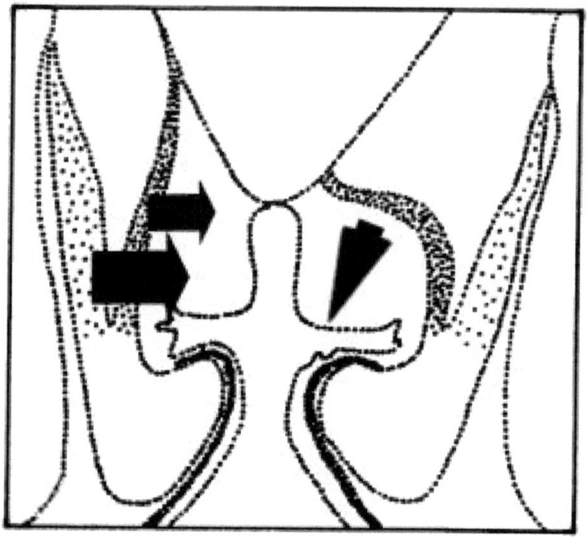

Figure 2.2: Suggested mechanism during medial contraction of the VTFs (after Reidenbach, 1998b: 367), frontal section of the larynx: "contraction of the anterolateral(ALM; single dots) and antero-medial muscular system (AMM; dense dots) pushes the entire tissue mass of the vestibular fold medially (arrows, left side). In addition, the AMM may exert a downward pressure on the vestibular fold (arrowhead, right side)."

Ventricular Fold Phonation and Ventricular Fold-Vocal Fold-Phonation
Ventricular voice or ventricular fold phonation (VTFV) appears in the clinical literature mostly within two contexts: first as a result of tissue disturbances as *dysphonia ventricularis*, second as an extreme of hyperfunctional voice production (sometimes also called dysphonia ventricularis). The latter was also determined to occur as intended ('desired') ventricular phonation, but only in cases of VF paralysis or after a cordectomy. Ventricular phonation would then count as a compensatory phonational process or VPT. In carrying out voice pathology diagnoses, (Colton and Casper, 1997: 309) also suggested that the descriptive term

ventricular phonation be used instead of dysphonia plica ventricularis in order to remain neutral as to the underlying etiology of behaviour. Ventricular phonation as intended voice register has been acknowledged only recently in the context of observations on ThS or ThS-like simulations (Fuks et al., 1998; Lindestad et al., 2001, 2004). In this connection a ventricular fold-vocal fold phonation type has been described, where VTFs and VFs oscillated either in phase or in a double-cycle pattern of a conjoined VTF-VF cycle and single VF cycle. Thus, the two pathological appearances point to the three (or possibly four) ways of involvement of the VTFs in the context of ThS: The first would be a separate (pure) VTF phonation type or "register" - which is probably hard to prove -, the second would be a VTF-VF phonation type, which has already been observed and described, and the third would be the supraglottic sphincter, indicating a joint vibration of AEFs, VTFs, and (possibly) VFs; the fourth possibility would involve the approximated ventricular folds serving as a specific configuration of the lowest part of the vocal tract. Besides of a possible involvement of the VTF in phonation types (whisper, creak) or vocal registers (vocal fry) and more recently in connection with VQ in certain register tones (see chapter 2.5) VTFs are relatively seldom addressed in the phonetic literature (Hirose, 1997; Hollien and Michel, 1968).

2.2.3 Aryepiglottic Fold (*plica aryepiglottica*)

The aryepiglottic folds (AEF) are "mucosal folds connecting the arytenoid cartilages and the lateral margins of the epiglottis dorsally separated by the interarytenoid notchĚ the posterior part of each aryepiglottic fold is bulged by a corniculate and a cuneiforme tubercle, caused by the corniculate and the cuneiforme cartilage." (Williams et al., 1989: 1644) Muscular constituents include, or are supposed to include, fibres emerging from the arytenoids (*m. arytenoideus pars aryepiglotticus, m. stylopharyngeus*, and *m. palato-pharyngeus*) in a longitudinal direction, and transversely, fibres reaching from the thyroid upwards as lateral fibres of *m. thyroarytenoideus.* In one of the few recent anatomical studies Reidenbach (1998a) points to a "lack of agreement" among clinicians regarding the alledged diagnostic redundancy of the aryepiglottic folds, because although the AEFs are intimately involved in laryngeal closure mechanisms, e.g. during swallowing, and in pathological conditions such as inspiratory stridor, descriptions on the normal topography of the aryepiglottic folds are very rare and in part controversial (cf. Reidenbach, 1998a: 224). And since for example the relation and proportion of muscular tissue to adjacent mucosal tissue had been left out of focus by most investigators, Reidenbach (1998a,c) reinvestigated the region in serial whole-organ sections of 25 plastinated normal adult human larynges.

Visual inspection shows that the aryepiglottic folds are also ventrally adjacent to the peri-epiglottic adipose tissue. According to Reidenbach both regions are clearly separated by several layers of transversely oriented collagenous fiber layers. The muscular component of the aryepiglottic folds is only poorly developed, and in her study no muscle fibres were found to insert at the epiglottis. Looking for an underlying framework, Reidenbach had to state that a coherent quadrangular membrane representing a ligamentous 'skeleton' of the aryepiglottic folds was absent. Only a "conspicuous collagenous fiber layer" was found as a factor that could strengthen the free dorsal margin of the fold. Both muscular and ligamentous components "may render the aryepiglottic folds sufficiently tense as to resist inspiratory inward suction in normal cases". However, Reidenbach also suggests that "pliability must be preserved to guarantee adequate folding in approximation of the aryepiglottic folds during deglutition. Thereby, the posterior part of the laryngeal inlet is closed, whereas the anterior part is probably closed by independent inward bulging of the peri-epiglottic adipose tissue"(223).

2.2.4 Aryepiglottic Sphincter (AES)

There are several terms for this structure in the literature, e.g. *anterior-posterior compression* (Koufman et al., 1996) in vocology or *aryepiglottic sphincter* (Grawunder, 2003b) or *laryngeal sphincter* (Esling, 2002b; Traill, 1986) in phonetics. Sometimes it is also found paraphrased as (*anterior-to-posterior* vs. *medial*[2]) *supraglottic activity* (Stager et al., 2000) or *supraglottal (laryngeal) constriction* (Hirose, 1997). Unfortunately descriptions of the actual mechanism of the AES are very scarce and poor in quality, especially in the phonetic literature (Gauffin, 1977).

[2] "Medial supraglottic activity is characterized by adduction of the false vocal folds..."Stager et al. (2000)

This structure has mainly been described in order to explain mechanisms of deglutition. Nevertheless, Grawunder (2003b) also pointed out this analogy to the AES configuration in ThS (see also 2.3.1.3).

It seems to be widely accepted that the thyroepiglottic and aryepiglottic muscle fibers rather contract to make the AEFs tense. In addition Reidenbach (1998a) suggests that "these muscles may mediate an adequate folding and approximation of the AEFs to cover the dorsal part of the laryngeal entrance during deglutition, whereas the lowering of the epiglottis is probably brought about by other than muscular forces." It may also be plausible that a mechanically induced pressure is involved, exerted onto the elevated larynx by the tongue root. The pressure would be also transferred to the periepiglottic space (PES), which borders the anterolateral part of the laryngeal vestibule. "When the peri-epiglottic adipose tissue is compressed, it probably bulges toward the adjoining ventral portion of the airway lumen, eventually obliterating it."(Reidenbach, 1998a)

In conclusion the approximation of the AEFs results in the closure of the dorsal portion of the airway lumen which is connected to a forward and inward movement of the arytenoid cartilage (Ardran and Kemp, 1967; Reidenbach, 1998a: after). And since Reidenbach's studies showed a clear separation of the lateral parts of the periepiglottic space and the AEFs by several coherent collagenous fiber sheets, the pressure exerted on the PES is probably not transmitted to the AEFs; rather, it results exclusively in a bulging of the PES and closure of the ventral part of the laryngeal vestibule. "However, inward movements of the AEFs may not affect the adjacent PES and result in closure of the dorsal part of the laryngeal vestibule only." (232) Regarding neural control it seems also that especially that regarding the aryepiglottic folds is not yet distinguished in detail, since branches of both laryngeal nerves (SLN and RLN) course towards this area (Sanders et al., 1993; Sanders and Mu, 1998).

Supplementary it needs to be added, that with respect to supraglottic constriction (Hirose, 1997: 133) reports about the fact that "...in laryngeal EMG, it has been observed that LCA appears to show a high degree of activity for this particular gesture together with activation of TA." Besides that PCA "continues to be active and the thyropharyngeal activation is also observed..." (133). Though it contrasts with a possible assumption of *m. aryepiglotticus* and *m. thyroepiglotticus* as only sphincter muscles, it also reveals/points at the involvement of other intrinsic muscles (for tilting of arytenoids cartilages) and their nervous control of to the constriction.

2.3 Physical Examination of the Lower Vocal Tract in Throat Singing

What do we know about Throat Singing (ThS)? What do we know about the physiology of ThS? What do we assume? In some works ThS techniques like *kargyraa* and *kai* are sometimes quickly and superficially categorized as simply ventricular voice (false folds voice) (Tsai, 2003), sometimes, just as quickly as *strohbass, Kehlbass* or pulse register or creaky voice (Kob, 2002). Other styles (*sygyt, enzeŋgileer, xöömej*) have been associated with "tensed" and "pressed voice", implying here also the physiological appearance of tensed or stiff vocal folds (Sakakibara et al., 2002b; Trân, 1991). Unfortunately there is very little relevant original material that's really available to the scientific community (see compilation in Table 2.8). Some has never been published (X-ray investigation of overtone singing by Wendler and colleagues, 1988, presented at the *1st Stuttgarter Stimmtage* conference, 1996, and cited in Seidner and Wendler (1997) as Wendler, U., Cebulla, M., Voelker, L. (1988): Production of isolated overtones during normal phonation. Video, Umatic, 6 min.). Some has never even been made available to the scientific community, (e.g. Zoja Kyrgys (2002) reports on the unpublished fibre endoscopic examination of a Tuvan ThSinger (Boris Xarly) (Grawunder, 1999: 56) which was carried out at the in Roosevelt Hospital New York University in 1994.

2.3.1 Preliminary Laryngoscopic Examination of Throat Singing

Surveying the literature one can clearly see the recent improvements in the techniques of equipment used for such visual inspection of the laryngeal and hypopharyngeal structures in live and phonating subjects. Whereas earlier researchers

AUTHORS/RESEARCHERS	YEAR of recording	METHOD/TECHNIQUE	TYPES	STYLES	SINGERS
Maslov/Černov	1982	laryngeal mirror, tomography	ThS	*xöömej*, xai	4 native singers
Wendler	1988	X-ray	OtS	(???)	unknown subject
Trân/Guillou	1989	X-ray	OtS	style TQH	Trân Quan Hai
Keidar/Shanom/Kyrgys	1994	rigid endoscope	ThS	*xöömej* and ???	Boris Xarli
Fuks/Hammarberg	1998	rigid endoscope	ThS	dzo-ke (???) style Fuks	Fuks
Grawunder/Gall	1998	fibre endoscope, rigid endoscope	ThS	*xöömej*, *kargyraa*	Grawunder
Adachi & Yamada	1999	MRI	OtS	"xoomij"	subject S.K.
Bless, Edgerton	1999	X-ray (video fluoroscopy), fibre endoscope	ThS and OtS	*xöömej*, *sygyt*, *kargyraa*	4 native singers
Lindestad/Merker	2000	rigid endoscope, high-speed camera	ThS	Simulated	Merker
Neuschäfer-Rube/Saus	2001	fibre endoscope, sonograph	OtS	style Saus	Saus
Sakakibara	2002	fibre endoscope, high-speed camera	ThS	*xöömej*(???), *kargyraa*	Sakakibara

Table 2.8: Prior investigations on ThS (/OtS) using image-producing techniques; (???) indicates a lack of certainty in labeling the investigated voice production in terms of style

since Garcia (1855) and Czermak (1879) had only the laryngeal mirror (Dmitriev et al., 1992) or rigid endoscopes, nowadays fibre endoscopes are used. All recent investigations have been made within the short time period of approximately the last 10 years. In the following all published laryngoscopic investigations which have been made specifically on either Throat singers or Overtone singers will be introduced.

2.3.1.1 Dmitriev, Černov, Maslov (1980)

As mentioned above, probably the first physiological examinations and descriptions of native Siberian "double-voice singing" [двухголосная фонация] were made by Soviet scientists, L.B. Dmitriev, B.P. Černov, and V.T. Maslov, in the 1970s (Dmitriev et al., 1983, 1992; Maslov and Černov, 1980; Chernov and Maslov, 1987). Amazingly the authors still felt impelled to prove that this kind of singing is not conditioned by an anatomical deviation or mutation of the VT or larynx of these Siberian natives. According to the only known publication in the 'West' in the course of this research project, a number of recording techniques were used: filming, indirect laryngoscopy, "tomography of the larynx", and "tele-X-ray cinematography" on "a large group of folk singers skilled in this art". Thus recordings "of various styles of double voice singing" were supposed to have been made, but (Dmitriev et al., 1983: 193) concretely investigated only Tuvan *xöömej*. The publications (in Russian) vary also regarding the number of subjects investigated, some mentioning 2 singers (one Tuvan and one Hakas)(Maslov and Černov, 1980) and some 3 singers (all Tuvan)(Dmitriev et al., 1992).

In their descriptions of the laryngeal behaviour Dmitriev and colleagues observed the tubercle of the arytenoids cartilages moving towards the tubercle of the epiglottis. The "tops of the arytenoids cartilages and the margins of false vocal folds in action in forming a narrow opening to the larynx like a small passage or nozzle."(Dmitriev et al., 1983) As the majority of direct laryngoscopic photographs reveal, the VTFs remain visible, and apparently the VFs as well, leaving a posterior gap; this indicates an aryepiglottic sphincter activity with an almost complete A-P compression and a less strong medial component. Regarding the x-ray cinematography obtained during a modal to AES-VF transition, an immediate raising of the larynx and a steeply upright position of the epiglottis blade "with the tongue not being stretched at all" are described. Tomography of an approximately mid-lateral layer illustrates highly compressed vocal folds whith a large contact surface, hence with a strongly compressed supraglottal structure with a large empty ventricle and open *rec. piriformis* clearly visible. In the publication of Maslov and Černov (1980) the authors also reported on a "single-voiced" throat singing of a Hakas singer. The completely different configuration here is constituted by the vibrating vestibular folds and the simultaneously vibrating VFs below, which sometimes become visible. The direct laryngoscopic photograph illustrates the adducted VTFs with a slight posterior divergence.

2.3.1.2 Edgerton, Bless et al. (1999)

Edgerton, Bless and colleagues (Edgerton et al., 2003) have undertaken presumably the most extensive original study of Siberian throat singers. The acoustic, endoscopic and videofluoroscopic examinations were carried out on 4 native ThSs from Tuva (two of whom presumably also took part in the present study: XK and AK) and on 5 other overtone singers or throat singers (2 France, 3 USA). "All subjects were asked to sing ascending and descending reinforced harmonic scales on both a low and high fundamental frequency for each style that the singer was proficient in." Further "...each subject was additionally asked to produce a facsimile of the double source phonation found in the Tuvan/Mongolian *kargyraa* style (or as found in Tibetan chant)." The endoscopic examination showed for two subjects that the epiglottis "swung anteriorly for the higher harmonics, while the base of the tongue and epiglottis retracted near the posterior pharyngeal wall for the low harmonics. Generally, for all styles and subjects the epiglottis featured much movement." In order to produce a, as the authors call it, "double source phenomena", the subjects used two different phonation types: Either a "supraglottal oscillation (involving the false folds, arytenoids and aryepiglottic folds)" or an "asymmetrical vocal fold vibration". Unfortunately it remains unclear if these "methods "were applied by members of both groups ('Western' and Tuvan) or were kept separate. In either case one would assume that the "supraglottic oscillation" was (mainly) used by Tuvan singers. In regard to the Tuvan subjects in particular, supraglottal medial approximation (involving the false folds, arytenoids and aryepiglottic folds) was then used to adjust the timbre characteristics during reinforced harmonic production. The authors also observed that the velopharyngeal passage and velum "featured significant movement with some subjects during the reinforcement of higher harmonics".

2.3.1.3 Grawunder, Gall (1998)

In a preliminary joint study by Volker Gall and Dr. Yvonne Stelzig, Clinics of Phoniatrics and Paedaudiology, University Clinics Frankfurt/Main, and the present author (Grawunder, 1999) some basic observations regarding laryngeal configuration during different ThS styles were made. The author served as subject demonstrating the Tuvan ThS styles *sygyt, xöömej* and *kargyraa*, and a pulse register similar to vocal fry. As mentioned above, the analogy of supraglottic sphincters before phonation was found to be comparable to the mechanism which is induced by the faucial reflex (gagging) or swallowing (see also 2.2.4). In addition a variant of *kargyraa* involving A-P compression with an AEF-VF phonation had been demonstrated. In this phonation type the approximated AEF formed unilaterally a pseudoglottis together with the dorsal surface of the epiglottis root (*tubercel epiglotticum*) (Figure 2.3).

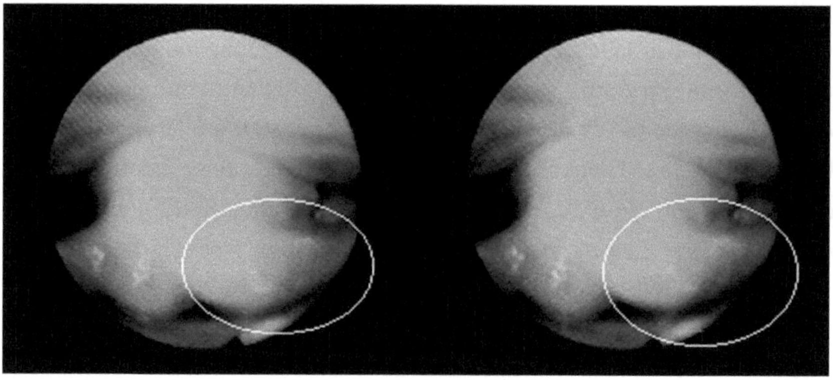

Figure 2.3: Left AEF as phonatory source, building a pseudoglottis at the epiglottis (Grawunder, 2003b)

For the styles *sygyt* and *xöömej* a similar aryepiglottic constriction with contact to the *petiolus* was observed (Figure 2.3), whereas only a small opening at the shifted *incisura interarytenoidea* persisted and underlying structures were obscured by the tubercle cuneiformis.

2.3.1.4 Fuks and Hammarberg (1998)

In the work of Leonardo Fuks, Britta Hammarberg and Johan Sundberg (Fuks et al., 1998) the authors present a series of highspeed images made during L.F.'s own imitation of Tibetan dzo-ke, which had been approved by a Tibetan chant master. The subject switched from a modal voice one octave (F0/2) and sometimes two octaves deeper (F0/3). The images, taken via a rigid endoscope, depict according to Fuks et al. a regular pattern of ventricular folds closing symmetrically at every second cycle of the vocal folds. The authors call this pattern a pulse like vocal-ventricular mode (VVM).

2.3.1.5 Esling (2002)

An extraordinary and unique investigation of unparalleled relevance was carried out by John Esling and colleagues in 1999. They succeeded in recording and examining a "33-year-old Tibetan lama, chant master from Ganden Jangtse Norling Monastery in Madras, India". At present this is still the only known original study of this kind. Images were obtained by means of a S-VHS recording device attached to a light source and fibreoptic nasendoscope. The focus during the investigation was on the behaviour of the lower pharynx vis-à-vis the high/low tonal register distinctions occurring as phonemic contrasts in Tibetan. Additionally two principal forms of singing were elicited, a "high" chant mode and a "deep" chant mode, which appeared to differ substantially in articulation (laryngeal setting). The videoendoscopic pictures show an extreme turned-V-shape of the subject's epiglottis, with the lateral edges bent back (posteriorly); in the medial part an upright even incisure remains as a straight passage through the aditus. Aside from this unusual epiglottis shape the larynx shows normal parameters. In the onset of deep chant the posterior parts of the aryepiglottic folds, reaching *incisura arytenoidea* to *tuberculum cuneiformis* come together and move further in a ventral direction, so that the anterior parts of the AEFs form a half ring around the epiglottis. The other half ring consists of adipose tissue in the pre-epiglottal space, also known as "corpus adiposum pre-epiglotticum" (Williams et al., 1989: 1248), which is superimposed on the VTFs and comes into view as clearly involved in the vibration. For the duration of the VTFs adduction of two-thirds of the anterior comissure, there remains a posterior gap and the VFs below sometimes become visible. During "deep chant" the vallecula and rec. piriformis remain open, while larynx height is normal (i.e. not raised). For high chant register the pharyngeal constriction increases, while also the aryepiglottic constriction continues. The pharyngeal space is quite narrow, so that the bent epiglottis margins actually touch the posterior pharynx wall. The vallecula become invisible and rec. pirifomis become somewhat filled. The vestibule of the additus is only visible during onset and offset. The phonation of the high chant appears as a deep tensed modal voice with a slight rough and breathy component. Crosslinguistic parallels to "non-standard phonation types" have been found by a number of authors (see chapter 2.5). John Eslings' own additional work on Yi and Bai (Esling, 2002b) supports the idea of the laryngeal sphincter (AES) as an articulator.

2.3.1.6 Lindestad (2001,2004)

Lindestad, Södersten, Merker, and Granqvist (Lindestad et al., 2001) used a high-speed image technique consisting of a high-speed camera attached to a fibre endoscope in order to observe a single subject (B. Merker), who was as a professional performer able to produce a "very low-pitched basstype singing technique in Mongolia called Kargyraa". For the high-speed imaging they describe "co-existing low-amplitude ventricular fold vibration with incomplete closures and with the same frequency and in the same phase as the vocal fold vibrations". The authors also note increasingly irregular onsets: "During a period of approximately 0.12 second (corresponding to the interval between 0.67 and 0.79 second in the narrow-band spectrogram) the irregularity persisted until the vibrations suddenly assumed a very regular pattern with the ventricular folds vibrating at the same frequency as the vocal folds but closing only every second vibration". Regarding the closure of the VTF oscillation the high-speed images disclose a remaining “chink in the posterior third”, whereas the vibration amplitude along the anterior two-thirds was large. This may be specifically to the subject’s individual technique. Also noteworthy seems to be “that the opening phase of the ventricular folds appeared faster than the closing phase. ”On the other hand the vocal folds showed a fast closing phase and a long and complete closed phase. This appears not very surprisingly and may be due to the “slightly pressed” character of the voice. Regarding the coordination of the two oscillations it is observed that the “closure of the ventricular folds did not coincide with vocal fold closure but preceded it. Thus the open phase and following closing phase of every second vocal fold vibratory cycle were concealed. At ventricular fold opening the vocal folds remained closed for a moment before opening. The ventricular fold vibrations between closures were of low amplitude and simultaneous with the unconcealed vocal fold closures. They also appeared somewhat shorter than those with complete closure.”

2.3.1.7 Sakakibara (2002 – 2004)

Sakakibara Ken-ichi (Sakakibara et al., 2002b) from NTT communication science laboratories, Japan, carried out another recording of high-speed images of a ventricular voice as used specifically in ThS. A, at that time, brand-new technique involving a high-energy light source connected to a fibre endoscope was applied. Sakakibara (Sakakibara et al., 2002b,c) reports on two manners of VTF-VF vibration which differ in narrowness of the constriction and in oscillation pattern. Thus he describes the modus of a “squeezed voice”(by S.K.) composed of approximate VTFs vibrating in the same frequency and opposite phase and a *kargyraa* voice (by S.K.) wherein VTFs are “…assumed to close once for very two periods of closure of the VFs and contribute to the generation…” of subharmonics. A more recent study Sakakibara et al. (2004b) present additional material of high-speed images which clearly reveal a persistant adduction of the dorsal part of the VTFs for a “drone voice”, which is supposed to be “the basic voice for singing with whistle-like high overtones”. For *kargyraa* Sakakibara et al. (2002b) claims “strongly adducted” VTFs but they are “looser than that in the case of the drone voice”.

2.3.1.8 Neuschaefer-Rube and Saus (2001)

As a contrast or comparison to ThS it was considered to be appropriate to include also a report on fibre endoscopic observations of overtone singing. One study has been undertaken by C. Neuschaefer-Rube, G. Matern, S. Klajman and M. Kob from the Clinics of Phoniatry, Paedaudiology and Communication Disorders (University Hospital of RWHT Aachen) with the German overtone singer Wolfgang Saus serving as subject (Kob et al., 2001; Matern et al., 2001; Neuschaefer-Rube et al., 2001). The singer uses an articulation strategy involving a fix tongue position at the palate and a forward-moving tongue root. Endoscopic images illustrate, concomitantly with the ascending enhanced overtones, an anterior displacement of the tongue root, a widening of the pharynx, larynx elevation and an anterior shift of the epiglottis. The velum constantly remained slightly open. Mouth opening was observed to increase at the beginning of the sequence and then to persist in the same position. Additional observations by the author showed the U-shape of the singer's epiglottis and a slight opening of the rec. piriformis aligning with the pharynx expansion, with the pharynx width in its ultimate configuration still remaining relatively narrow. And somewhat surprisingly, a supraglottal constriction with an A-P compression component becomes increasingly visible over the sequence. The findings support statements mentioning an "unusual pharyngeal constriction "by other singers (explicitly by OtS teachers such as M. Vetter in his OM overtone singing school).

2.3.2 Additional Recordings of Fibre Endoscopic Examination of Throat Singing

2.3.2.1 Subject

In association with the discussion about adequate subject recruitment (see also section 3.2.5) the issues of the subject's qualification, acceptability and applicability ought to be considered. van Tongeren (1994), Grawunder (2003b) and Edgerton et al. (2003) have already pointed out that even within the groups of Siberian ThSingers (Mongolian, Tuvan, Altai, Bashkyr, Hakas) individual singers' personal characteristics of style components, phonation modes and types, articulation strategies (even the visible ones), timbre etc. are quite variable. This leads to the assumption that even if a 'Westerner's' or Non-Native Siberian's singing is judged to be equivalent or similar to native's singing, there could be no certainty of true identity, especially for invisible pharyngeal and laryngeal procedures. In the transfer situation, a Western adept shares with his Tuvan 'classmate' the problem of having to rely only on auditive and visual cues, perhaps supplemented by the comments and advices of a teacher. The same should apply to an individual single singer from South Siberia[3]. Would a European or 'Western' singer who learnt ThS in Siberia be as typical as a Siberian who learnt OtS? Given the lack of subjects on the one hand and of available portable techniques (fibre endoscopic) on the other, those subjects are especially considerable who have received an a positive judgement or evaluation by native singers, singing teachers and experts.

2.3.2.2 Research Questions

How do *kargyraa* 1 (VTF-VF phonation) and *kargyraa 2* (AEF-VF phonation) differ from each other, in terms of pharynx constriction, epiglottis position, or piriformis sinus width? How can the AES meachanism for ThS be described, possibly in contrast to the sphincter behaviour during deglutition? Is there a difference in tension (approximation or A-P compression) between *xöömej* and *sygyt* (PM1 AT2 andPM1 AT1)?

2.3.2.3 Method

The recordings were made by the Dr. med. Ernst Röpke and Dr. med. Cornelia Welzel in 2002 at the Phoniatric Department of the Clinics for Otorhinolaryngology of the University Clinics in Halle. During endoscopic inspection the subject (the author) produced sequences of sustained stable voicing in the different voice production types: modal voice, *sygyt, xöömej, kargyaa*, and pulse register voice. The setup, including the singing subject, was filmed with a DV-camera SONY DCR-PC 100 by Christoph Walther. The singer was not given a

[3] In fact, there are cases where individual Mongol, Tuvan, Hakas or Altai singers differ so much in their interpretation of ThS from others of their own group that these singers are evaluated by the native audience as un-typical or at least non-traditional.

synchronous visual feedback. Subsequently the resulting material was subjected to a frame-by-frame analysis by means of SoundForge 7.0 Sonic Foundry software. The description of the different VPTs was made according to a grid pattern of laryngeal parameters introduced by Painter (1991). The observations and description were carried out on a single subject (the author). They were formulated in terms of the following 12 parameters: In the mediolateral dimension (medial components): "glottal width (distance between VFs)" (GW); "false folds width, ventricular folds width (VTFW)"; "the distance between the cuneiform apices" (ICW); "the distance between the arytenoids apices" (IAW); "epiglottic width as measured between the junction with the superior ridge of the aryepiglottic fold on each side" (counting shadow but not firm contact) (EW). In the anteroposterior dimension (A-P components): "glottic length" (GL); "epiglottic blade position as 'measured' from the posterior wall of the pharynx at midline to the furthest posterior part of the epiglottis excluding the tubercle" (EBP); "epiglottic tip position as measured from the posterior wall of the pharynx at the midline to the highlight of the tip" (ETP); "cuneiform fronting as measured from the posterior wall of the pharynx at the midline to the plane drawn between the cuneiform apices" (CFF); "aryepiglottic fold length as measured from the apex of the arytenoids to the junction with the epiglottis"(AEFL); "piriformis sinus width at its maximum" (SPW); "aryepiglottic fold angle, as measured between the line drawn from the apex of the arytenoids to the cuneiform apex and the line drawn from the cuneiform apex to the junction with the lateral pharyngo-epiglottic fold" (AFA)

Some parameters may overlap in their 'explanatory coverage'. To disentangle the effects of these is impossible with just a single subject; hence this issue can only be sensibly discussed after recruiting a larger number of subjects.

2.3.2.4 Findings

Fibre endoscopic video recordings were obtained of several techniques of Tuvan provenience: *xöömej* (PM1a), *sygyt* (PM1b), *xöömej-sygyt*-transition (AES-VF), *kargyraa* (variant 1: AEF-VF) (PM2b) and *kargyraa* (variant 2: VTF-VF) (PM2a). During performance of *sygyt* the epiglottis (EP) appeared as upright standing, valleculae were mostly 'free' and rec. piriformis empty. For *xöömej*-

sygyt-transition can be stated that in the course of the transition and afterwards no further constriction appears, as one might assume on the basis of the evaluations regarding more tension in *sygyt* (cf. Grawunder, 2003b; Kyrgys, 2002; van Tongeren, 1994). Small-ranged epiglottis movements can be observed during so called leaps, pulsing overtones caused by accordingly pulsed anterior tongue movements (cf. van Tongeren, 1994). These increase in range anterior posterior movements during overtone articulation or shifting. In the course of phonation of *kargyraa* variant 1 (PM2a), the more pulse like phonation, inward bulging of periepiglottic adipose tissue and subsequently approximation of ventricular folds was observed. Unfortunately the subject was not able to produce a clear observable and stable equivalent of VF-VTF phonation. Nonetheless *kargyraa* variant 2 (growl like, PM2b) showed an almost complete closure which also involved a strong epiglottis retraction so that the actual examination of moving AEF was not repeatable (cf. 2.3). Additionally observations could be made during the onset phase of the VTF here the velum closure was observed and could be evaluated as not fully closed.

	GW	GL	EBP	ICW	IAW	VTFW	EW	AFA	ETP	SPW	CFF	EAFL
PM1a	4	5	1	1	4	3	4	4	2	2	4	4
PM1b	4	5	2	1	4	3	4	4	3	2	4	4
PM2a	4	5	3	2	4	4	4	3	3,4	4	4	4
PM2b	5	5	4,5	2	4	4,5	4	4	4,5	4	4	4

Table 2.9: Fibre endoscopic findings according to selected parameters (after Painter, 1991); numbers represent a rating on a scale of 0 to 4; (0 = normal; wide; unaffected; 4 = extreme; narrow; tight; 5 invisible); the abbreviation in the head row refer to those parameters at page 58.

2.4 Vocal Tract Shape Investigations – Articulation of "Reinforced Harmonics" in Throat Singing

2.4.1 Observable Techniques or Methods of "Overtone Articulation"

Based on introspection and interviews with throat singers and throat singing teachers the following categories of articulation strategies are suggested. They will also be referred to as overtone articulation types (AT)[4], given their function of formant shifting for melodic articulation of reinforced harmonics:

AT1 consists of a relatively fix tongue tip (*apex linguae*) at postalveolar position ("[j]"), so that the airstream flows mid-sagitally through or laterally ("[l]") around the constriction. The tongue root is coronally approximated towards the palate and the medial (and dorsal) part of the tongue varies in height according to formant height. The lips are protruded and rounding is adjusted to the reinforced harmonics height (formant height).

AT2 For this AT the tongue tip is kept low, while the anteromedial part of the tongue (AT2a) or the posterior part (*dorsum*) is moved up towards the velum (AT2b). Besides a coronal closure for AT2a in the highest position ("[j]") in both cases, no sagital closure is achieved. Lips are nearly closed, lip protrusion and rounding are aligned to the higher reinforced harmonics but change only very slightly. The airstream flows mid-sagitally. This type also includes the Tuvan style *borbaŋnaadyr* (AT2c), involving a rapid rocking-movement in either direction.

AT3 consists basically of pronounced (Tuvan and non-Tuvan) vowels along the second formant height, where preferentially either a front or back vowel row is used. The vowels are articulated with a relatively open clear quality.

Another strategy subsequently was added as an additional (O)AT:

[4] For the decision making whether articulation strategy, articulation technique or articulation type would here be most appropriate the crucial point lays in the reflectedness of the process. Insofar a reflected auditory goal is seeked to be accomplished the term *technique* would be sufficient. But as far as observed, do singers not always reflect the exact articulation movement, which then could be named strategy, since this would within the field of phonetics not imply conscious behaviour. Besides that 'strategy' focuses very detailed on articulatory behaviour. The term articulation type or overtone articulation type tries to get around this dilemma.

AT4 encompasses constant velar lowering (AT4a), i.e. opening, or intermittent 'coupling' of nasal resonance (AT4b). This is used in a number of styles like *ezeŋgileer, dumčuktaar, xamryn xoomij*, which are in part also explicitly named after the nose (*xamryn* (M), *dumčuk* (T) 'nose, nostril').

More clearly of a supplementary character is the following strategy:
AT5 - Strong lip protrusion and/or mandibular protrusion (masseter muscle) produce a clonus which results in *byrlaŋnaadyr* ('glimmer, flare'), a style featuring a 'glimmering', whirring, thrilling timbre (ca. 10-12 cps).
AT6 and **AT7** appear, if at all, only very rarely (e.g. in Mongolian xoomij) as a distinct type of overtone articulation, which serves as preparatory step in learning to perform AT1.
AT6 can be simply described as a maximally prolonged alveolar trill, and
AT7 represents in analogy to AT6 a prolonged uvular trill.

Table 2.10 demonstrates how the ATs correspond to the styles defined by the native Tuvan ThS terms:

PHONATION MODUS 1 (single-cycle modus) *xöömej*-voice type	PHONATION MODUS 2 (double or non-single-cycle modus) *kargyraa*-voice type
AT1 - *sygyt* AT2 - *(sygyrdyp) xöömej* AT3 - *xöömej*	AT1 - *čylandyk* AT2 - *xöömej kargyraazy* AT3 - *kargyraa*

Table 2.10: Suggested overtone articulation types (strategies) in combination with phonation modes applied to Tuvan style terms

An additional parameter is the modus of degree of oral (labial) opening/closure in ThS, featuring either a closed or a nearly closed or an open mouth. The closed mode would reproduce the style *xamryn, dumčuktaar* (see above AT4). The progression from AT3 to AT1 would be considered a progression of increasing closure (tongue-alveoles; tongue-palate), whereby the closure (articulated obstacle position) is: AT1 (permanent) alveolar; AT2 alveolar and palatovelar; and AT3 palatovelar.

Following the classification of Zemp and Trân (Zemp and Trân, 1991) AT3 would correspond to the one-cavity technique and AT1 and AT2 would correspond to the dual- or two-cavity technique (see also van Tongeren, 2002).

2.4.2 Phonation Modes and Articulation Types in Throat Singing

In continuation of the observations on articulatory strategies such a grid pattern (table 2.10) could be illustrated by examples, so that a general impression of the variety encompassed could arise. This may have only appeared in chapter 4.1.4, but is given here already as illustration for the various forms and styles appearing in South Siberian ThS (Grawunder, 2003b).

2.4.2.1 PM1 AT1

Tuvan *sygyt* (IK), or Mongolian *taglain xoomij* (HS) are presumably regarded as 'default' throat singing (overtone singing) styles, with a prominent whistling F2 as almost singular appearing melodic sound in the spectrum.

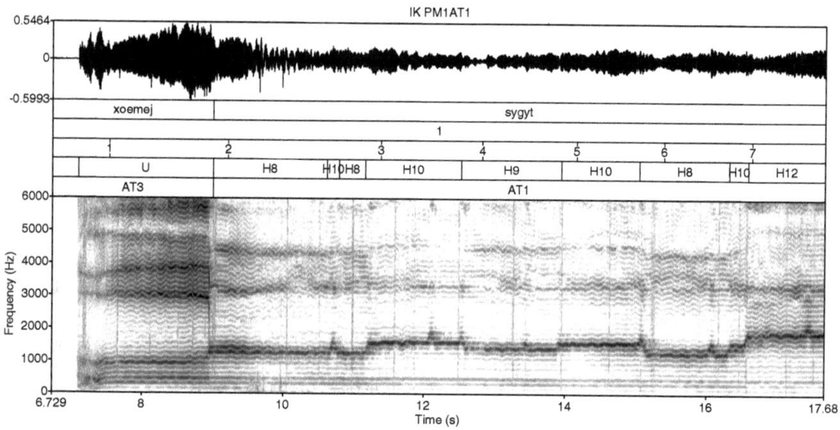

Figure 2.4: Tuvan *sygyt* (singer IK) illustrating PM1 AT1; the second tier refers to phonation mode (1); the third tier contains the numbered measure points (starting point of measurement) ; the fourth tier contains interval labels regarding the sung vowel or reinforced harmonic; horizontal stripes and bars are due to quantization error in the recording

We find, F1 and F0 are damped strongly in most of the cases. We see also an immediate damping and merging of F3 and F4, aside from an increase of F2 intensity and as well as bandwidth. As typical appears a pulsating beat punctuation in terms of a short raising (approx. 90ms) of one or two harmonics (in the interval of about a second) described by van Tongeren (1994) as "leaping technique" involving a small scale anterior movement of tongue body.

2.4.2.2 PM1 AT2

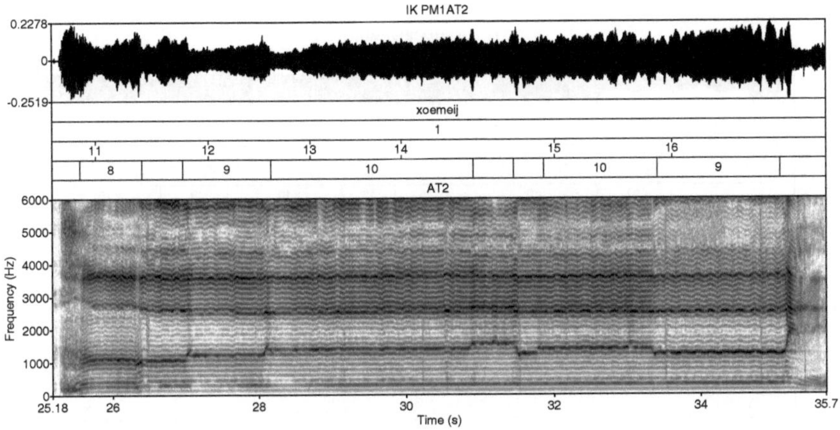

Figure 2.5: Singer IK (T); Tuvan *xöömej* PM1AT2

The examples of Tuvan *xöömej*(IK) or Mongolian *čedžnij xoomij* (HS) allow already the acknowledgment of diffuse vowel qualities. But a prominent F2 is superimposed. Good singers (like OK) are able to change articulation types/techniques within one phrase and continue the same musical line of notes just in the other technique (see Figure 2.6). The transition would be different from the usual onset (as in Figure 2.4.2.1) being not as abrupt. F3 and F4 appear in a dense energy band, that contributes to the typical timbre of *xöömej*. Overtone singing styles lack this band. F0 stays usually at the same height and would be only altered if a melodic overtone would need to be reached. This is especially also true for PM1AT1 where an F0 shift usually is highly marked as 'improfessional', i.e. not desirable for most styles of this sort in Southern Siberia. Mongolian performers (e.g. T4) instead do sometimes use F0-movement as special stylistic nuance which indeed reveals high proficiency and excellence in the command of ThS techniques. As another feature of high-qualty performance serves the carrying out of one musical phrase onto one breath(-group).

Since the highest tongue position of AT2 enables a transition in to AT1 (tongue tip at the alveolar ridge), we find this in fact in many performances. Tuvan and Hakas singers use AT2 in this way as intermediate technique from AT3 to AT1.

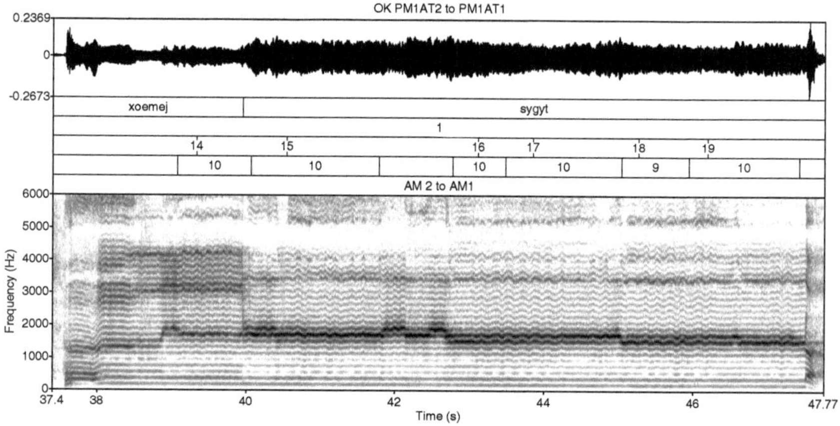

Figure 2.6: Transition from AT2 to AT1 (*xöömej* to *sygyt*) within one musical phrase and breath, and on the same musical note; sample from a Tuvan singer (OK)

Kyrgys (2002: 84) refers to the Tuvan *xöömej* as "basic style" which employs the specific PM1 with PM1AT2 and PM1AT3 as main techniques for reinforced harmonic articulation. The harmonics are not as prominent as in the other *sygyt*-like PM1AT1 styles and phrasing derives often of prolonged 'non-sense' elements in the *libretto*.

2.4.2.3 PM1 AT3

Within the present corpus mainly Tuvan *xöömej* and Hakas *xai* employ this combination.

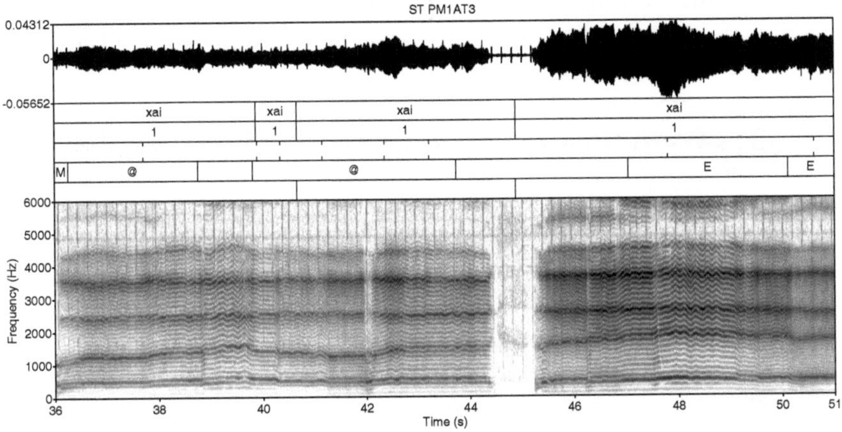

Figure 2.7: Vowel and pitch change in PM1AT3; singer ST (H)

AT3 often not only involves vowel changes as F2 strategy for melodical phrases, it also comes along with changes in pitch (fundamental frequency), as a kind of 'transition into singing'. It is a special feature of Tuvan ThS to use this form of functional non-sense (cf. Grawunder, 1999) usually in two ways, either with a row of front vowels or a row of back vowels (Grawunder, 2003b) but also in a mixed row like [u]-[o]-[ø]-[y]-[i] (cf. Grawunder, 1999). In transfer situation this technique is usually taught first, since on the one hand it allows to control tongue height in a explicit way and on the other hand it allows to control the intended 'timbre' (i.e. voice quality). In the example in Figure 2.7 again the full resonant voice timbre is supported by high-intensity of F3 and F4.

2.4.2.4 PM2 AT1

We find examples for AT1 in phonation mode 2 as Tuvan *čylandyk* (singer IK) (Figure 2.8 but also in Mongolian *xarxiraa* singing. This technique is considered to be one of the most difficult and demanding, since a singers needs to control the 'overtone articulation' as well as sustaining the phonation mode of *kargyraa*.

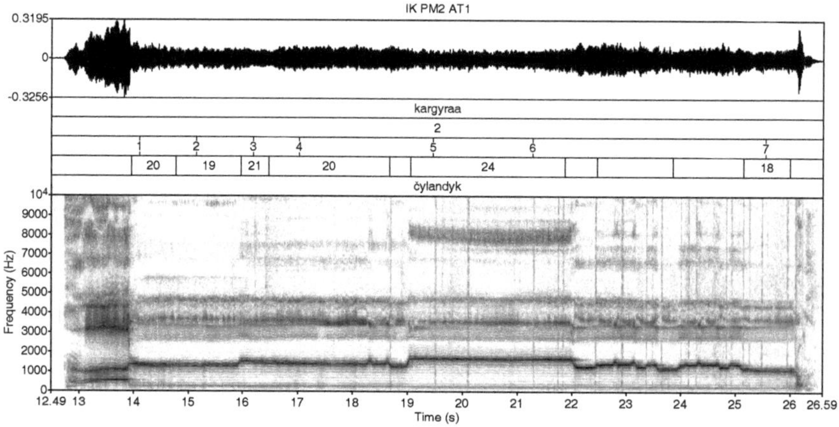

Figure 2.8: *sygydyŋ kargyraazy* or *čylandyk* of singer IK (T) as example for PM2AT1; the vertical stripes in the spectrogram result from quantization errors during the recording

Interestingly the sample of PM2AT1 in Figure 2.8 shows that even the 3kHz energy band is damped in support of enhancement of F2. The non-harmonic band at about 8kHz during the highest harmonic in that phrase corresponds to an auditory impression of breathiness of the fundamental but also an impression of broadening the 'overtone' formant. Again the 'leaping' in terms of small-scale tongue body protrusions works as rhythmical punctuation.

2.4.2.5 PM2 AT2

The example in Figure 2.9 is taken Tuvan *xöömej kargyraa* performed by singer IK. Within the corpus of recordings of Mongolian *xarxiraa* it seems to appear more often (e.g. by HS, see B.2.1 [A 65]), but still it demands a high command of the PM2 production from the singer, since the medial compression of PM2 and dorsal tongue raising seems to contradict impede each other (at least to some degree).

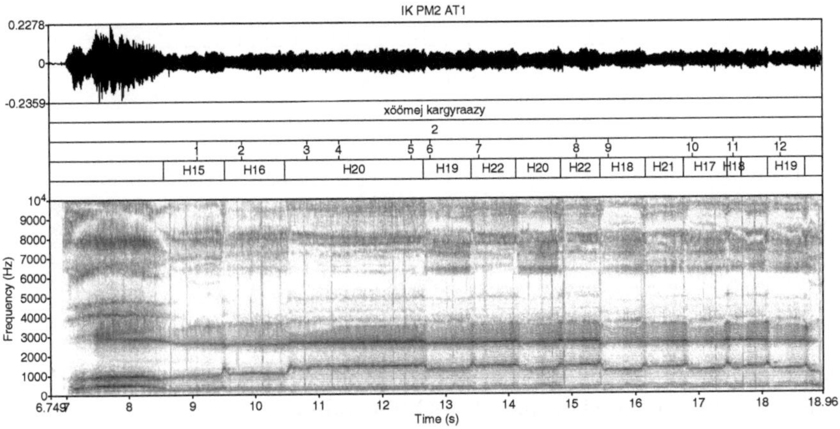

Figure 2.9: Example for Tuvan *xöömej kargyraazy* (PM2AT2) by singer IK; the short vertical stripes in the spectrogram result from quantization errors in the recording

2.4.2.6 PM2 AT3

The combination of PM2 plus prolonged vowel articulation serves as basic element of Tuvan *kargyraa*, Mongolian *xaxiraa*, Altaian low register *kai*, and Hakas low register *xai*. For a large number of singers a constant ostination in terms of a "ringing" quality or accompanying formant at about 3000Hz can be described (see 2.10 and see 4.1.6).

By looking at higher frequency ranges one can observe that after a consistent energy dent or dip in the range 4.5-4.9kHz other specific areas of energy bands appear only very weakly.

Especially the Tuvan *kargyraa* and its Hakas pendant use the vowel scale according to F2 height. Here the back vowel row, including [m],[n] and [ŋ], is usually preferred. Nonetheless, the example in Figure 2.10 reveals that also open front

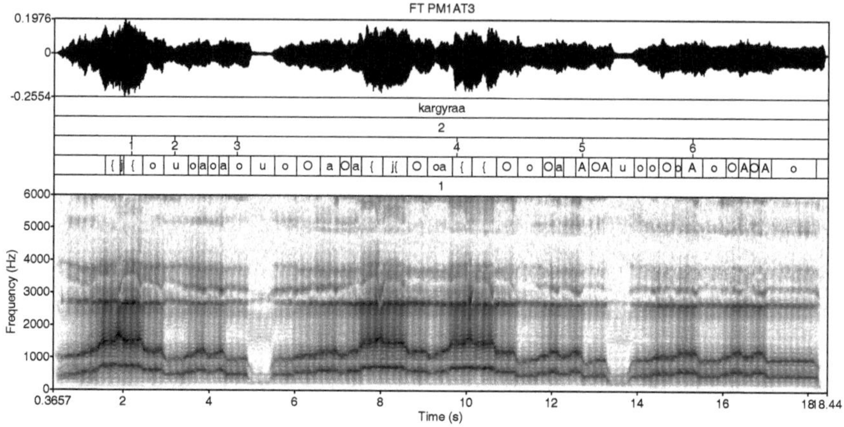

Figure 2.10: Example for PM2AT3, *kargyraa* of singer FT (T); the fourth tier contains annotation of vowel qualities (XSAMPA coding)

vowels like [æ(= {)] and [ɛ(= E)] are used.

In other sub-styles of Tuvan *kargyraa* (usually in terms of PM2AT3) the voice quality appears as very rough and its spectral properties resemble those the aryepiglottic voice production produced by the author (Grawunder, 1999, 2003a). In the sample from IK in Figure 2.11 vowel articulation becomes fairly diffuse and 'imprecise'.

2.4.2.7 Tuvan *ezeŋgileer* as example of PM1 AT2+AT4

Ezeŋgileer ('stirrup') shows a strong rhythmically structured behaviour, where there sudden switch on of nasal resonance (*nasopharynx*) can be observed. The syncopic alternation between melodic overtone and nasal accompaniment in the sample (Figure 2.12) allows the observation of a F3/F4 but also F1 enhancement during the nasal passages. The prominence of the reinforced harmonics (H8-H10) seems to be uninfluenced. Kyrgys (2002: 91) and van Tongeren (1994: 24) observe an usual overtone ambitus ranging from H7/H8 to H13, which suggests that a number of singers also use AT1.

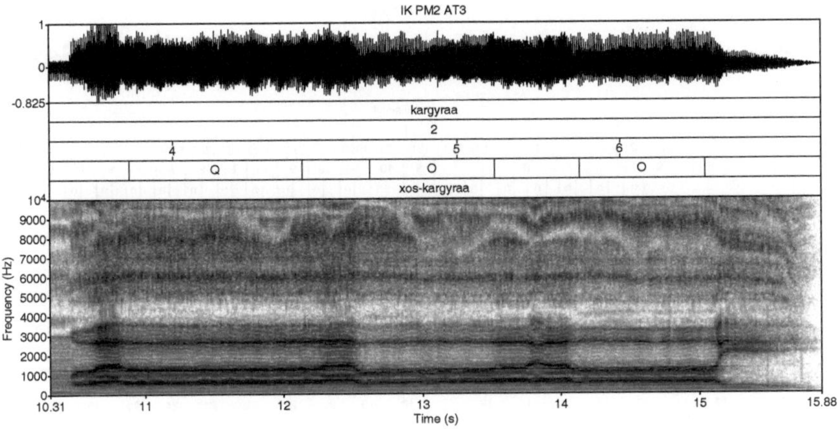

Figure 2.11: Singer IK (T) demonstrating a very rough, open ("xos") *kargyraa*

2.4.2.8 Tuvan *borbaŋnaadyr* (PM1 AT2ab+AT2c)

The various interpretations of *borbaŋnaadyr* are reflected in a number of techniques which all aim to create the impression of a "rolling, waltzing" sound. The specific mimesis of a rolling stone at the bottom of a creek translates for many singers into an articulatory 'waltzing' of the tongue body in a piston-rod like movement. Levin and Süzükei (2006: 58-62) describe this "timbre oriented" musical concept of Tuvan music specifically by using *borbaŋnaadyr* as example.

In the example of the singer AD(T) a secondary nasal component comes into play. And van Tongeren (1994: 24) emphasizes an almost closed lip aperture. Additionally, older recordings (see reference B.2 [A1]) of *ezeŋgileer* and *borbaŋnaadyr* suggest a specific lower layer of PM1 but also a combination with PM2.

2.4.2.9 Trill(AT7)

The trilled '*borbaŋ*' of the Mongolian Singer BO appears to be reminiscent of the Tuvan *birlaŋnaadyr* ('whirr, glimm')', since here too a fast (ca. 25Hz) vibrating modulator comes into play. Whereas here the uvula serves as additional modulator, *birlaŋnaadyr* as performed e.g. by KX (T) is using a muscular tremor of the

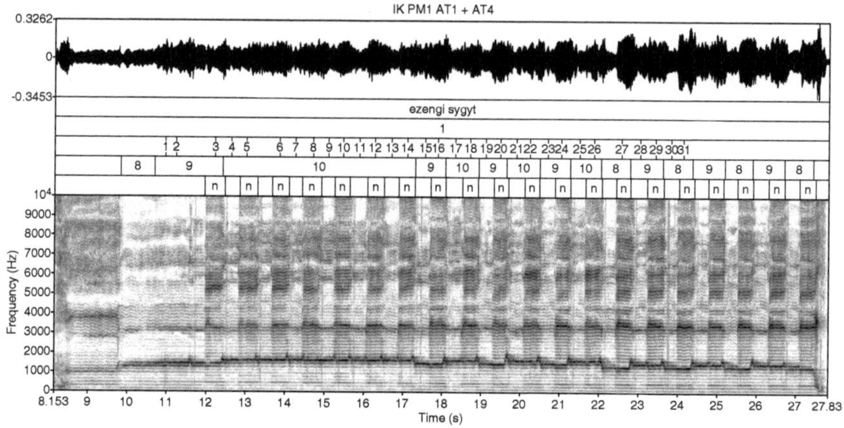

Figure 2.12: Example of Tuvan *ezeŋgileer* (PM1AT1+AT4) by singer IK; the lowest tier marks the nasal passages with "n"

lower jaw muscles including oral facial muscles.

The examples of a uvular trill as overtone AT may be unique to the singer BO. Nevertheless all other ThS features as tensed VQ and prominent formants are present. In the example in Figure 2.14 the trill is performed with PM1. The specialty lies in the fact that the singer has to coordinate also the oral airstream. This special technique resembles another individual sample of a singer from Rajasthan, as presented in the documentary by Hugo Zemp and Trân Quan Hai (see B.2.2 [F1]).

The last examples illustrate the 'degree of freedom' that lies in the individual performance and interpretation of a particular style by one singer. In this way the individual flavour, i.e. artistic singularity, would be expressed through an articulatory setting adding a particular 'timbre'.

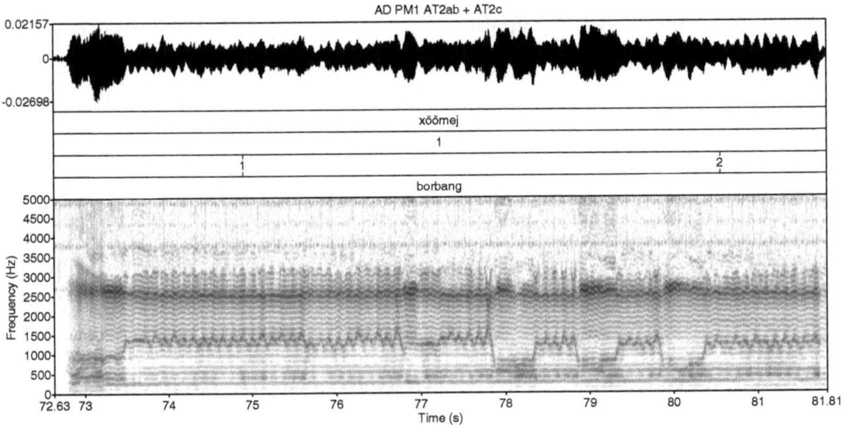

Figure 2.13: Example for Tuvan *borbaŋnaadyr* by singer AD (PM1 AT2c)

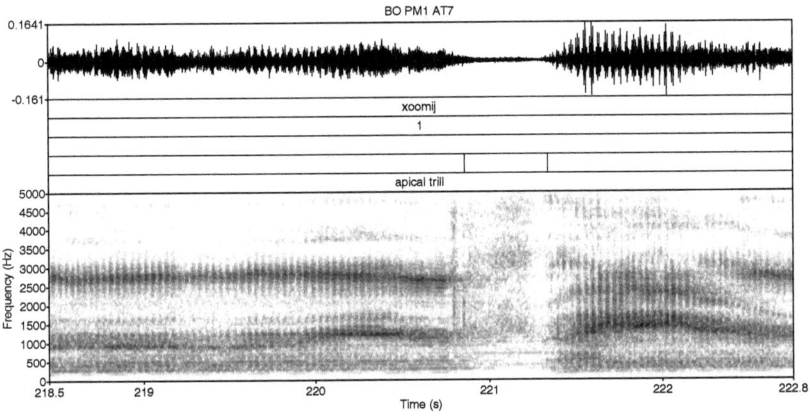

Figure 2.14: AT7 as demonstrated by the Mongolian singer BO

2.4.3 Physical Observations on Singers

Purely visual inspection and palpation of throat-singing individuals may provide preliminary observations of subjects. The following description is essentially a summary of collected observations and should convey a general idea of visually observable articulatory behaviour in ThS.

Larynx position: The larynx appears to be kept in a raised and fixed position for VTF-VF and AEF-VF VPT. For AES-VF VPT this seems not to be the case. This is supported by Edgerton et al. (2003): "Reinforced harmonic singers, when examined through external visual observations and endoscopy tended to raise the larynx as the fundamental frequency rose, thus shortening the tract and raising all formant frequencies."

Head position: Sometimes the singers tend to lean their heads to one side, especially during *kargyraa*. This could be assumed to be an ancillary mechanism for VTF approximation.

Jaw: The *mandibula* in some cases exhibits an extreme protrusion in AT1, slightly opened in AT1/2, more open in AT3.

Lips: Lip protrusion depends on formant height and serves as an rHs-adjustment. Regarding general (muscle) tension, as seen e.g. through the degree of lip protrusion, imposing of jugular tendons and also neck and temple veins, as well as other visible signs of muscular effort, the tension is considerably higher evaluated in Mongolian singers than in Tuvan, and higher in Altai than in Xakas singers.

2.4.4 Investigations using X-ray Videofluoroscopy

Using videofluoroscopy Edgerton et al. (2003) (see 2.3.1.2) describe "four distinct methods of articulation during the production of a reinforced harmonic melody": *Method 1* shifted the dominant formant to align with the harmonic to be reinforced by slightly opening and closing the mouth, such that as the mouth widened, the harmonic melody rose. *Method 2* shifted the formant to align with the reinforced harmonic by retaining the tongue tip near the alveolar ridge while raising the mid-tongue as the reinforced harmonic melody rose. *Method 3* shifted the formant the reinforced harmonic to align with the tongue low and back, similar to an /o/ for the lower harmonic. As the reinforced harmonic melody rose, the tongue moved anterior towards an /i/. *Method 4* shifted the formant to align with the reinforced harmonic by movement in the pharyngeal cavity, with little to no movement in the oral cavity. Specifically, the tongue blade remains on or near the hard palate, while the tongue root/epiglottis nearly touches the posterior pharyngeal wall for the lowest harmonics. As the harmonic melody rises the tongue root and epiglottis move anterior until the middle harmonics, when a large gap appears in the *vallecula* (or space between tongue root and epiglottis). For the highest harmonics the tongue root continues to move forward while the epiglottis swings forward to close the *vallecula* (cf. Edgerton et al., 2003).

The now well known Scientific American article of Levin and Edgerton (Levin and Edgerton, 1999) "The Throat Singers of Tuva" encompasses in its online version five short sequences of the videofluoroscopic recordings which originate in the investigations described in the unpublished article by Edgerton, Bless et al. (Edgerton et al., 2003). Unfortunately video-sound alignments as well as time resolution were degraded because of the necessary data compression. This has considerable negative impact on the fluency of the articulation that can be observed. Despite this degradation, the above published sources contain usable data for one Tuvan subject performing three different styles, reflecting three different overtone (reinforced harmonics) articulation types (PM1 AT1, PM1 AT2, PM3 AT3), as described in Table 2.11.

Velar closure is hard to judge on and the label "closed" is only indicating that there is no visible space between elevated velum and posterior pharynx wall.

VT shape feature style singer	PM1 AT1 sygyt S4	PM1 AT2 xöömej S4	PM2 AT3 kargyraa S4
larynx height	elevated	slightly elevated	elevated
epiglottis declination	according to the formant height, but relatively upright	upright, 'open', sometimes EP is even tilted anteriorly	constant position, slightly tilted posteriorly
tongue root position	vallecula open,	vallecula open, non retracted tongue root	retracted, close to EP, vallecula invisible
meso pharynx width	very wide	very wide	slightly narrowed
hypo pharynx width	ETP very wide, aditus sometimes visible (narrowed)	ETP very wide, aditus sometimes visible narrowed	ETP wide, aditus narrowed
epilaryngeal width	very narrow	very narrow	almost no visible space
velar closure / declination	elevated ('closed')	elevated ('closed')	elevated besides /m, ŋ/
tongue tip position/ movement in *sygyt* type ThS	alveolar	low, rocking movement	low, not raised

Table 2.11: Observations based on the video-fluoroscopic images of a single Tuvan subject (S4) presented in Levin and Edgerton (1999); ETP = space between epiglottis tip and posterior pharynx wall

2.4.5 Investigations using Ultrasound

Neuschaefer-Rube et al. (2001) had applied ultrasound imaging in order to monitor tongue movement during overtone singing. Unfortunately time resolution as well as appropriate image-tracing technology for fast-moving structures is at the moment still in an early stage of development. Nevertheless certain observations of OtS were possible. When singing an ascending scale of reenhanced overtones the tongue root is moved forward and turned steeply. At the end of the sequence a step-like configuration of the tongue has been created due to the forward progressing of the tongue root. The investigation also points out the importance of examining of VT shape variation with respect to another parameter: the shape of the cross-section area. Here the ultrasound images reveal a u-shaped sagittal kerf or groove in the dorsal part of tongue, whose depth increases with the ascending scale.

2.4.6 MRI Investigation

Adachi and Yamada (1999) investigated an amateur "Xöömij" singer by means of MRI technology. The samples of mid-sagittal VT slices depicted show a wide epilaryngeal tube, also during so-called 'pressed singing'. When performing an ascending scale of reinforced harmonics the singer used an articulatory strategy which had not yet been observed on south-Siberian singers, although it is a technique developed and introduced by Trân Quan Hai for OtS (cf. Trân, 1991)[5]. For a pitch-raising overtone formant the singer moves the tongue tip from an alveolar position backward towards the palate into a more retroflex position. The VT calculations that were based on these images were used for further experiments on the synthesis of overtone singing.

[5] This would also explain why the authors use the misleading term *biphonic singing*: Trân himself uses to the terms *chant diphonique* or *chant biphonique* (Trân, 1991; Zemp and Trân, 1991).

2.5 Discussion of VPTs and Laryngeal Settings in Throat Singing

The deductions from field observations in particular (van Tongeren, 2002) give rise to further questions regarding across individuals variability. For example, it is already apparent just from the auditive and visual observations that there exists a wide range of possibilities in the actual articulation of enhanced overtones, hence in the techniques and strategies within one single ThS style (Grawunder, 2003b; van Tongeren, 1994, 2002). This should not be surprising since we are dealing here to a considerable extent with a true living folk art. The same variability seems to hold for the occurrence of laryngeal settings in actual VP.

2.5.1 Posterior-Anterior Compression, Supraglottal Constriction

Endoscopic examination of ThS reveals for PM1 a constriction of the *aditus larynges*, also described as posterior-anterior (A-P) compression or aryepiglottic sphincter (AES) movement. This constriction is physiologically involved in basic laryngeal functions like swallowing, choking or gagging. During deglutition "the ventral part of the laryngeal vestibule is closed by bulging of the adipose tissue of the lateral parts of the peri-epiglottic space toward the airway lumen. The dorsal part of the laryngeal vestibule is closed by approximation and folding of the aryepiglottic folds. In addition, the access to the caudal airways is probably protected by coverage of the lowered epiglottis"(Reidenbach, 1998a). In ThS is often a raised larynx observed, but not a lowered epiglottis. Such larynx elevation could be interpreted as a secondary auxiliary mechanism of A-P compression, involving the stylopharyngeal muscle chain (espec. *m. pharyngeus, m. stylopharyngeus*). It should also be noted that supraglottal constrictions with an almost complete anterior-posterior narrowing toward the *petiolus* (MT3, after Koufman et al., 1996) in addition to medial compression was not observed on all (Tuvan) singers (M. Edgerton, personal communication, Berlin, Spring 2002); in such cases a medial component (VTFs) and pharyngeal tightness were observed, but not an anterior-posterior compression. This marks an import fact since Dmitriev et al. (1992) were generalizing for sygyt-like styles there a nozzle-like function of the AES would play the major role as source for the melodic whistle-like tone.

Sphinctering and Compression in Singing Clinicians have usually not considered supraglottic constriction to be normal, at least for speech or singing. "Anterior-Posterior and Medial Compression of the Supraglottis: Signs of Nonorganic Dysphonia or Normal Postures?" was the question asked by Behrman et al. (2003) in the title of their paper, and the same question was asked by Stager et al. (2000): "Supraglottic activity: evidence of vocal hyperfunction or laryngeal articulation?" In 1989 Eiji Yanagisawa, John Estill, and colleagues, citing a 19th-century report by Manuel P. Garcia to the Royal Society of London, characterized aryepiglottic constriction as a resonance strategy for a "ringing" voice quality (Yanagisawa et al., 1989). In 1855 Garcia (cited after Yanagisawa et al., 1989) had already described such aryepiglottic constriction:

> "'Various simultaneous causes modify the qualities of the voice : 1, according as the glottis partially or entirely closes the passes between the explosions, it produces veiled or brilliant sound; 2, the tube which surmounts and surrounds it also greatly affects the quality of the voice, by its contractions it gives brilliancy to it and by its widening volume; 3, the epiglottis also plays a very important part, for every time it lowers itself, and nearly closes the orifice of the larynx, the voice gains in brilliancy; and when, on the other hand, it is drawn up, the voice immediately becomes veiled.'"

Yanagisawa and colleagues investigated 5 professional singers performing the task of a *messa di voce* for 2 song passages in 6 different voice qualities (speech, falsetto, sob, twang, belting, and opera). They observed aryepiglottic constriction accompanying the three loudest qualities (belting, twang, and opera). So Garcia's observation was fully confirmed. Susequently Koufman et al. (1996) investigated muscular tension patterns involving supraglottic constriction for various degrees of A-P compression in 100 singing subjects of different proficiencies (48 professional and 52 amateur), proveniences, backgrounds, genders, and race. A-P contraction of the supraglottis during singing was acknowledged as the "most common biomechanical alteration", representing step 3 (the third-highest) in a four-graded scale of muscle tension scores. The results of Behrman et al. (2003) are similar in a group of 40 patients with nonorganic dysphonia, a greater degree of A-P compression was found than in the (normal) control group, but no significant difference emerged for medial compression. Hence medial (ventricular) compression was stated to be a possible normal laryngeal posture and thus clearly not an indicator of laryngeal dysfunction; A-P compression, however, also failed to be a reliable indicator of dysfunction. These findings would also allow the hypothesis of a gradual adjustment of the epilaryngeal resonator, which would be supported by the findings in OtS of Neuschaefer-Rube et al. (2001)(see section2.3.1.8). Such effortful 'laryngeal work' in singing which bear the usual risk of overexertion and laryngeal fatigue followed by mucosa lesions and tissue conversion/rebuilding, not only for normal singers but also for throat singers. This risk must be evaluated in terms of the different phenomena involved, especially the extensiveness and frequency, the transfer situations, and over a long term (life time) perspective. But the aryepiglottal or ventricular component in certain (paralinguisticaly and linguisticaly relevant) voice qualities and sounds also must be considered with regard to a general tendencies of voice usage in those particular speaker communities.

In the context of throat singing the excitation/stimulation of the AES towards an vibratory pattern of the AEFs was taken into consideration for voice usage ("growl voice") of various singings in "ethnic and pop styles" by Sakakibara et al. (2004a) and Grawunder (2003a,b). Edgerton et al. (2003) had also observed that also the margins of the AES are sometimes visibly vibrating. A "pure" AEF-voice would, strictly speaking, have to be determined not only as distinctive phonation type but also as "para-phonation" since it is comparable to other supplementary mechanisms of phonation (or voice production resp.) (cf. Ptok, 993a; Ptok et al., 1993).

The 'linguistic bridge': AES as source and articulator in linguistic context A number of findings on supraglottic phonetic features that serve as phonemic function reveal another argument towards the role and nerval control of the lower

VT, not only as resonator but also as articulator in a not inconsiderable number of languages: Along the study of Tibetan voice quality in tones and chant registers (see above 2.3.1.5) Esling (2002a) had also observed very similar laryngeal (supraglottic) behaviour in the Sino-Tibetan language Bai. In Bai a harsh voice quality aligns with a "tensed" register tone that has a medial (ventricular) compression component. Another Sino-Tibetan language, Yi, contrasts "tense" register with a (sphinctered) raised-larynx and "lax" register with an "open pharynx". The supraglottic laryngeal constriction in the Tibetan "high chant" thus resembles "tense" register in Yi, while the deep chant resembles 'tense/harsh/low-tone' register in Bai. Other recent studies (Apiluck, 2003; Carlson and Esling, 2003; Edmondson, 2004) point to similar involvement of the laryngeal constriction (including A-P and medial compression) e.g. in Amis, Chong, Nuuchahnulth, and Ket. Consequently Esling (1996, 1999, 2002b) pointed to the aryepiglottal constriction as epiglottal vs. pharyngeal articulation, indicating that the epiglottis or aryepiglottic sphincter is a more often used articulator and used in a wider range of articulatory modes (sphincter, stop, fricative, "trill", source) than has been thought heretofore (cf. Laufer and Condax, 1979, 1981). Esling's "pharyngeal trill" (Esling, 1996) in its A-P approximation and vibration of AEFs resembles most the described AEF-VF phonation (Grawunder, 1999, 2003b; Sakakibara et al., 2004a). Anthony Traill (1986) described "the laryngeal sphincter as a phonatory mechanism in !Xóõ Bushman", a so-called KhoiSan-language in southwestern Botswana. !Xóõ differentiates four distinctive phonation types: normal voicing, creaky or laryngealized voice, murmur and an unusual "sphincteric" phonation type. This appears as an extremely rough and noisy voice quality having an almost aperiodic waveform with only sporadic low-amplitude low-frequency components and a spectrogram that contains almost no harmonic. Endoscopic examination showed different degrees of supraglottic A-P and medial constriction, so that VTFs sometimes imposes as medially approximated. Additionally obtained lateral xerograms also reveal a pharyngeal constriction and a raised larynx. The coincidence of such phonetic phenomena along geographically close to the Xhosa *umxube* and *umŋqokolo* singing demands a more detailed investigation. Grawunder (1999, 2003a,b) had suggested for Xhosa ThS a AEF-VF phonation type which would require a laryngeal configuration similar to that found in !Xóõ "sphinctered" voice or "strident vowels" (Ladefoged and Maddieson, 1996: 310). It should be (re-)emphasized that it is not always transparent, on some of the investigated recordings of ThS, which specific phonatory mechanism is present. The one or the other mechanism may ultimately turn out later to be identified as AES-VF VPT. This cross-linguistic and cross-genre perspective seems very promising for reconnecting and assessing theories of how specific articulatory features are involved in phonological processes.

2.5.2 Ventricular Fold Mechanism (VTF) – Medial Compression of Supraglottal Constriction

For PM2 in ThS an approximation of the ventricular folds has also been observed. Within the ventricular fold tissue, posterolateral, anterolateral and anteromedial muscle layers can be found, detached from TA muscle, and are "...presumed to exert a downward pressure on the vestibular folds in addition to an adductor function. According to clinical experience, adductor movements of the vestibular folds can be trained, even in cases with a recurrent laryngeal nerve lesion, in order to produce a compensatory voice" (Reidenbach, 1998b: 365). Considering these mechanisms, the observation of a free line of sight down to VFs while the VTFs are approximated seems to be explicable. Medial compression could be then treated as a separate and independent component of the supraglottic constriction. The observation in ThS of a relatively raised larynx but upright epiglottis and non reduced pharynx width would support this idea of an independent mechanism. Nasri et al. (1996) reported on a mucosal traveling wave in/at a patient with ventricular dysphonia, which would indicate a certain degree of tension in the observed VTFs. In a comparative study Lindestad et al. (2004) compared the ventricular fold vibration of a patient with hypertrophic VTFs and chronic laryngitis with the phonation of a vocally healthy person who was "simulating a hyperfunctional, breathy voice "by means of VTF vibration. The comparison was carried out using high-speed imaging, including kymographic, acoustic and perceptual analysis. 'True' ventricular voice appeared as aperiodical, with large amplitudes and complete closure sometime without the vocal folds whereas the simulated voice showed fairly regular features involving simultaneous vibration at the ventricular and VF level. Laryngoscopic photos as also high speed images (Fuks et al., 1998; Lindestad et al., 2001; Maslov and Černov, 1980; Sakakibara et al., 2002b) of VTF vibrations in ThS reveal a posterior chink in the 'rima ventricularis'. This phenomenon aligns with the histo-anatomical observations of the ventricular folds (Reidenbach, 1998b) (see also 2.2.3). Since this implies an incomplete closure it is expected to find also correspondences in glottal flow data.

Role of the VFs in "growl" and "*kargyraa*" In a remarkable study Sakakibara et al. (2004b) have recently attempted to elucidate the role of *m. aryepiglotticus*, *m. thyroepiglotticus* and *m. vocalis* using EMG techniques. The research questions were suggested by prior observations on imitated throat singing. Hooked wire electrodes were inserted perorally under endoscopic control. Muscle activity was measured while the phonatory task of producing "drone" voice (*xöömej*), *kargyraa*, growl, vocal fry, falsetto and modal voice was carried out. Unfortunately, but not very surprisingly, it proved very difficult to insert the electrode in the AEF area, and the electrode would not stay in place. Hence the results could not be used for discussion. However, the measured potential for *m. thyroepiglotticus* showed higher activity during such phonation types when supraglottic constriction was present ("pressed type 'drone'", *kargyraa*, growl). Unfortunately, here too a "contamination" by LCA activity could not be completely ruled out. Nevertheless the study gives information about VF activity during *kargyraa* (VTF-VF phonation) and growl (AEF-VF phonation). The measurements show the highest activity for *m. vocalis* during VTF-VF (*kargyraa*) and AEF-VF (growl) phonation, but also a raised level of activity for Sakakibara's "pressed type". For *m. thyroepiglotticus*, vocal fry phonation is also included in the group of high-activity VPTs, although *kargyraa* shows a slightly lower level of activity within this group.

2.5.3 Double Source Phonation or Diplophonic Phonation in Throat Singing

Pulse register, vocal fry and creaky voice Such non-modal phonation, reidentified as pulse, fry or creak, has often been described as diplophonic or double source phonation (cf. Gerratt and Kreiman, 2001).

The terms vocal fry, pulse register and creaky voice are often used synonymously (cf. Gerratt and Kreiman, 2001; Henton and Bladon, 1988; Laver, 2002: 194)and attempts to separate them have very seldomly made, beyond a growing tendency to use creak or creaky voice as descriptive category in the phonetic (linguistic) literature and vocal fry (or vocal pulse) register for general voice analysis of speech and singing (cf. Crystal, 1992; Titze, 1994b). Laryngoscopic examination of creaky voice "illustrates a reduced antero-posterior dimension"(Esling, 1984) and the "arytenoids cartilages are tightly together, so that the vocal cords can vibrate only at the other end" (Ladefoged, 1975: 123). As Henton and Bladon (1988) summarize, in creaky voice[6] the VFs appear as thick and compressed, and the VTFs are "also somewhat adducted, may 'load' the vocal folds"; the VFs "are somewhat relaxed"; the arytenoids "are tightly together, with only a small length of the ligamental vocal folds able to vibrate"; the closed phase of the glottal cycle is "considerably longer than the opening, open and closing phases"; and "creak may be characterized by either a single or double glottal pulse". For pulse register (vocal fry) Allen and Hollien (1973) described in a laminographic study that, in contrast to modal register, in pulse no dependence or correlation of fundamental frequency and VF-thickness could be detected. Changes in thickness appeared to be unpatterned. But in all cases the ventricle (space) "was smaller than in modal register, indicating ventricular fold impingement." The involvement of the ventricular folds in the production of vocal fry has also been assumed, inter alia by Blomgren et al. (1998).

Hypothetical VPTs in ThS Table 2.5.3 has been assembled as a step towards constructing a hypothesis on possible voice production mechanisms which could occur in ThS styles.

Other possible variants, suggested by analogy to substitutional phonation mechanisms, e.g. a pseudo-glottis 'created' by the epiglottis and lateral or posterior pharyngeal walls (cf. Ptok et al., 1993; Ptok, 993a), are not included here; although presumably very rare, they cannot be ruled out a priori. AEF- and VTF-phonation as well as AEF-VF- or AEF-VTF-phonation are here of purely hypo-

[6] Apparently studies of vocal fry were also included in the summary.

	AES-VF	AEF-VTF	AEF-VF	AEF	AES-VTF-VF	AEF-VTF-VF	VTF	VTF-VF	VF-VF
o	single source	double source	double source	single source	double source	triple source	single source	double source	single
c	single cycle	non-single-cycle	non-single-cycle	non-single-cycle	non-single-cycle	non-single-cycle	(non-) single-cycle	double cycle	double cycle
p	PM1	PM2	PM2	PM2	PM1	PM2	PM2	PM2	PM2
s	*xöömej, sygyt, xoomij, özlyau, sygyrtyp*	*xos-kargyraa, xarxiraa*	*kargyraa, umŋqokolo*	*kargyraa, umŋqokolo*	*tespeŋ-xöömej*	*tespeŋ-kargyraa, umŋqokolo*	*xos-kargyraa xarxiraa*	*kargyraa, xai dzo-ke xarxiraa*	*ün-kargyraa, dzo-ke Strohbass*

Table 2.12: Hypothetical variants of laryngeal oscillation types/mechanisms in different ThS variations. Several styles (s) appear twice or more since auditory representation (p) and physical appearance may differ and overlap. Source refers to the number of oscillators (o), hence it says nothing about the symmetry or linearity of oscillation (bifurcation etc.). Cycle (c) predicts the kind of cycle that will be present in the glottal flow/EGG curve; grey backgrounded are those where such VPT is most unlikely to appear in ThS.

thetical character because the involvement or absence of VF or VTF cannot be proved or disproved by direct visual inspection, since AEF/AES mostly covering and occlude all structures below them. The possible (oscillating) involvement of VTFs or VFs below the closed or oscillating AEFs, as well as the vibration (pattern) of the VFs below the oscillating VTFs, seems difficult to clarify by means of other (i.e. non-direct visual) methods. Besides "conventional" laminographic tracings (Agarwal et al., 2003) this ultimately may prove feasible only by high-speed endoscopic or stroboscopic examination, or perhaps by MRI or ultrasound sonography. Here it must be born in mind that a fibre endoscopic intrusion into the relevant (probably constricted) area creates, not only physically but also acoustically and aerodynamically a massive obstacle which must be tolerated and compensated for by the subject. "Plain" fibre endoscopic video recording (Esling, 2002a) or video fluoroscopic images as presented by Levin and Edgerton (1999) thus could not reveal any activity of the involved laryngeal structures, let alone any vibrational pattern. The choice of an electrophysiological acoustic study is partially motivated by the desire to employ a less invasive technique than laryngoscopy still is at the present time (see for further discussion section 3.2.3).

Organic variability Histo-anatomical studies reveal the variable and unstable disposition of ventricular and aryepiglottal tissue composition across individuals. Consequently there will be a dependence of articulatory strategies for medialization (medial approximation) of VTF on the (supra-) laryngeal morphology of different individuals, such as

- ventricle size,
- shape of the epiglottis (blade),
- AEF tissue (relation musc.-mucos.-adipose tissue),
- VTF tissue, or
- "adipose peri-epiglottal bulges".

This dependence must also be taken into account with regard to observations of supralaryngeal articulation strategies across individuals, and likewise with regard to velo-pharyngeal structures (palatal shape, velar shape) and oral structures (maxilla size, mandibula size, and dentition). The discussion (see above) about the fraction of muscular fibre present in the tissue of VTFs could probably only be carried further by extensive histo-anatomical investigation, in terms of both basic research into the anatomy of the larynx and specifically into the anatomy of professional singers (not necessarily of ThSingers). Such unique research as that of Sakakibara et al. (2004b) clearly needs to be continued, but its high demands on both investigator and subject make it rather unlikely to be carried out on a large number of singers. Empirical testing of whether there is also a change in subcortical structures or nervous control of AES or VTF manoeuvres, as presumed by Chen-Gia Tsai Tsai (2003), seems to be even more unfeasible at the moment. These congenitally predefined structures and preconditions, which can nonetheless be influenced or moulded by recurrent use, should also be kept in mind when discussing the concepts of "giftedness" or talent as (ThS) singer. A highly interesting point that remains to explore concerns the not unlikely physiological changes resulting from a lengthy or lifelong practice of ThS (not to mention the alleged healing effects (de la Breteque, 1988; Goldmann, 1992).

2.5.4 Discussion of Vocal Tract Articulation

The supraglottic constriction in ThS, especially in AES-VF phonation needs to be acknowledged as a specific shape feature of the VT tract. Though this configuration has also been described for singing types other than ThS, it seems to be a significant and distinctive component of ThS. Other specific voice source characteristics very likely remain to be discovered.

Methods or strategies of re-enhanced harmonics articulation The five methods for enhanced harmonics suggested by Edgerton (Edgerton et al., 2003; Edgerton, 2005) have been revised here to yield a (somewhat) simpler three-way matrix. This should hopefully suffice to encompass the main articulation strategies occurring in south-Siberian ThS. These strategies refer to basic VT shape tendencies, which affect the perceived timbre differences between styles. The matrix can easily be extended in both dimensions allowing further subcategories to be introduced for later specifications. The OAT column represents the three basic articulation strategies for formant shifting over harmonics, which thereby

	OAT	PM1		PM2						
VPT	AT	VF	VF-AES	VF-VF	VF-VTF	VTF	VF-AEF	VTF-AEF	VF-VTF-AEF	AEF
AM1		+	+	+	+	+	+	+	+	+
	3	+	+	+	+	+	+	+	+	+
		+	+	+	+	+	+	+	+	+
	1	+	+	+	+	+	+	+	+	+
AM2		+	+	+	+	+	+	+	+	+
	2	+	+	+	+	+	+	+	+	+

Table 2.13: Basic combination matrix of articulatory and phonatory modes;

become reinforced. AT1 is composed of a narrowed VT with a constant anterior (prepalatal/postalveolar) constriction. AT2 is composed of a VT with a narrowed VT with alternating and changing posterior (velar/postdorsal) and anterior (alveolar, prepalatal/predorsal) constrictions. AM represents the lip tuning modus (which could probably also be separated into the three parameters of jaw/mouth opening, lip rounding and lip protrusion)

Of course there are styles like *türlegt xoomij* or *byga xöömej*, which do not fit into the above-described systematization. As emphasized in chapter 2.1.1 it is not the ultimate goal here to create a system that will cover all existing styles. Such an enterprise would be illusionary and unrealizable since style terminology and concepts reflect not only voice production and overtone articulation, but factors such as timbre, ornamentation, rhythm, application (use/purpose), emotional expression, mimesis and other musical aspects (see 2.1.1). Instead the matrix (in Table 2.13) tries to abstract the essential oral articulation strategies from the multiple VT adjustments which of course interact with the source (PM1/PM2) in question.

General tendencies of VT shape 'behaviour' Despite the fact that there is of course a large variety of singer-specific individual differences due to individual interpretation and adaptation, some general tendencies of VT settings for all VPT in ThS are listed here:

(1) larynx position (height) slightly raised

This is supported by reports about larynx height vis-à-vis vowel height (tongue height), tension and nasal coupling (velar declination).

(2) epiglottal movement aligned with formant movement

Note, however, that instead of a 'covering' function of the epiglottis, an upright position of the epiglottis more often is observed.

(3) dorsal tongue height aligned with formant height

Main strategy of F2 shifting for melodic articulation

(4) lips rounded and protruded, adjustment of rounding specifically with rHs.

2.6 HYPOTHESES & Expectations

Based on existing primer research by different authors (Baken and Orlikoff, 2000; Kent and Ball, 2000) show the following selection of possible biased values in acoustic measure. Unfortunately most parameters show a high variance, if obtained by different research groups, so that even ranges of correlations could not be established yet. More often discussed in singing are sob, ring, twang VQ (Colton and Estill, 1981; Titze, 2001; Yanagisawa et al., 1989). Here at least the resonant, "ringing" voice should serve as subject-matter of comparison. A rough summary of expectations on acoustic and electrophysiological correlates is given in Table 2.14.

One of the main hypotheses formulated here is that of an area specific characteristic of voice production in acoustics terms within the south-Siberian area of throat-singing. It reflects the ethno-musicological / ethnographical record of a genre specific and singer specific characteristic of the

1. Rejecting the null-hypothesis of a homogeneous appearance of voice production in the different areas of south-Siberian throat singing, it is assumed that significant differences will be seen in over the population of measured values along certain selected parameters of Vx and Lx signals.

2. The null-hypothesis of a homogeneous appearance of voice source parameters is rejected with regard to the three suggested articulation types.

Acoustic Characteristics	single-cycle phonation mode 1 – PM1	double-cycle phonation mode 2 – PM2
Similarity to	tensed VQ, resonant VQ, ringing voice	harshness/ throatiness, breathiness
perturbation	Low shimmer rates, Low jitter rates	Higher shimmer rates, Higher jitter rates
Spectral slope/tilt	Enhanced	Enhanced
Noise component	Less noisy component, but higher prominence of harmonics	Higher noise, not as prominent harmonics
Spectral components	Damped F1 area Higher energy in	Higher energy around 3kHz and 4.8kHz
Electro-glottographic Characteristics	PM1	PM2
EGG patterns	Single cycle rhythm	Non-single cycle rhythm (double or triple)
EGG quotients	Short CP similar to tensed voice (Marasek, 1997)	Longer OP and CP than in PM1

Table 2.14: Expected impacts of PMs in ThS on acoustic parameters

3. It is also assumed that correlations will be observed

   (a) between certain acoustic parameters, especially perturbation parameters which gradually express the specific characteristics of ThS voices

   (b) between group variables (area, articulation type) and certain acoustic and electro-physiological parameters (jitter, shimmer, HNR, H1-H2)

4. AES-VF phonation and VTF-VF phonation are assumed

   (a) to be the most extensively used VPT in south-Siberian Ths for phonation mode 1 (AES-VF) and phonation mode 2 (VTF-VF), respectively

   (b) to be significantly different in their voice-source characteristics from modal phonation, involving a specific single-cycle mode for AES-VF

VPT (PM1) and a specific double cycle mode for VFT-VF VPT (PM2)

5. Thus presumably both the characteristics of Vx and of Lx would significantly indicate an (individual) occurence of aberrant VPT within a given phonational mode
   (a) This would include variation between AES-VF voice and (VF-)modal voice in PM1.
   (b) This would include AEF-VF/ AEF-VTF-VF/AEF-VTF/AEF voice production and VTF-VF/ VTF or VF-VF (pulse) voice in PM2.

Chapter 3

METHOD – Physioacoustical Analysis of Voice Production in Throat Singing

3.1 Preliminary Considerations – Why do we need field data of ThS?

Previous acoustic, aerodynamic, and electro-physiological analysis of ThS have been based on laboratory data from single-subject experiments (Bloothooft et al., 1991; Fuks et al., 1998; Lindestad et al., 2001; Sakakibara et al., 2002b,c, 2004b), as well as (Edgerton et al., 2003), which is based on simulated or imitated ThS. Single-subject experiments usually involve 5-6 subjects and have, generally speaking, the potential for good validity since they demand the "use of absolute baselines in raw data measures with little or no variance"(Shearer, 1997). But of course such experiments have the problem of representativeness: they may not represent a sensible, relevant group average. Hence it appeared to be reasonable to set as one task for this study the acquisition of data on a larger number of singers. In addition, valid data needs to be collected on the variational range of several phenomena, notably those involving more than just the acoustic signal.

Since it is neither practicable nor realistic to achieve data standards that will encompass all the characteristics of voice physiology, the description of the field data will focus only on certain aspects, such as acoustic properties (short-term analysis), glottal function and subglottal resonance (formant influence). In addition such factors as feasibility of the method in a field situation, subject recruitment, environment, and 'invasivity' had to be considered. Additional data gathered in a more controlled experimental setting, will be considered for supplementary analysis.

3.2 Specific Non-Invasive Methodology for Voice Investigation in Field Work

3.2.1 Field Work within Voice Research

Given the typical field ambience of talking people, barking dogs, crying children and roaring rattling motorcycles in the background of every scene, the investigator often has to deal with an acoustic environment (wind, rain noise, or insects buzzing around the microphone) which is anything but controllable and 'shieldable'. In addition the experimenter typically has to adapt on mostly improvised setups for instrumental techniques, and s/he mostly has to employ a foreign language to convince and instruct possible informants (subjects) about the experiment, not to mention unexpected cultural tabus which have to be respected (e.g. 'swallowing' anything during daytime in Ramadan is forbidden in Islam).

Vocology experiments are generally carried out in the quiet surroundings of a clinic or in a phonetics lab. The number of vocology experiments performed in a fieldwork situation appears to be quite small in the literature; if at all, they appear in the context of phonetic fieldwork. Of course, the standards governing data acquisition, recording quality and applied methods, and the demand for reliability and validity of measurements, should not be compromised if at all possible. But there are certain factors that cannot be avoided. Ladefoged (2003) seems to be optimistic enough to assume that a researcher can have control over those factors,

laboratory experiment	field experiment
in order to prove a hypothesis (on specific parameters)	in order to broaden one's data base on a certain phenomenon; exploratory experiment hence prior to lab experiments
smaller number of dependent (predicted) variables (also not monovariate)	larger number of dependent variables, due to larger corpus and varying environment (multivariate) Ű unexpected variability due to inhomogeneity of all sorts
larger number of independent (controlled) variables (mostly because of a smaller corpus (mostly smaller numbers of subjects, but also more repetitions)) -	fewer independent (controlled) variables Ű larger corpus (in terms of subjects; perhaps smaller number of repetitions)
definite (relatively small) number of confounding variables: controlled environment (however, there might still remain variables which one is not aware of)	indefinite number of confounding variables; environment less controlled and controllable, even if one follows the advice of experienced fieldworkers

Table 3.1: Rough comparison of the characteristics of laboratory experiments and field experiments (as they are applied in the present study)

which is presumably possible to a certain extent. Greisbach (2001), discussing the theoretical framework of phonetic experiments, addresses the feasibility of perception experiments in a free field situation (which he of course rejects). But except for the experiments in speech sciences by Shearer (1997) such items as value of measured field data, of measurement errors, acceptable variance and probability etc. are relatively unaddressed questions (cf. Ladefoged, 2003; Lass, 1974, 1996). So it could be predicted not all the acoustic standards as they are recommended e.g. by Gibbon (2000: 314-317) are met, or can be met, in the present study. On the other hand, some of these negative factors will be partly compensated for by corpus size. Table 3.1 provides a rough confrontation of laboratory and field experiments as they are designed and applied in the present study.

3.2.2 Field Conditions in Southern Siberia

South-central Siberia has a continental climate, featuring a very arid atmosphere with a summer-winter-temperature difference of sometimes as much as 90° K (-50° C – +40° C). These extremes of temperature, as well as the nearly ubiquitous dust, impose requirements of insulation, durability and robustness on any electronic (and electric) field equipment. Other factors that must be taken into consideration include bulkiness, manipulability and manageability of transport via airplane, train, bus, car, and on foot. Data media must be not only durable and big in terms of data capacity, but also small in terms of size. In this way it would allow not only to acquire large amounts of (raw) data which then could encompass longer sessions, but it would also allow necessary backups. Especially in rural areas but even in towns, a reliable self-contained power supply is very important in order to stay rather independent from the local electricity network and possible current fluctuations. This then demands equipment that can operate on accumulator batteries. Another aspect one should consider is the availability of alternative equipment, spare parts and tools, in case of a breakdown. And finally, concerns of robustness and simplicity of the chosen technique and the need for backup must be weighed against the concatenated costs, either for travel or equipment. Transporting such equipment over distances as great as 6000 km by the variety of means of transportation already mentioned is costly in terms of both time and money [involves not only additional expense in the form of overweight baggage fees, but also requires additional time].

3.2.3 Invasivity, Manageability, and Costs

Influence on the subject (phonation) by the method (invasivity)

For field research it seems not only plausible to keep as advantage recording of people in their habitual everyday environment. But also to allow the singer to perform in an unhindered singing position seems to be expedient. Unfortunately this leads to the exclusion of a number of significant and interesting objective methods, at least as they are carried out in a lab. For example, in the context of ThS, obtaining measurements of the very interesting and promising parameter of subglottal pressure would only be possible by means of relatively invasive methods. Direct subglottal pressure measurement involves either a "hypodermic needle" punctured into the trachea (Ishiki, 1964) or "a transnasal inserted miniature pressure transducers placed" directly under and above the glottis (Schutte and Miller, 1988). And according to Schutte and Cranen (Cranen and Boves, 1985) it is also very unlikely that one might find enough subjects who could tolerate an esophageally placed catheter, which would be the third (indirect) method of pressure measurement. For analogous reasons other 'desirable' techniques like fibre endoscopy also had to be excluded from this study. Not only would medical assistance probably be necessary for such invasive measurement, it is also highly doubtful that a significant number of subjects could be convinced to take part in the investigation. Ladefoged himself states about the method of direct subglottal pressure measurement that it "is not a procedure that can be carried out in fieldwork situations" (Ladefoged, 2003: 59). The author also had to decide against airflow measures because of high equipment costs and insufficient durability. And since this would also have required an additional recording channel, it would have made it necessary to conduct a second run in the experiment, too. Moreover, most apparatuses of this kind are very sensitive and need to be calibrated with an extra (bulky) gadget. Consideration of all the above factors (see chapter 3.2.1) argued in favour of omitting certain measurements, and focusing instead on robust, cost-effective, available and approved measurement techniques.

3.2.4 3-Channel-Recording of Voice, EGG, and Subglottal Pressure (Inverse Filtering)

In order to acquire as much relevant data as possible with a non-invasive methodology another measuring technique had to be devised for use in the field. A number of descriptions of ThSingers in the field and elsewhere (Grawunder, 1999; van Tongeren, 1994; Zemp and Trân, 1991) mention strong chest wall vibrations which can be perceived (i.e. hand sensation at sterno-clavicular joint) by another person. Teachers and singers emphasize that there is a "chest(y) tone" which is essential for a good *xöömej* voice. In particular Kyrgys (2002: 79) assumes that this is not only belonging to the basic concept for ThS in Tuva, but also that the chesty tone has a physiological compound or correlate. Whereas the sensation of chest wall vibrations (by the singing person him/herself, or by someone else) has been acknowledged for a long time (cf. Nadoleczny, 1923: 27, Ranke and Lullies, 1953: 207), it was not assumed to be a real resonance phenomenon (Sundberg, 1983).

Hence ThS seemed to be a highly suitable context for studying such a phenomenon, since, as mentioned above, ThS involves a strong coupling of subglottal tract and source. Observations in the field had already pointed to the relevance of breath support (but also of chest wall vibrations as a factors contributing to a good resonance feeling, indicating a 'good' technique in the 'chest'-voice (xöömej but also kargyraa) (see chapter 1). It was assumed that, due to the supraglottal constriction and enhanced excitation in the source, the so-called chest resonator (i.e. the subglottal space) (Gall and Berg, 1998) would also be more strongly excited. Drawing on an ongoing discourse about the relevance of subglottal pressure waves for vocal fold vibration, which has also become relevant as subglottal formant discussion (Cranen and Boves, 1987), Don Miller and Harm Schutte in 1988 succeeded in recording sub- and supraglottal pressure signals in a professional singer directly via a miniature transducer (Schutte and Miller, 1988).

Gall, Berg, and Stelzig (Augsten and Gall, 1997; Gall and Berg, 1998; Gall and Stelzig, 1997; Stelzig et al., 1999) introduced a non-invasive way of recording 'subglottal resonance', interpreting the signal as a derived and filtered mapping of subglottal pressure waves. The procedure consists of a 3-channel recording of the voice (Vx), the electroglottographic signal (Lx), and Sx. Sx stands here for subglottal pressure waveform and represents the signal of a small microphone placed directly on the skin of the *fossa jugularis* (suprasternal notch). Complementary recordings of simultaneous direct (intratracheal) and indirect (contact microphone) measurements (Neumann et al., 2001, 2003) showed good agreement between the two signals. The term "subglottal pressure waves" may be misleading in that it would suppose either direct or indirect measurement of pressure as a function of vibrational support. Neumann et al. (2001) showed a rough correlation between the contact-microphone signal (Sx) and a direct measurement of subglottal (intratracheal) pressure waves obtained at the trachea stoma of a voice-normal patient. Accordingly, as a reasonable alternative, it was decided to use the non-invasive method of subglottal pressure wave recording including electroglottography and voice signal recording.

Field Recording Settings

In the field work situation the method described above was carried out using two stereo recording devices. The voice channel (Vx) served as synchronization signal. Altogether three different equipment settings were used. For Setting 1 and 2 (in the field situation) a hyperbolic condenser microphone (AKG 1000 S) was used, positioned in an approximately 15 to 20cm from the subject's mouth. Another electrets microphone (H&H EM100N, or H&H EMV 200) placed at the jugular fossa served as low-cost accelerometer. As a third measuring device an electroglottograph (Laryngograph Ltd. 1) was used, with the electrodes placed as usual on the skin over the thyroid cartilage. In all cases contact gel was used in order to compensate for possible resistance due to unshaven skin, etc.

The signal of the first (mouth-) microphone was split onto two stereo mini jacks, on the left channel in each case. The right channel was supplied with the laryngographic signal and the signal of the (second) contact microphone (see Figure 3.1). A portable DAT-Recorder TD-100 SONY and a laptop Notebook Dell Latitude CPx with an ESS maestro 2E onboard sound card served as recording devices. Both devices recorded at a sample rate of 44.1 kHz (16bit) in a frequency range from 20 Hz to 18 000 Hz. Alternatively in Setting 2 a portable Digital Compact Cassette Recorder Philips DCC 170 was used in the same way (44.1 kHz, 16 bit). With respect to the data reduction in dcc-format, this was considered to be acceptable for low-frequency signals, like Lx and Sx.

Setting 3 was used to obtain additional data with a single singer (the author) in the supplementary experiments (section 4.4). Here either a multichannel tape recorder (Tascam PORTASTUDIO 414MKII) or the M-Audio Firewire 1814 external soundcard was used for recording purposes. For postprocessing the raw data (DAT/DCC tapes) into soundfiles (*.WAV) a Marian-Digi-4 sound-card was used with an optical SPDIF connection. The software products Goldwave v5.06 (Goldwave Inc., `www.goldwave.com`) and Audacity (GNU, open source, `www.audacity.de`) were utilized to control the recording, for data editing and for raw-signal processing (analysis preparation) (see 3.3.1).

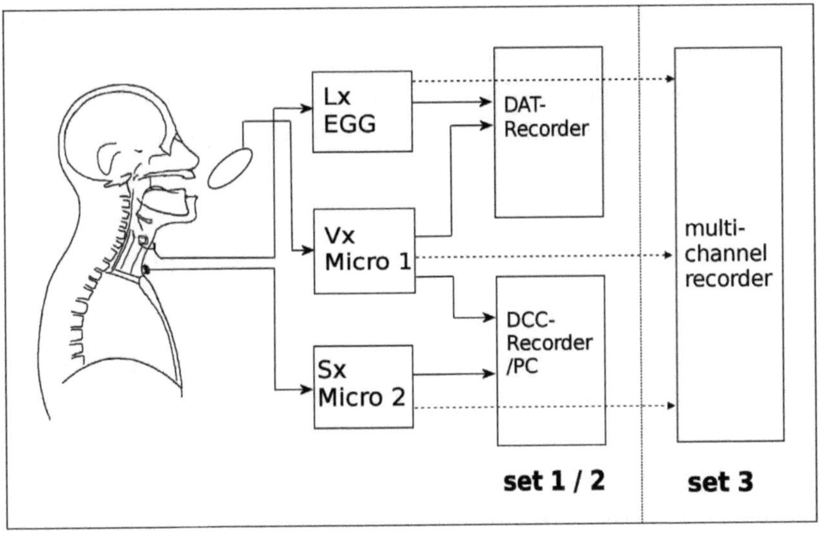

Figure 3.1: Recording scheme illustrating the three different recording settings

3.2.5 Subject Recruitment

Given the importance of the socio-cultural context and of functional comprehension (according to motor theory, incl. Carpenter effect etc.), Siberian ThSingers whose biographies include exposure to ThS from their early youth should be selected. Some of the subjects in the present study had started to sing very early indeed (IK, AM at the age of 5/6). For the most part, too, they have been throat singing for a longer period than their European 'ThS-colleagues'. But there are also Tuvan, Mongolian, Hakas and Altai singers, who have received training in classical (European) music, and sometimes even classical singing ('Russian school'). Despite a reflection of musical features, a 'foreign' influence on the singing techniques can not be ruled out, especially regarding arpeggio and vibrato. A useful size for the dataset was considered to be at least 10 singers per area group. To ensure a high level of proficiency it was decided to include only singers from the age of 18 to 60, and only semi-professionals and professionals, i.e. to exclude amateurs or adepts. High proficiency was thought to be an appropriate indicator of good approved technique. Such a 'good' technique should not cause any paresthesia, i.e. “strained voice” feeling after longer periods of singing, and should guarantee a certain degree of accomodability to the novelty of the experimental situation. But since the investigation needed to look at a range of different techniques in a variety of styles, this variety was not restricted in any way, except for instrumental accompaniment.

3.2.6 Subject Tasks and Raw Data Corpus Description

Singers were asked to produce longer passages in various styles, preferably all the styles they commanded. They were told that the passages should preferably be sung without text (at least these were the passages afterwards chosen for analysis). The tasks that the singers had to perform were deliberately kept uncomplicated in order to keep the situation as ‘normal’ as possible, given that the subjects had to tolerate EGG-electrodes and the microphone at the jugular fossa, as well as the fact that they were asked not to play their instrument (*čatxan* (H); *topšur, tošpulur, igil,* or *čanzy* (T); *morin xuur* (M)) while singing. The recruited subjects (singers) were recorded over the course of two field trips to the republics of Hakassia and Tuva in 2000 (March-May; November).

The data corpus obtained (approx. 5 GB) consists of approx. 200 wav-files comprising a length of approximately 7,5 hours. The lack of a channel-mixing tool for amplitude (recording level) adjustment and of a monitor that would display the recording in real time posed serious problems for both the laryngographic signal and the ‘jugularis’ microphone signal. In fact, it turned out that there was only one complete set from among the 3-channel field recordings (singer SI). All the other sets contained a distorted signal either of EGG or of microphone 2. This fairly discouraging result led to a re-design of multi-channel recordings of this kind.

The number of valid recordings of Vx-Lx or Vx-Sx tracks was counted as 9 for SxLx and 20 for VxLx. Accordingly, it was decided to include in the corpus an additional collection of audio recordings (approx. 2.5 hours) for Vx-only analysis. This extra material was collected over the years of 1993-2000 by Mark van Tongeren, Sven Grawunder, Ludek Brož, Zoja Kyrgys, and Mariata Sundui. In order to increase the number of Altaian and Mongolian singers in the corpus, professional audio recordings of available Audio-CDs or broadcast radio features were also included for Vx-anlysis; these consisted partly of field recordings and partly of studio recordings.

Corpus 1		Corpus 2	
non-single-channel tracks		single channel tracks (audio only)	
Field data of SG	30 singers	Field data (SG) + selection of Vx in corpus1 (SG) + additional field rec. (other) + Audio-CD material	44 singers
1 Vx, Lx, Sx of 1 singer 62 Vx Lx of 15 singers 11 Vx Sx of 9 singers	74 tracks	77 Vx of 44 singers	77 tracks

Table 3.2: Data corpora scheme (Vx=voice signal, Lx=laryngographic signal, Sx=suglottal resonance signal); SG=material collected by the author); see B.3 for complete list of subjects; see B.2 for explicit list of analyzed recordings

Although this would appear to be a fairly large amount of recorded material, in fact there was not enough material to serve for gender comparison or for a long-term study of individual singers. Both these factors ought to be assessed for a comprehensive OtS-ThS comparison. This remains for further research.

3.3 Voice (Source) Analysis Design

The framework design was informed by several previous investigations on the acoustical and electro-physiological correlates of vocal qualities, e.g. Kent and Ball (2000) as well as Baken and Orlikoff (2000), Anders (1997), and Blomgren et al. (1998), but also Colton and Estill (1981) and Klasmeyer (1999).

3.3.1 Preparation and Data Pre-Analysis

Given the large amount of data and the need for them to be processed and analyzed automatically and semi-automatically, the software PRAAT (version 4.2.16-4.3.02) (Boersma and Weenink, 2005) served as the tool of choice. Tokens for

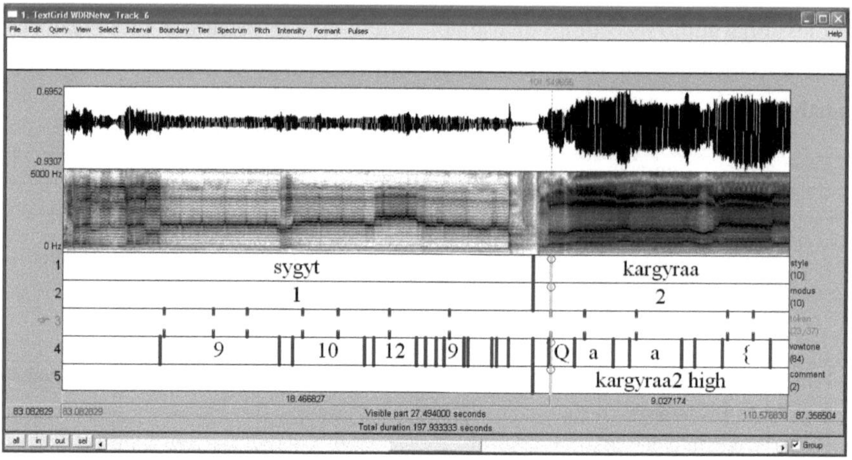

Figure 3.2: Data pre-analysis for all analyzed tracks; 5 tiers have been used to describe the ThS passage in terms of the analysis: style, phonation mode, token (measure point = begin of measurement interval), vowel quality or perceivable 'melody harmonic' according to articulation type (AT1, AT2 or AT3), and comment

signal measure were chosen out of the sung phrase (minimum 3 to maximum 5 tokens per musical phrase) depending on (breath-grouped) phrase length and length of the recording. Preliminary analysis and tests, which are not included here, were carried out using the Multidimensional Voice Analysis Program MDVP (KAY Elemetrics Ltd.). The parameters to be applied were developed on the basis of the MDVP Manual (KAY-ELEMETRICS-CORP., 1993) and the PRAAT manual (Boersma and Weenink, 2005). Further statistical analysis of data was carried out using MS Excel 2003 and SPSS 12. For raw signal preparation of Vx, Lx or Sx, such as dc-offset adjustment, left-to-right channel switch or polarity change, the software Goldwave (Goldwave Inc.) was used. Filtering (band-pass 25 - 2500 Hz) was applied to Lx in some cases in order to reduce high-frequency noise in the raw signal. Observations of Gx in these cases could therefore only be made prior to filtering. After transforming the DAT/DCC tapes into wave-files, these were cut into individual takes of sessions with each singer. Subsequently each take was evaluated and categorized in terms of style, phonation mode, and either vowel or ordinal number of the reinforced harmonic for each individual section (measure sequence). For the defined sequences a measure point was (manually) set, which would define the beginning of the measurement sequence.

3.3.2 Physio-Acoustic Analysis Methods

3.3.2.1 Waveform Shape and Pattern Analysis

The first step in waveform analysis even prior to inspection of the spectrum, must be an examination of the raw acoustic signal. This is especially important in the case of certain ATs that force the waveform into a superperiodic behaviour, which reveals the dominance of a frequency range in the spectrum or may cause difficulties in period detection. As for PM2 in ThS Grawunder (2003a,b) has described different non-single-cycle patterns, which would in Vx appear as very aperiodic in a short term perspective. Only longer time frame would reveal a systematic pattern, which could of course also bear additional supraperiodic patterns.

3.3.2.2 Vx (Lx) - Perturbation, F0

Given the variability of perceptual ratings (see Table 2.5) one could already expect a certain degree of aperiodicity or irregularity in the glottal cycle and acoustic waveform, especially for PM2. Such irregularity could be described by terms like perturbation, fluctuation or variability. Variability would just refer to the ability of an entity to vary (by accident or by design), whereas fluctuation already indicates a systemic instability, involving irregular movements of a disturbed pattern (cf. Titze, 1994b). The term perturbation on the other hand describes a "minor disturbance, or a temporary change, from an expected behaviour" (Titze, 1994b).

Signal (Perturbation) Parameters Perturbation analysis relies heavily on periodicity analysis of the signal. For reasons of accuracy the method of pitch detection or acoustic periodicity detection applied in PRAAT is based on forward crosscorrelation algorithms, instead of the generally used autocorrelation algorithm, where a (windowed) sequence of the signal would be compared (correlated) to the signal itself. For the crosscorrelation method as computed in PRAAT this would involve a pre-determined analysis window or frame that is moved forward with a time step of 0.25/(pitch floor). The time step represents the frame duration of the measurement interval in seconds. The pitch floor was defined depending on the phonation mode, as 50Hz for PM2 or 80Hz for PM1 (although this had to be adjusted manually in some cases). This would mean that for PM2 (0.25/50s-1=0.005s) 500 pitch values per second would be computed. The length of the analysis window makes also reference to the defined pitch floor value, since it will be exactly the same as the longest period. For PM2 this would mean that the window length will be 1/50s-1=0.02s (cf. PRAAT Manual, 2005, Boersma and Weenink, 2005). For acoustical perturbation analysis of Vx but also of Lx, period, jitter and shimmer analysis were carried out using the following parameters:

(1) Information on fundamental frequency variation: F0mn, the mean value of fundamental frequency, and F0md, the median value of F0, are obtained through the processing of a PRAAT PointProcess object. This was used in order to more directly arrive at the mean period length (period mn). The standard deviation of the period length within the current measurement period was also calculated (period sd).

(2) Short-term period perturbation measurement: Jitter, the cycle-to-cycle variation of the fundamental period, is associated with stability of the glottal cycle (Titze, 1994b).

There are different methods for jitter calculation: The absolute jitter (in μ s) or local, absolute Jitter, as it is called in PRAAT, is the average absolute difference of lengths between consecutive periods. MDVP calls this parameter Jita. Since in the data acquisition the fundamental tone was not constrained or stipulated, it made no sense to obtain absolute values. Therefore the selection of methods focused on relative jitter measurement: Relative jitter, jitter factor, or local jitter, as it will be referred to in this study, is often given in percent, since it expresses the percentage of period perturbation of the average period. Local Jitter is calculated as the average absolute difference between consecutive periods, divided by the average period (see equation 3.1). MDVP calls this parameter Jitt.

$$jitterLoc = \frac{\frac{1}{N-1}\sum_{k=1}^{N-1}|T_k - T_{k+1}|}{\frac{1}{N}\sum_{k=1}^{N} T_k} \tag{3.1}$$

RAP stands for relative average perturbation and equals the Jitt "smoothed" over 3 periods (ppq3 in PRAAT). It will be referred to here as jitter RAP. This Relative Average Perturbation is calculated as the average absolute difference between a period and the average of it and its two neighbours, divided by the average period (see equation (3.1)).

$$RAP = \frac{\frac{1}{N-2}\sum_{k=2}^{N-1}\left|\frac{T_{k-1}+T_k+T_{k+1}}{3} - T_i\right|}{\frac{1}{N}\sum_{k=1}^{N-1} T} \tag{3.2}$$

By analogy to the smoothing in RAP, a general "smoothed perturbation quotient" has been developed, sPPQ, as it is called in MDVP. Its calculation derives directly from the jitter calculation of local jitter and jitter RAP (see equation (3.2)). In this way jitter RAP could also be called PPQ3, and a smoothed ppq over 5 periods would similar be ppq5. ppq5 is the 'default' PPQ in MDVP, but of course the smoothing factor (sf) could be 7, 11 or even 55. Equation (3.3) determines the smoothed period perturbation quotient in a general form; sf is the smoothing factor and must be an odd integer greater than one, and $m = (sf - 1)/2$ (Kent and Ball, 2000: 141)

$$ppq = \frac{\frac{1}{N-sf+1}\sum_{k=1}^{N-sf+1}\left|\frac{1}{sf}\sum_{r=0}^{sf-1}(T_{i+r} - T_{i+m})\right|}{\frac{1}{N}\sum_{k=1}^{N} T_k} \tag{3.3}$$

Jitter (ppq5) [PRAAT] "is the five-point Period Perturbation Quotient, the average absolute difference between a period and the average of it and its four closest neighbours, divided by the average period. MDVP calls this parameter PPQ..." (PRAAT Manual, 2005) Additionally, the measurement of jitter (ddp)

[PRAAT] was considered, which is calculated as the average absolute difference between consecutive differences between consecutive periods, divided by the average period (see equation (3.4)). This value is three times the RAP value (cf. PRAAT Manual, 2005, Boersma and Weenink, 2005).

$$jitter(ddp) = \frac{\sum_{k=2}^{N-1} |2T_k - T_{k-1} - T_{k+1}|}{\sum_{k=2}^{N-1} T_k} \tag{3.4}$$

(3) Short-term Amplitude Perturbation Measurement: The absolute shimmer (dB) (ShdB in MDVP) represents the mean value of absolute amplitude differences between two adjacent periods. In PRAAT this is called shimmer (local, dB). The present study focuses on relative amplitude perturbation measures, and therefore the relative shimmer [Shimmer (local) in PRAAT] or shimmer factor was chosen. Shim, as this parameter is called in MDVP, is basically the percentage rate of the mean amplitude value (see equation (3.5)):

$$shim = \frac{\frac{1}{N-1}\sum_{k=1}^{N-1} |A_k - A_{k+1}|}{\frac{1}{N}\sum_{k=1}^{N} A_k} \tag{3.5}$$

The amplitude perturbation quotient (APQ) follows the same algorithm as the PPQ. This method is provided by PRAAT as smoothed APQ over 3, 5 and 11 periods - Shimmer (apq5), Shimmer (apq3), Shimmer (apq11), respectively (see (3.6)).

$$apq = \frac{\frac{1}{N-sf+1}\sum_{k=1}^{N-sf+1} \left| \frac{1}{sf}\sum_{r=0}^{sf-1} A_{k+r} - A_{k+m} \right|}{\frac{1}{N}\sum_{k=1}^{N} A_k} \tag{3.6}$$

Analogous to sPPQ, sf is the smoothing factor and must be an odd integer greater than one, and $m = (sf - 1)/2$ (Kent and Ball, 2000: 141). Baken and Orlikoff (2000: 194) consider a minimum of 30 consecutive periods as needed "to ensure a valid sample for normal voice". In order to keep the influence of the variance of a larger sample as low as possible they also recommend a minimum of 110 periods for disordered speech. Assuming an average pitch of 90 Hz for all perturbation analyses an approximate minimal interval of 0.5sec, corresponding to 45 periods, was chosen for the present study.

(4) Short-term Additive Noise Measurement: Harmonics-to-Noise Ratio (HNR) – This ratio represents the degree of acoustic periodicity and is given in dB. Somewhat simplified it could be expressed as:

$$HNR = 10 \times \log_{10}\left(\frac{harmonicEnergiePortion}{non - harmonicEnergiePortion}\right) dB \qquad (3.7)$$

A HNR of 0dB would thus mean that the energy in the noise and the energy in the harmonics are equal (cf. Manual of PRAAT (Boersma and Weenink, 2005)). In terms of signal analysis it would be more appropriate to speak of a relationship of periodic vs. non-periodic or non-stationary components (cf. Boersma, 1993). The HNR algorithm uses the forward crosscorrelation method for periodicity analysis. The applied procedure exploits PRAAT's "Harmonicity (cc)" analysis, where HNR mean values and standard deviation values over a pre-defined time interval were calculated. The beginning point of the period is defined in terms of the measure points pre-set during data pre-analysis.

3.3.2.3 Spectral Components (NHR, Band Energy Differences, Slope)

Noise-to-Harmonics Ratio (NHR) The noise-to-harmonics ratio constitutes a ratio of inharmonic components to harmonic spectral magnitudes (cf. Buder, 2000: 188). Higher rates of NHR have been highly associated with breathy and rough voice, e.g. in connection with VF lesions, and with dysphonia evaluations (cf. Pereira Jotz et al., 2002). According to the MDVP manual, Noise-to-Harmonics Ratio (NHR) refers to the relationship or ratio of inharmonic to harmonic spectral magnitudes, i.e. the ratio of nonharmonic energy (frequency range: 1500Hz - 4500Hz) to harmonic energy (frequency range: 70Hz - 4500Hz) in the spectrum. NHR in MDVP is computed using a pitch-synchronous frequency-domain method with algorithm functions that can be expressed in general terms as follows: After the analyzed signal is divided into windows of 81.92ms (4096 points at 50kHz sampling rate or 2048 points at 25kHz), for every window, the following steps apply:

> "1. Low-pass filtering at 6000Hz (order 22) with Hamming window, downsampling of the signal data down to 12.5kHz and conversion of the real signal into an analytical one using the Hilbert transform.
> 2. 1024-points complex Fast Fourier Transform (FFT) on the analytical signal (corresponding to a 2048-points FFT on real data).
> 3. Computation of the power spectrum from the FFT.
> 4. Calculation of the average fundamental frequency within the window synchronously with the pitch extraction results...
> 5. Harmonic/in-harmonic separation of the current spectrum synchronously with the current window fundamental frequency.
> 6. Computation of the Noise-to-Harmonic Ratio (NHR) of the current window. NHR is a ratio of the inharmonic (1500-4500 Hz) to the harmonic spectral energy (70-4500Hz)." (KAY-ELEMETRICS-CORP., 1993)

In order to process the data semi-automatically, NHR mean values drawn from PRAAT's voice profile analysis (Voice Report) were used. NHR measurement provided by PRAAT is supposed to not differ in principal from the one provided by MDVP, besides a corrected autocorrelation algorithm (cf. Boersma, 1993; Deliyski, 1993) and therefore a more reliable voicing detection, and it should insofar be comparable with other studies, however this makes sense or not.

Spectral Band Energy Difference (BED) Since NHR focuses on a specific ratio of spectral components in voice it aligns with other clinical parameters such as the Voice Turbulence Index (VTI) or the Soft Phonation Index (SPI). VTI refers to a "ratio of the spectral in-harmonic high-frequency energy (2800-5800Hz) to the spectral harmonic energy (70-4500Hz)" for a group of windows which "includes four non-contiguous windows, where the frequency and amplitude perturbations are the lowest for the signal"(Deliyski, 1993: 1971). SPI is described as the relation of low-frequency harmonic energy (frequency range: 70Hz - 1600Hz) to high-frequency harmonic energy (frequency range: 1600Hz - 4500Hz) (KAY-ELEMETRICS-CORP., 1993), and SPI is supposed to serve as an "evaluation of the poorness of high-frequency harmonic components that may be and indication of loosely adducted vocal folds"(Deliyski, 1993: 1971). By analogy to this Soft Phonation Index (SPI) in MDVP has been derived a similar quasi soft phonation index or just a spectral band energy difference (BED). In contrast the present study uses the 'simple' energy band difference as provided by PRAAT, meaning that it gives the 'plain' energy difference (in dB) without any low-pass filtering or downsampling involved. For the Vx corpus BED measurements were obtained in three different bands (0-2kHz, 2-5kHz, and 5-8kHz) by carrying out an energy extraction of a FFT spectrum slice from a spectrogram. In order to show differences between individual singers the results would have had to be normalized with respect to the component of noise (non-harmonic energy within these frequency bands), which was omitted for the present study, since here the investigation focuses just on group differences. Additionally, the spectral slope within the described frequency bands was also obtained. Theses spectral slopes are expected to correspond with the energy differences.

3.3.2.4 Formant structure (Fx, Bx, Hx)

(1) Formants Estimates of formant positions, their bandwidths and amplitudes were examined. Formant analysis in PRAAT is based on Burg algorithm (Boersma and Weenink, 2005; Childers, 1978; Press et al., 1992) for LPC with a frame length of 0.025sec and a pre-emphasis from 50Hz on. The corresponding vowel quality for each measured time-interval (of AT3) was evaluated (and transcribed) by the author during data pre-analysis. Because of the common occurrence of damping of F1, not only the obtaining of F1 but also of F5 in *sygyt* can therefore be a problem; only in a few cases was F5 actually successfully obtained. Such 'melting phenomena' of F2, F3, and F4 are problematic for automatic formant detection as well.

(2) Harmonics Like the vowel qualities for AT3, in AT1 and AT2 perceptually prominent harmonics were notated for each longer song passage which was relevant for analysis. Even in the stage of data pre-analysis, which is read straight out of the PRAAT TextGrid and refers to its time-related measure values, it was possible to point to the range of preferred rHs used in the creation of melodies. The pre-analysed harmonic data could later be used for a comparison of perceptual and acoustic prominence of reinforced harmonics.

(3) Reinforced Harmonics It is assumed in the perception of reinforced harmonics, the harmonics that are perceived as particularly prominent are those which have the highest amplitude within the ('melodic') formant. Here the data pre-analysis, including identification of reinforced harmonic ordinal numbers, was primarily based on auditory judgements. For the analysis the ordinal number of the central superimposing harmonics was obtained by dividing the frequency of the formant amplitude by F0 and calculating from this its harmonic neighbours (the next-lower and next-higher harmonics).

The formant structure itself was investigated in terms of the difference between the highest harmonic, in the center of the formant, and its adjacent lower and higher neighbours (Hmax, Hmax-1, and Hmax+1). Amplitude values were derived from a grid defined by bandwidth and formant center. The grid determined the analysis frame of the short- term spectral analysis, which was carried out via a spectral slice from a narrow-band spectrogram at each measurement point.

Formant and harmonic analysis, spectrum analysis, and formant structure analysis were assembled for every measurement point and recorded on a chart (see Appendix for more examples A.2.2).

3.3.2.5 Glottal Flow and Inverse Filtering of Vx

(1) Glottal Flow by Inverse Filtering Based on the method introduced by Miller (1959) and Miller and Mathews (1963), the glottal flow signal can be obtained by inverse filtering. Though there remain many questions regarding the interpretation of the output signal, it is assumed to be a valuable indicator of the glottal

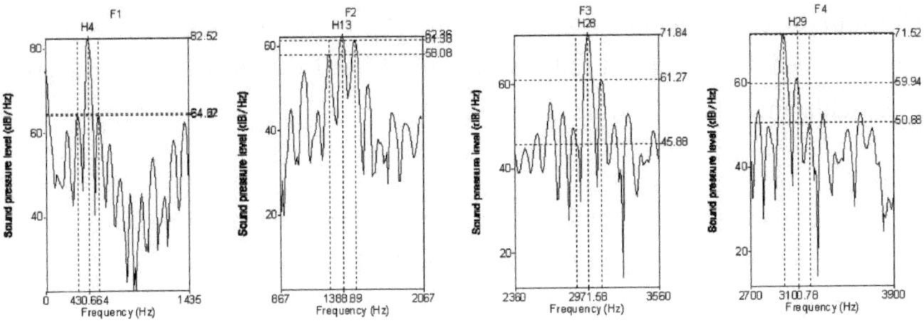

Figure 3.3: Analysis of formant center harmonics and neighbours; SK3 p3, PM1AT3, vowel [ə]

source action. Inverse filtering is a process of removing the vocal-tract transfer function from the speech wave and as a consequence regenerating a reproduction of the underlying source. For this procedure the VT filter function is estimated by a LPC algorithm. The result is applied inversely to the original voice signal. Especially the precise fine-tuning of the LPC curves as anti-resonance filter is problematic, and the method is highly dependent on the exactness of period detection (cf. Keller, 2004). In the glottal flow signal, which is supposed to closely resemble the glottal area function, we typically find an ascending part (T0→U0) that corresponds to glottal opening, and an immediately descending part corresponding to glottal closing (U0 → Tc). Both signal parts are determined and identified as open phase; the closed phase follows after the descending part, acting mostly as a flat sequence in the curve (Tc→T0) (see Figure 3.4).

(2) Voice Source Model / LF-Model For the voice source model of Liljencrants and Fant (LF-Model; 1985) a derivative of an idealized volume velocity waveform was used, whose specific shape has undergone revisions by a number of authors (Rosenberg, Fant, Hedelin, Ananthapadmanabha) (see for an overview Fant, 1997; Ní Chasaide and Gobl, 1997). Analysis of the differentiated glottal flow [dUx or U'g(t)] reveals a number of landmarks and specific consistent shape patterns. These parts of the curve are thus easier to identify and in this way more reliable, especially for automatic detection, rather than the underived ('true') glottal flow. In the derived glottal flow curve a number of features or parameters have been described that are specifically associated with voice quality (cf. Keller, 2004; Ní Chasaide and Gobl, 1997)(see Figure 3.4)

(1) Fundamental Frequency(F0) as time between two maxima (Uo),
(2) Excitation strength (Ee, shown as -Ee): the excitation energy strength,
(3) Glottal frequency [(1/2Tp)/F0, or the inverse of twice the opening phase Tp normalized to fundamental frequency]. This parameter estimates the degree of enhancing found with some voices in the areas of the first and the second harmonic. (cf. Keller, 2004)
(4) Glottal (a)symmetry or skew [(Te-Tp)/(Tp-T0)] "specifies the relative duration of the rising and falling branch" (Keller, 2004). In general, glottal pulses tend to be right-skewed, and increased symmetry results in an enhancing of lower frequencies and a deepening of spectral dips (cf. Keller, 2004).
(5) Dynamic Leakage or return time [Ra = Ta/T0]: This parameter measures the sharpness of glottal closure, i.e., the time that the glottal folds require to accomplish closure. "In terms of the true glottal flow, the return phase shows up as a 'rounding of the corner' of the closing branch of the curve..." (Ní Chasaide and Gobl, 1997: 440). This in turn has a major effect on the slope of the glottal spectrum. Sharp closures are associated with increases of spectral amplitudes in the high frequencies (cf. Keller, 2004).
(6) Open Quotient [OQ = Te/Tc]: The open quotient as the relative measure of the proportion of open phase per period.
(7) Aspiration noise (AH): measurable in terms of periodicity of the signal (jitter, shimmer, HNR)

The present investigation makes use of such parameters only as a rough guideline for description, since the 'real' glottal flow curves are harder to interpret and a methodology for (semi-) automatic analysis of glottal flow signals of ThS (in particular PM2) has yet to be developed.

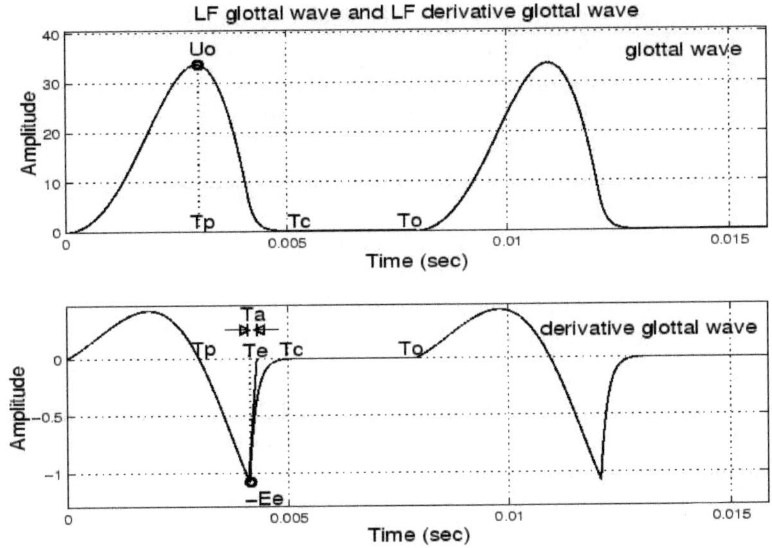

Figure 3.4: LF-model glottal flow wave and its derivative, after Fant (1997); Note that the determination of glottal instants and the use of symbols differs somewhat from those given by Titze (1994a: 115-116), where Uo(U0) would be the average flow, To (To) the opening point, Tp (Tp) the positive slope (T0-Tp), Tc=Tn the negative slope (Tp-Tc).

Investigating the glottal flow signal a number 'voice source parameters' (Ní Chasaide and Gobl, 1997: cf.) were described. Voice source variations were identified and correlated with evaluated vocal qualities by Ní Chasaide and Gobl (1997). A summary is given in Table 3.3. The observation and analysis of the inverse filtered Vx signal and its derivative was only done for examples which were obtained by means of the "Inverse filter programm" provided by the "UCLA Bureau of Glottal Affairs" (BoGA) [`http://www.surgery.medsch.ucla.edu/glottalaffairs/software_of_the_boga.htm`, retrieved 1/3/2005] (Jody Kreiman). A semi-automatic or automatic analysis of larger corpora would have required an adaptation of LPC formants and bandwidths. Since the BoGA software does not support such integration as a subdevice of PRAAT etc., inverse filtering was carried out using methods implemented in PRAAT (see Appendix A.3.3) .

tense	Very low RA, very low RK, small OQ, high RG
lax	Low RG, close to modal as (neutral) position
creaky	Alternation of two very different pulses: (A) high Ee (lower than for mod and lax); (B) Ee very low, RA very high; Both low OQ, low RK and a relatively high RG
breathy	Low RA; High RK reflecting greater symmetry; high open quotient values (OQ) reflect the looseness and gradualness of the glottal gesture; Aspiration noise (AH)

Table 3.3: Correlations/correspondences of glottal flow parameters contrasting and VQs with modal voice (cf. Keller, 2004; Ní Chasaide and Gobl, 1997); see page 109 for explication of parameters

(3) Spectral Characteristics of the Source By employing the LF-Model of the glottal source Klatt and Klatt (1990) were able to do a synthesis of various voice qualities, especially those related to the voice source (breathy voice). The KLSYN88-synthesis model is based on some 39 variables that can be specified. By using the synthesis model for creating voice qualities, spectral components also come into play. These can afterwards be reinvestigated in 'real' voices, assuming that such prominent characteristics of synthetic speech should also have a correspondent in a real signal. Stevens and Hanson (1995), Hanson (1997), and Hanson and Chuang (1999) showed that certain spectral parameters (H1, H2, F1, B1, A3) and their interrelations (H1-H2, H1-A3) correlate with evaluated degree of breathiness (or noisiness) in male, female and childrens' voices. H1-H2 as the difference of the amplitude of the first two harmonics serves as an indicator for open quotient (cf. Fant, 1997; Hanson, 1997: 469; Ní Chasaide and Gobl, 1997). H1-A1, the difference between the amplitude of the first harmonic and the amplitude of the first formant, is taken as an approximate measure of the first formant bandwidth and is insofar interesting for cases of F1 damping and close F1 and F2, e.g. in non-high back vowels. H1-A3, as the difference between the amplitude of the first harmonic and the amplitude of the third formant, serves as an equivalent measure of the spectral tilt. A larger spectral tilt, i.e. a 'greater' H1-A3 should appear in such cases of a glottal chink corresponding to an energy loss caused by this incomplete closure. In addition H1-H3 was investigated, since progressively increasing amplitudes of the first three harmonics were found after initial visual inspection of the spectra.

Stevens and Hanson (1995) also suggested a normalisation regarding the vowels and formant levels of different persons, which has been omitted in order to attempt to observe exactly this dependency of source and vocal tract (here articulation type). Otherwise an adjustment of the different loudness levels of individual subjects need to be considered for the interpretation of results. Assuming that a possible influence of the observed glottal and ventricular chink shows up on the resulting Vx signal, the chosen parameters should show some effect of this. So it would be expected to find such effects especially in samples of the phonation mode 2, at least as a feature of an individual singer. These findings would then need to be correlated with evaluations of breathiness or 'noisiness' of the individual sample.

3.3.2.6 Lx, Gx - shape, patterns, and quotients

(1) Lx technique As Childers and Krishnamurthy (1985) state in their "critical review" of the electro-glottography (EGG): The ultimate goal was an instrument to help detect "subtle changes that signal incipient disease". Though expectations had to be lowered somewhat over the decades, EGG is still a highly valuable technique which has found applications in many fields of speech processing, voice diagnostics and phonetic research. Preliminary progress in the development of the technique of electroglottography is based on the work of such researchers as Fabre (in 1957), Frøjaer-Jensen (1968 to 1970), Fourcin (in 1974), Teaney (Synchrovoice; in 1981), and Rothenberg (in 1981).

Basically the electroglottograph or laryngograph measures the impedance of a low high-frequency alternating current which is applied to the front of the neck by means of two electrodes. The derivation of the impedance variation is displayed as time varying signal. The usual characteristics of the AC are an alternation frequency of 300kHz to 5MHz, a flow of up to 10mA, and depending on tissue impedance, a voltage of about 0.5V. Following (Baken and Orlikoff, 2000: 416) the early theory of Fabre (1958) was ultimately confirmed, which states that the device is affected by the amount of vocal fold contact, i.e., lateral vocal fold contact area (VFCA). Consequently, the electroglottogram does not reflect a direct measure of glottal area, but a derivation or transduction of the vocal fold contact area. Since the glottal area is obtained by measuring the area of the glottis, or the opening between the vocal folds, it is the perilaryngeal tissue that provides the path for the electric current and which thus has a certain impact on the impedance function. The competitor theory to the VFCA theory was that of Smith (1981), who argued that EGG should work as a kind of microphone which reflects in its signal the compression of the perilaryngeal tissue excited by the soundpressure waves within the vocal tract (Baken and Orlikoff, 2000). It must be stressed here that the precise derivation of tissue impedance including the current flow is not fully understood.

A fortiori the impedance or current deflection has to do with two different vibrating tissues, like those of the vocal folds and the ventricular folds, which are different regarding (1) mass and potential contact area (cross-section area of the folds) (2) tissue structure (muscle fibres, collagenous fibres, adipose tissue, intercellular density, mucosa lubrication, etc.) (3) positioned at different heights vis-à-vis the placed electrodes Besides a considerable shunt impedance another specific problem concerns DC offset and Low-Frequency (Gx) component, since Baken and Orlikoff (2000: 423) have also shown that an increase in Lx shape triangularity is forced by keeping the cutoff frequency too high during post-processing. Consequently Lx has to be only considered as an impedance signal that is related to summarized or added contact area of all moving larynx areas that come into question (VF, VTF, AEF, peri-epiglottic adipose tissue, intercartilage tissue). Though it would be more precise to speak of a contacting phase and decontacting phase in the present study the widely used terms open phase and closed phase are applied synonymously. Since the components of medial (cranial-caudal) and longitudinal (ventral-dorsal) contact are hardly to separate these terms bear a lack of precision anyway.

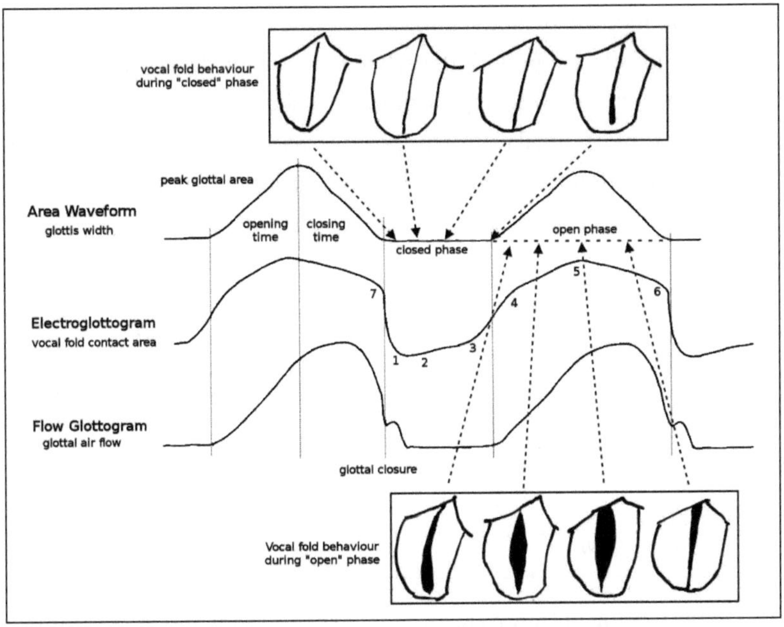

Figure 3.5: Estimate relation of the glottal air flow signal, vocal fold contact area signal of the electroglottograph (Hertegard and Gauffin, 1995) and glottal cycle (Fourcin et al., 2000); the margins in the EGG signal refer to those in (Rothenberg, 1979)

(2) Shapes and Patterns in Lx Usually descriptions of EGG-signal shapes are oriented towards features of the curves which stay relatively stable. Although general agreement exists on the gross segmentation and interpretation of the Lx signal into four segments (cf. Figure 3.5), it must be emphasized that the landmarks in the glottal flow signal and the contact area signal do not (necessarily) coincide, as been clearly shown by Bear et al. (1983). The four segments are (1) a flat segment representing the minimal contact, interpreted as glottal open phase which corresponds to a peak in glottal air flow (5-6), (2) a mostly short phase of rapid impedance fall implying a growing contact area ('closing') and an abruption of the glottal flow (6-1), (3) a short phase of 'maximal contact' or 'closed phase' marked by an impedance peak; no glottal flow is assumed (1-2), and (4) a generally longer phase of 'losing contact' or 'opening phase' which corresponds to a reinitiation and increase of glottal flow.

In relation to adjacent periods the actual curve shape deviations will be considered in terms of peak widening (width), peak skewing, ramping of the shape (including a possible triangularity of the positive[1] part) (Baken and Orlikoff, 2000: 422) and skirt elevation (bulging etc.) (see for illustration Figure 3.6).

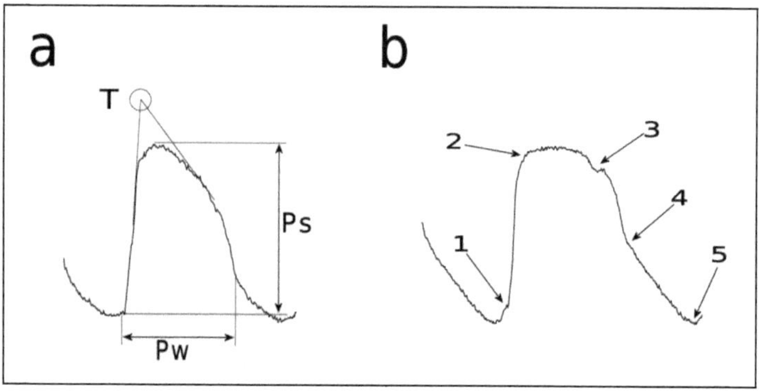

Figure 3.6: Illustration of Lx waveform geometry variations and their parameters: a) triangularity (T), peak widening (Pw), and peak skewing (Ps); b) skirt bulging at typical places (1-5)

Deviations from normal regarding oscillation (cycle) pattern or shape as shown by Childers and Krishnamurthy (1985) or Baken and Orlikoff (2000), also comprise complex pattern modes which become apparent only over a (longer) sequence of cycles. On the basis of previous observations and research in ThS the following possible basic patterns are expected in the corpus: a) cycle type 1: single-cycle pattern b) cycle type 2: double-cycle pattern as observed by Edgerton et al. (2003), Fuks et al. (1998), Grawunder (2003a), and Lindestad et al. (2004) c) cycle type 3: triple-cycle pattern, as observed in Grawunder (2003a). Similar observations were made on vocal fry by Blomgren et al. (1998).

(3) Gx In addition to Lx could be also observed Gx, the so called global signal, which refers to the baseline of Lx. As Rothenberg (1992) showed, neither a clearly

[1]It seems to be an almost fixed convention to position the area which contains the bow of maximal glottal closure in the positive (upper) part of the diagram.

absolute nor a relative measurement is possible, however Gx might allow an estimation of relative larynx height movements. Several attempts have been made to use EGG also as a non-invasive monitor for swallowing movements (Firmin et al., 1997). It seems clear that a 'relative measuring' of Gx, i.e. a description of relative ranges on the basis of Lx baseline of unfortunately, otherwise high-pass filtering to avoid any deviation that could confound Vx measures (e.g. on perturbation). But Gx does provide a basis for evaluation of stability of larynx position during singing. A description of Gx is also expected to be relevant in transitional phases of different VPTs as well as in on- and offset phases.

(4) Derivation of EGG (DEGG) For a better evaluation of the instant of glottal closure Henrich et al. (2004) have suggested - on the basis of an earlier observation of Cranen (1991) - that it would be useful to also use the derivative of Lx, called DEGG, dLx or Lx'. For purposes of the corpus analysis DEGG was computed based on the high-pass filtered Lx (cut-off 25Hz) by means of the formula function for signal manipulation supplied by PRAAT.

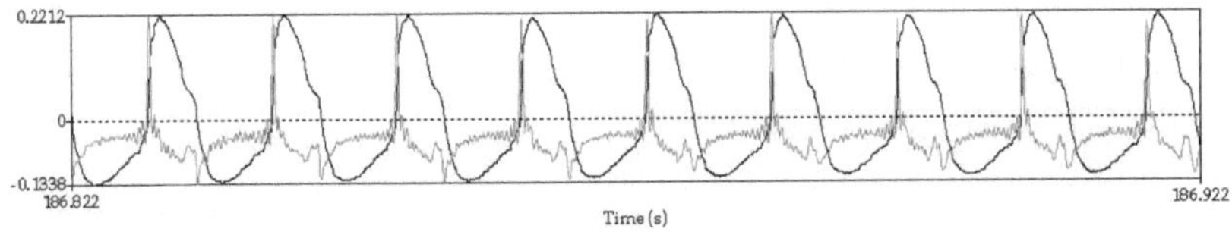

Figure 3.7: EGG (black) signal and its derivative DEGG (gray)

(5) Electroglottographic Perturbation Parameters Perturbation in Lx is primarily measured in the same way as perturbation measures of Vx, Parameters which have been considered are therefore, for F0: (F0mn, md, sd), for Jitter: jitter (loc), RAP and ppq5, and for shimmer: shimmer (loc), apq3, apq11. These have been adapted for cases of double-cycle phonation modes, so there are now values measured for each cycle and values measured for every second cycle (named jitterRAP2, shimmer apq32 etc.). Lx perturbation measurements are expected to provide a more direct and clear mapping of 'glottal' activity with minimal VT influence.

(6) EGG - Quotients Analogous to the analysis of the glottal flow signal but also specific to the nature of the Lx signal a number of quotients have been suggested. These quotients concern the relative contact duration of the VFs, relative contact rise time and contact symmetry (cf. Baken and Orlikoff, 2000: 426-427). All in all, due to a determination of glottal contact area phases which cannot rely on constant invariable landmarks, EGG-quotients are difficult to obtain. In relative terms the following quotients can be computed:

1. Contact Quotient or closed quotient (CQ) is calculated as the length (duration) of the closure phase, or better the contact phase (including impedance fall and peak), divided by the duration of the period. CQ is defined as the portion of the entire vibratory cycle wherein contact area is greater than some 'minimal level' (cf. Baken and Orlikoff, 2000: 426)

2. Closing quotient (CiQ) as a distinct quotient from CQ is a measure of relative contact rise time. It is considered since the closing phase (time of abrupt impedance fall) is marked more concisely than the other phases in the EGG curve (Marasek, 1997).

3. Open Quotient (OQ): defined by duration of open phase or minimal contact phase (flat sequence of high impedance) divided by the period

4. Quasi-Open-Quotient (QOQ) is a specific Lx signal-based quotient and defines the (quasi-)open phase simply by the negative component in the EGG curve (cf. Böhme and Gross, 2001; Hacki, 1996: 140-141)

5. Skewing quotient (SQ) (aka speed quotient, symmetry quotient, open slope, or slope quotient) is calculated as duration of closing phase divided by duration of opening phase (phase of increasing impedance) (cf. Marasek, 1997: 90).

6. Contact index (CI), another measure of symmetry, "is the time difference between the contacting and decontacting phases devided by the duration

of the full contact phase. CI will vary between -1 (for a negligibly short contacting phase) and 1 (for a negligibly short decontacting phase), such that CI=0 represents perfectly symmetrical contact phase" (Baken and Orlikoff, 2000: 427).

The usage of DEGG seems to be an appropriate way to ensure the detection of certain landmarks, so that pitch and period (PRAAT PointProcess) procedures were also carried out on dLx. For the double-cycle phonation modes, alternating periods (cycles) were expected which should each possibly be reidentified as either a single VF cycle or a joint VTF-VF cycle. In order to describe the two functions especially with regard to their relative contact area here it was necessary here to adapt the method used for phase and quotient obtainment. Accordingly, within the time-determined sequences for each pair of two cycles and their following right neighbours counted from a manually set measure point, 15 markers (by means of a PRAAT PointProcess object) were detected automatically. The point determination was supported by pitch detection which was based on maxima in the DEGG signal (t2 and t10). All other points were set by referring either to the adjacent minima or to the maxima in a separate minima-based or maxima-based PRAAT point process. So e.g. for the first sequence of the double cycle ta2 was defined as the adjacent minimum before the highest maximum (pitch process point) and, analogous, t2a was defined as the adjacent minimum after the highest maximum in the DEGG (t2).

Zero crossings would then be used as the reliable starting and ending points of the phase. It is quite apparent that this method is strongly dependent on an absent dc-offset and that it is not a very good indicator of real closing or opening times as they are potentially reflected by Lx. Nevertheless these quasi-closed and quasi-open phases are easy to detect and give a rough estimate of the cycle proportion. Fourcin et al. (2000) also determined QOQ as a quasi-closed quotient, which then of course would be simply an inversion of the open phase into its complement.

Regarding the different methods of automatic processing, closing quotients are calculated in two different ways, because the closing phase was either defined by t2a – ta2 or t3 – t1, analogously t6a – ta6 or t7 – t5b. Therefore the speed quotient refers only to ratio of the "moving" phases or "rising and falling" parts of the

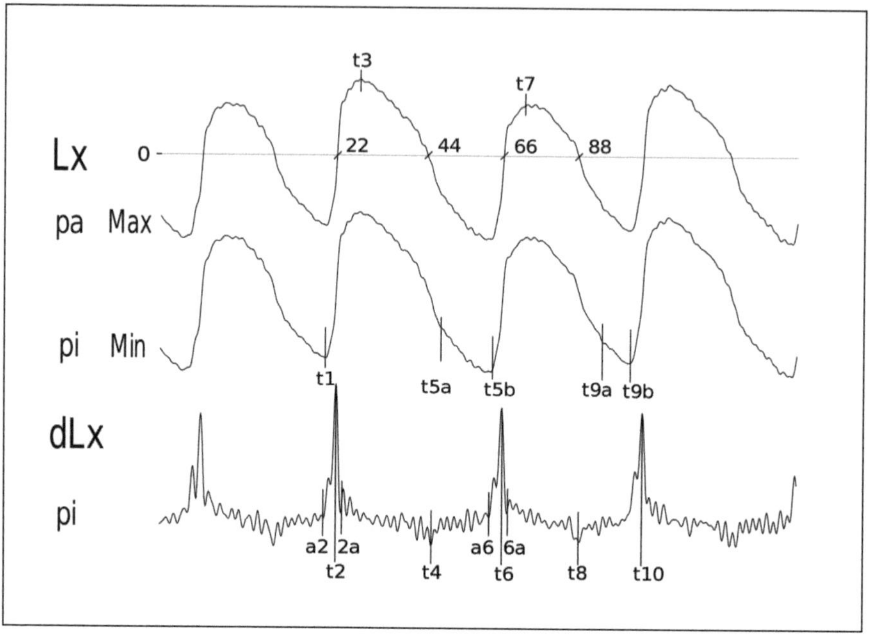

Figure 3.8: Sketch of the quotient obtaining method EGG and DEGG of double-cycle signal (PM2); the segmentation and subsequent point determination follows on the bases of landmarks in the EGG signal and its derivative; lowercase letters mark alternative definitions

signal. Contaxt index calculation was based on t2 (and t6) in dLx since it should be identical to the zero crossing points of Lx (see for point determination Figure 3.8 and for an overview of calculation methods Table 3.4). A possible description of VQ using the Lx signal, regarding especially linguistically relevant VQs, was investigated by Marasek (1997).

3.3.2.7 Sx - subglottal pressure waves

As described above for several reasons it was decided to apply a non-invasive methodology that includes, along with the recording of the voice signal and the EGG, another signal which originates in a contact microphone serving as low-cost accelerometer placed in the midline of the suprasternal notch (*fossa jugu-*

PARAMETER	NAME	METHOD	FIRST CYCLE	SECOND CYCLE
OQ	Open Quotient	$\frac{OpenPhase}{Period}$	$\frac{(t5b-t5a)}{t\_pd}$	$\frac{(t9b-t9a)}{t\_pd2}$
QOQ	Quasi Open Quotient	$\frac{QuasiOpenPhase}{Period}$	$\frac{(t6-t4)}{t\_pd}$	$\frac{(t10-t8)}{t\_pd2}$
CiQ1	Closing Quotient	$\frac{ClosingPhase}{Period}$	$\frac{(t3-t1)}{t\_pd}$	$\frac{(t7-t5b)}{t\_pd2}$
CiQ2	Closing Quotient	$\frac{ClosingPhase}{Period}$	$\frac{(t2a-ta2)}{t\_pd}$	$\frac{(t6a-ta6)}{t\_pd2}$
SQ	Skewing Quotient	$\frac{ClosingPhase}{OpeningPhase}$	$\frac{(t5a-t3)}{(t3-t1)}$	$\frac{(t9a-t7)}{(t7-t5b)}$
CI	Contact Index	$\frac{QCiP-QOiP}{QCP}$	$\frac{((t3-t2)-(t4-t3))}{(t4-t2)}$	$\frac{((t7-t6)-(t8-t7))}{(t8-t6)}$

Table 3.4: Equations for EGG quotients; the equations and variables appear as in the scripts (see Appendix 7.5); see 3.8 for point determination (tx); read e.g. t10mt8 as distance of t10 minus t8

laris). The abbreviation Sx refers to subglottal pressure waves as a time signal, sometimes also called the subglottal resonance signal (Neumann et al., 2003, 2001: cf.). Analysis of Sx was based on the Vx-Lx-Sx relation, and was carried out by means of signal comparison (cascades, interlinearisation, cohorting) and spectral analysis (Gall and Berg, 1998; Henke, 1974; Neumann et al., 2003). Since Lx-Sx relation and correlation analysis is only hardly supported with data the period segmentation has to be based on period detection of either Vx or Sx. Otherwise Lx could serve as the 'tool' for synchronization, as it was intended for.

Chapter 4

RESULTS

4.1 Analysis and Findings in the Voice Signal (Vx)

4.1.1 Vx-signal Corpus Description

For the analysis of the audio signal (Vx) 1617 cases (measure points) were processed comprising 71 files of 44 singers (3 Altai, 6 Hakas, 24 Tuvan, and 11 Mongolian). 1582 cases have finally been entered into (statistical) analysis.

Vx measures	Atype	Pmodus	N (cases)
Jitter Loc,	1	1	368
Jitter RAP, Jitter ppq5,		2	32
Shimmer loc,	2	1	154
Shimmer apq3,		2	50
Shimmer apq11 etc.	3	1	180
		2	798
total	at1 399 (12.9 %) at2 204 (25.2 %) at3 979 (61.8 %)	pm1 701 (44.31 %) pm2 881 (55.69 %)	1582

Table 4.1: Numbers of analysed cases (defined measure intervals) for the defined groups (phonation modus 1 and 2; articulation type 1, 2, and 3)

The corpus sample itself was assembled on the basis of available material (unpublished recordings, including field recordings of the author and of other colleagues[1]; commercially distributed professional audio recordings, documentaries, radio features). The composition of the corpus regarding origin of the singers corresponds approximately to the estimated numbers of throat singers in the individual areas (see chapter 1.2). As regards other criteria (see chapter 3.2.5) the selection has followed strictly the situation in the field (male singers, age 20 - 50, semiprofessional to professional level). Personal information (date and place of birth) was not always available.

Area	Frequency	Percent	Cumulative Percent
altai	114	7.2	7.2
hakas	196	12.4	19.6
mongol	299	18.9	38.5
tyva	973	61.5	100
Total	1582	100	

Table 4.2: Numbers of analysed cases (defined measure intervals) for pre-defined groups (singer's origin)

Given the resource situation, the number of cases in each areal group was not consequently kept to an equal proportion of that group, but it was kept in a proportion to ThS singer frequency per area (Hakassia, Altai, Mongolia, Tuva; see chapter 1.2). Note that for Altai there are no samples of PM1AT2, PM2AT1, and PM2AT2, and for Hakas there are no samples of PM2AT1 and PM2AT2, or vice versa there are for PM1AT2 no Altai samples and for PM2AT1 and PM2AT2 neither Altai samples nor Hakas samples.

Since a modus1-modus2 difference in phonation seems to be clearly evident, statistical analysis has been focused on intra-mode differences and regional differences. Following the hypotheses 1 and 2 (chapter 2.6), rejecting the null-hypothesis regarding area and regarding, all cases have been basically grouped together by phonation mode, area and articulation type.

[1]I again thank Mark van Tongeren, Zoya Kyrgys and Ludek Brož for allowing me to use their recordings.

	Singer	Frequency	Percent	Cumulative Percent
1.	AK	7	0.4	0.4
2.	OT	7	0.4	0.9
3.	Y1	8	0.5	1.4
4.	SI	11	0.7	2.1
5.	VO	13	0.8	2.9
6.	BI	14	0.9	3.8
7.	ZS	15	0.9	4.7
8.	SS	17	1.1	5.8
9.	SE	19	1.2	7
10.	OS	20	1.3	8.3
11.	SU	20	1.3	9.5
12.	HS	21	1.3	10.9
13.	BO	23	1.5	12.3
14.	NH	24	1.5	13.8
15.	AM	26	1.6	15.5
16.	SH	26	1.6	17.1
17.	SA	28	1.8	18.9
18.	DB	29	1.8	20.7
19.	SK	30	1.9	22.6
20.	MS	32	2	24.7
21.	ST	32	2	26.7
22.	AA	33	2.1	28.8
23.	KO	34	2.1	30.9
24.	RM	34	2.1	33.1
25.	SO	34	2.1	35.2
26.	YT	36	2.3	37.5
27.	MA	38	2.4	39.9
28.	OB	39	2.5	42.4
29.	SV	39	2.5	44.8
30.	JT	41	2.6	47.4
31.	TG	41	2.6	50
32.	AD	42	2.7	52.7
33.	AS	46	2.9	55.6
34.	TK	47	3	58.5
35.	S2	49	3.1	61.6
36.	T4	50	3.2	64.8
37.	KX	52	3.3	68.1
38.	NS	53	3.4	71.4
39.	ZU	54	3.4	74.8
40.	ET	64	4	78.9
41.	OX	69	4.4	83.2
42.	IK	73	4.6	87.9
43.	OK	90	5.7	93.6
44.	KK	102	6.4	100
total		1582	100	

Table 4.3: Proportion of individual singers in the corpus

4.1.2 Vx Waveform Shapes and Patterns

Findings in Vx waveforms, as well as other parameters, are given as grouped after a grid of PM and AT, as discussed in chapter 2.4. Sonograms for each of the subtypes are given in 2.4.2.

4.1.2.1 Vx-waveform Shapes and Patterns in PM1 (single cycle mode) - AT 1 (Articulation type1)

Waveforms of AT1 are dominated by F2 and higher formant frequencies, thus producing a supra-periodical signal wherein a fundamental frequency is very hard to determine. In fact the sinusoidal shape reflects the whistle-like reinforced harmonic within the carrying formant (F2/F3) and also illustrates the almost complete damping of F0. Only supraperiodic ondulations indicate roughly the phases (Figure 4.1).

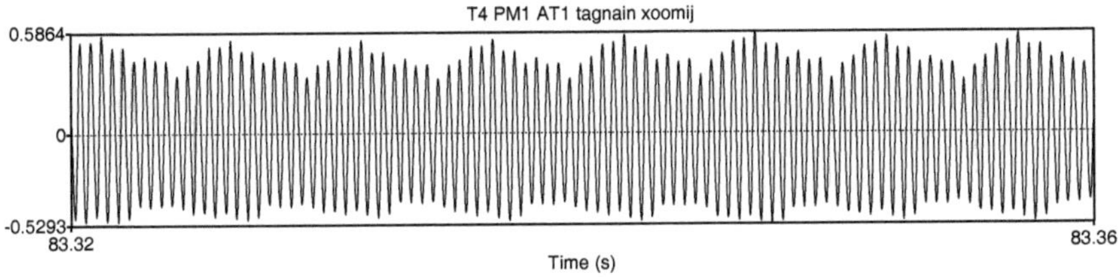

Figure 4.1: PM1AT1 sequence from *tagnain xöömij* performed by the Mongolian singer T4 (H20 prominent)

4.1.2.2 Vx-waveform Shapes and Patterns in PM1AT2

In waveforms of AT2 the influence of F1 is plainly visible (as a kind of carrier wave) but other higher formants (F2/F3) are clearly (super-)imposed on it. The amplitude is as high within the closed phase as within the open phase, revealing a high and long lasting VT excitation (Figure 4.2).

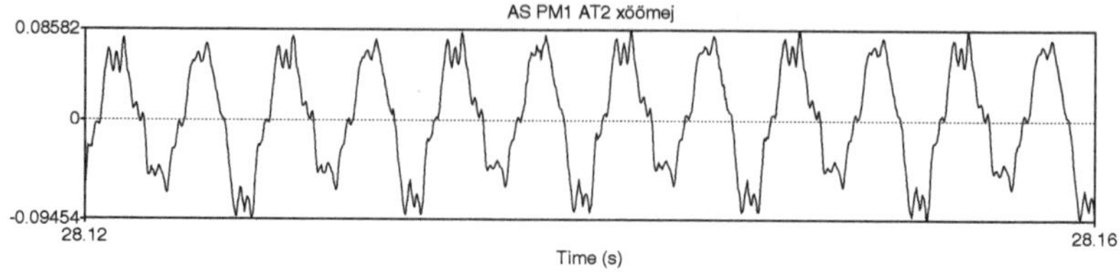

Figure 4.2: Example for PM1AT2; Tuvan *xoomej*; sequence with a neutral vowel quality [ə] and a prominent H10

4.1.2.3 Vx-waveform Shapes and Patterns in PM1AT3

AT3 waveforms clearly contain all the features of the individual vowel qualities and generally show a strong influence of the vowel's formant structure (Figure 4.3).

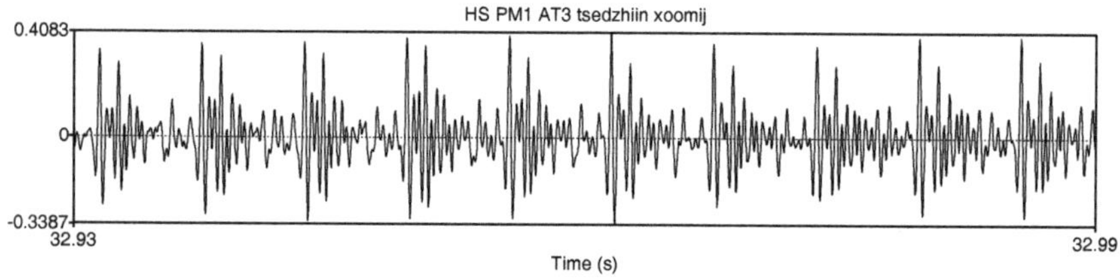

Figure 4.3: PM1 AT3 sequence of *tsedzhiin xoomij* by the Mongolian singer HS; [æ]-like vowel quality

4.1.2.4 Vx-waveform Shapes and Patterns in PM2(double cycle mode) - AT1

As stated above, supraperiodical effects are found in both phonation modes (PM1 and PM2) and complicate pitch detection. The superimposition of higher formants is also evident in PM2, though the underlying structure of the fundamental mostly remains visible (Figure 4.4).

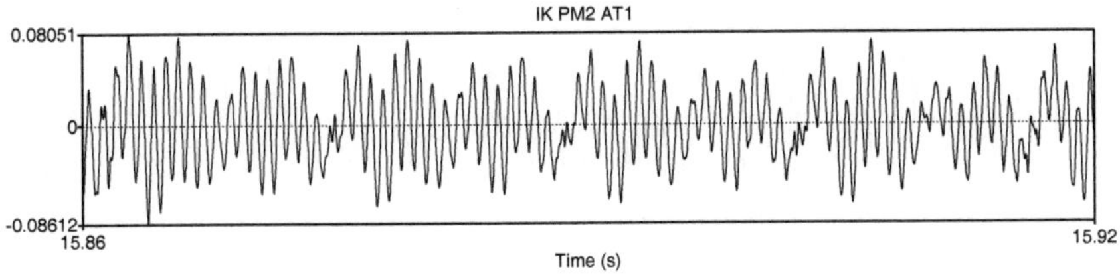

Figure 4.4: Example of PM2AT1; *čylandyk* or *sygyrtyy kargyraazy* of the Tuvan singer IK

4.1.2.5 Vx-waveform Shapes and Patterns in PM2AT2

Since in PM2 the period is longer, F1 and in particular the more prominent (energetic) F2 of approx.1500 to 2000Hz can superimpose on the closed phases (Figure 4.5). Thus the long double cycle mode becomes fully evident.

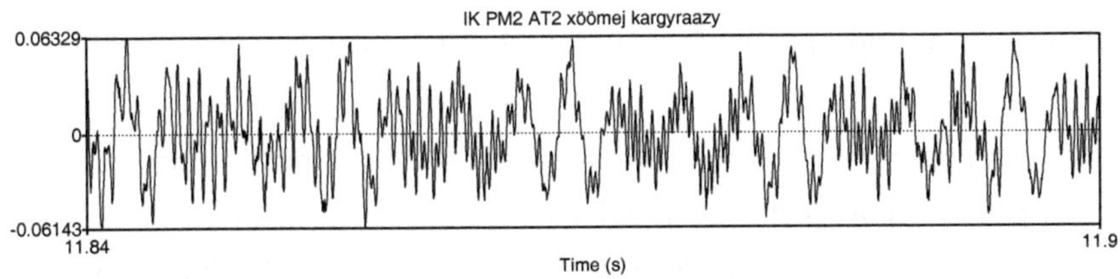

Figure 4.5: Waveform of PM2AT2: *xöömej kargyraazy* of singer IK (T) with prominent H18/19

4.1.2.6 Vx-waveform Shapes and Patterns in PM2AT3

Higher vowels can serve as a kind of 'transitional area' from AT3 to AT2. Especially [i], as can seen in Figure 4.6, shows similar patterns of high formant overlay to Figure 4.5.

The double cycle period structure, with both open and closed phases, is already visible with [i] but becomes clearer with a more open vowel ([ɔ]).

The example in Figure 4.9 shows very clearly the superimposition of formants

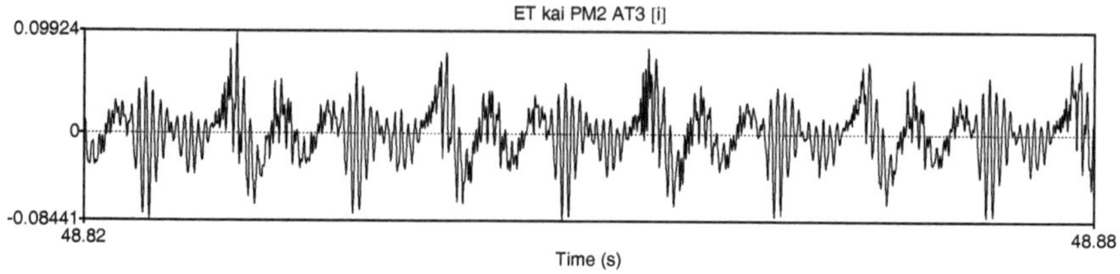

Figure 4.6: Waveform example for PM2AT3, Altaian *kai* singer ET; vowel [i]

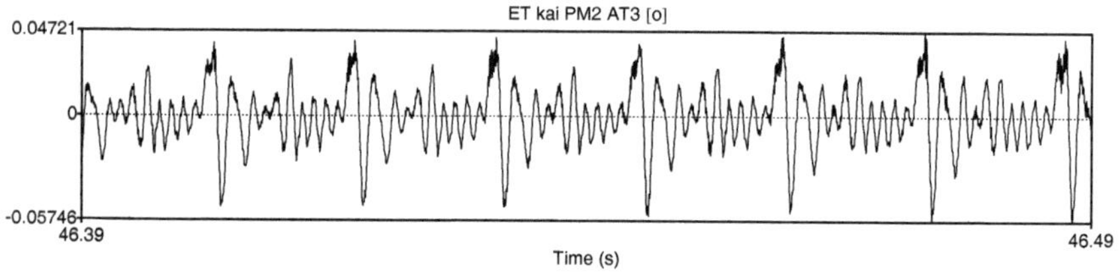

Figure 4.7: Waveform example for PM2AT3; Altaian *kai* singer ET; vowel [ɔ]

onto the double cycle wave. The wave was segmented into periods by the recurrent strongest amplitude maxima, so that the period starts right after the 'glottal' instant (closure), which shows signs of high-frequent (noise) components. At the beginning of the sequence (periods 2-15) F1 superimposes right in the closed phase, but with a lowering of F1 in the second half of the sequence (from period 21 on) F1 no longer fits twice into the closed phase. Hence it superimposes on the beginning of the open phase. The second cycle shows a more closed character but clearly with less energy than the first cycle. Nonetheless F2 and F3 are more prominent whereas F1 is overlaid.

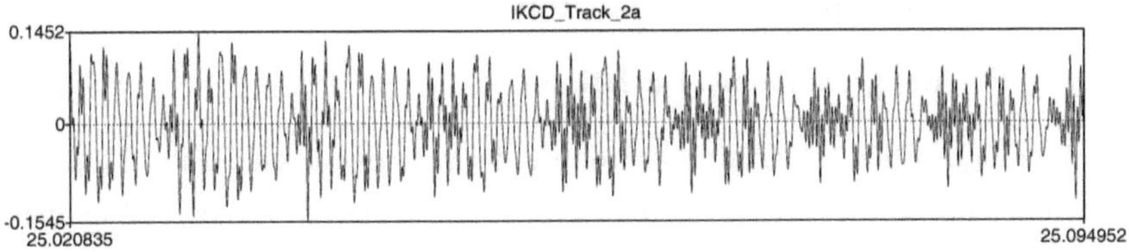

Figure 4.8: High pitched *kargyraa* by Tuvan singer IK; F0=107Hz; vowel [ɐ]

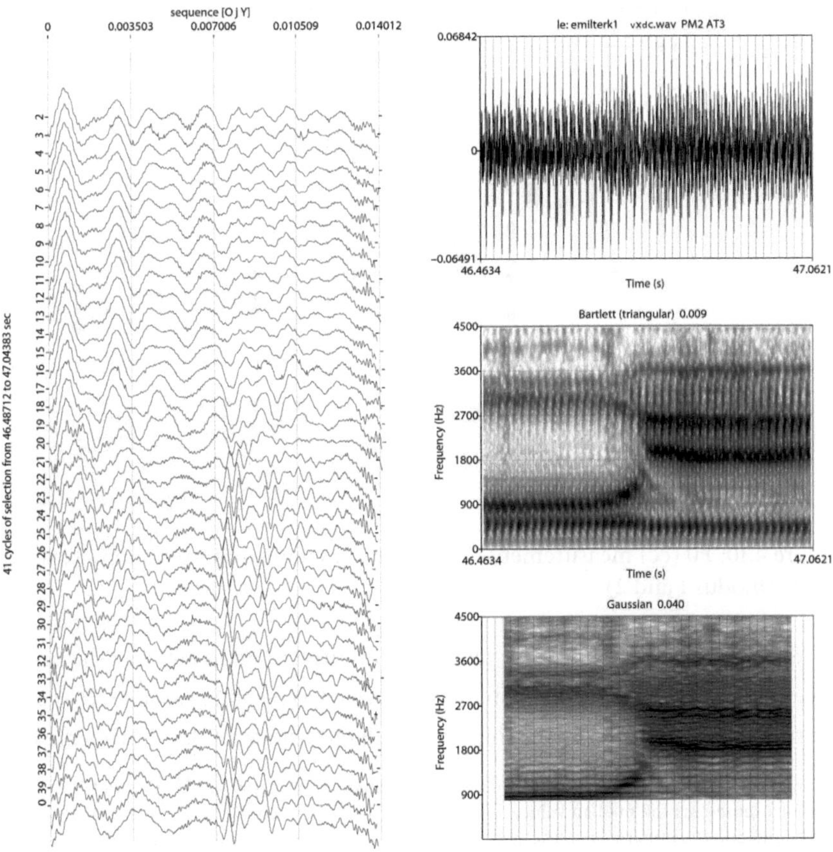

Figure 4.9: PM2AT3 - transition from [ɔ] over [j] to [ʏ]; *kai* singer ET (A)

4.1.3 Vx Waveform Perturbations

4.1.3.1 F0 - Range, Standard Deviation

The F0 range of the different phonation modes was investigated only as a group preference but not for the performance of single subjects. The overall tendencies of F0 can be described for both phonation modes as an increasing F0 going from articulation type 1 (AT1) to type 3 (AT3)(see figure 4.10)[2]. This finding is supported by the ethnomusicological observations in the fields (see table 2.3).

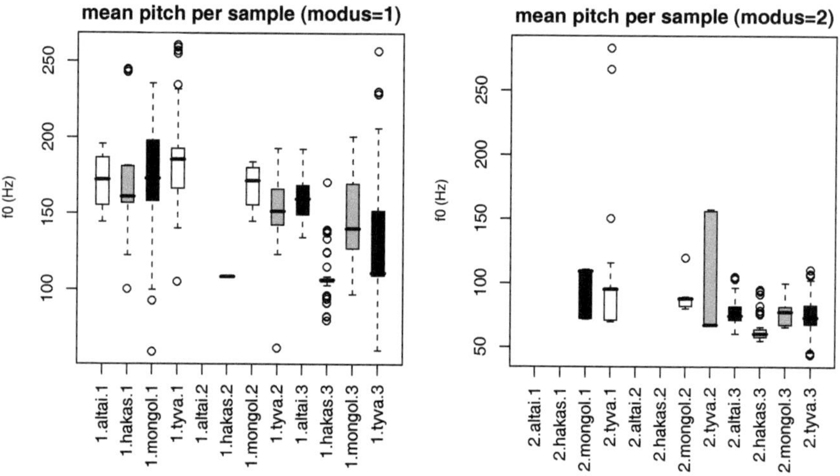

Figure 4.10: F0 (cc) measurements based on Vx; grouped by area and phonation mode (modus 1 and 2)

Since for the phonation task pitch was not prescribed in any way the differences between the area groups might be expected to be quite variable. However, the fundamental chosen by the singers in both phonatory modes shows a distinct

[2] In the presentation of results so-called modified boxplots are preferably used. The bold line within each box represents the median value; the lower edge of the box represents the first quartile (25%-percentile) and the upper edge represents the third quartile (75%-percentile). The upper and lower edges define the inner quartile range (IQR = Q3 - Q1). The so-called whisker line goes from the minimum value to the maximum value within the range of 1.5 of the IQR. Small circles represent both, the outliers greater than one and a half times the IQR *and* the outliers greater than three times the inner quartile range.

behaviour of the median value at least for the group of Hakas singers. Though of course the F0 mean values could be given (for PM1= 160.4Hz and for PM2 = 77.1Hz), the two period ranges (or F0 ranges with 201Hz for PM1 and approx. 100Hz for PM2) overlap, so that no absolute or discrete cut-off point between the two modes can be established. Hakas *xai* singers in particular show a very deep PM1 (especially singer ST). Outliers of over 150Hz in modus 2 are explicable by measurement failures, e.g. in *čylandyk* due to its deviant superperiodic waveform (see 4.1.2). To be sure, in the style *kargyraa* there exists a substyle, sometimes named after one of its best-known performers (Oidupa), in which we find very high-pitched (110-140Hz) *kargyraa* voices (see Figure 4.11). This style, however, was not included in the corpus. Results for pitch detection in PM2 had to be corrected anyway in a number of cases. An estimated upper limit of PM2 for pitch detection was therefore set at 90Hz as default.

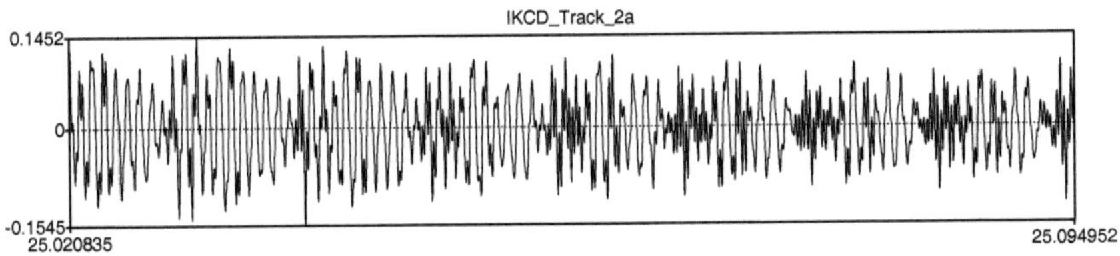

Figure 4.11: Example for a high-pitched (ca. 110Hz) PM2 (AT3) by the Tuvan *xöömej* singer IK

For F0 standard deviation all groups showed a very similar behaviour. It is not surprising that the largest number of outliers is found for Tuvan AT3, which simultaneously represents both the largest areal group and the largest A-type group. Here pitch tendencies inherent in the individual vowels may also perhaps come into play; these might be expected in particular for the high vowels. As seen in Figure 4.12 (right), however, this is not the case, since such outliers are reported for [ə], [ɑ], and [ɔ].

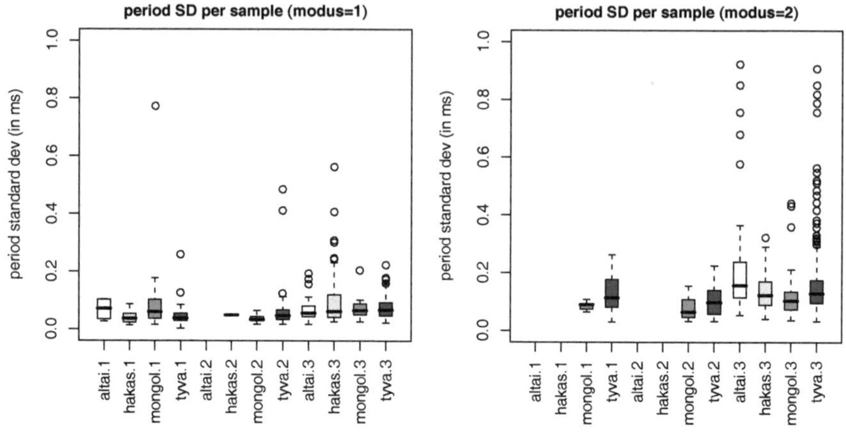

Figure 4.12: Period standard deviation within the measurement intervals of 0.5 sec; x-axis label refer to area and articulation type (AT)

4.1.3.2 Vx Jitter Measures

Since the different nature of voice production types used in phonation mode 1 and 2 have to be considered, for further presentation the results and findings will be shown separately for PM1 and PM2. Jitter measures are carried out within a time frame of 0.45 sec; depending on period length, this means that approximately 65 periods and 33 periods (in PM1 and PM2 respectively) were included in the analysis.

Vx Jitter in Phonation Mode 1 Jitter parameters in PM1 show a very low range of values. The RAP parameter illustrates this; it would be low compared to the RAP values for 'normal' voices given by, for example, Pützer (2001: 77) or Baken and Orlikoff (2000: 208). The MDVP manual gives for Jitt (local jitter) 1.040% as a threshold for pathology, which is clearly under-run by the values for PM1. One may wonder about such a threshold since it is higly unlikely to achieve acoustic parameters that would display a 'measure of pathology' in such a direct way. Jitter certainly can be associated (and also correlated) with voice qualities, such as roughness, but this is not sufficient enough to rely on jitter as a voice quality index as such (Kreiman and Gerratt, 2005; Rabinov et al., 1995).

	N	Range	Minimum	Maximum	Mean	Std. Dev.
jitterLoc	701	.047604	.000327	.047931	.002414	.0038200
jitterRAP	701	.017116	.000079	.017195	.000560	.0015005
jitterppq5	701	.041571	.000195	.041766	.001214	.0029510

Table 4.4: Descriptive statistics of Vx jitter values for PM1

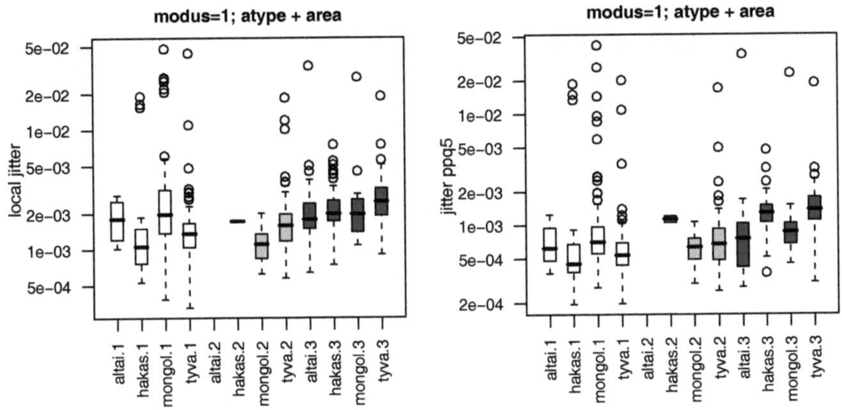

Figure 4.13: Local jitter values (left) and ppq5 values (right) marked after articulation types and clustered by area groups (styles); y-axis has been scaled exponentially

As seen for local jitter and ppq5 (in Figure 4.13), and for RAP (in Table 4.4 and Table A.1), jitter values seem to show a tendency to increase from AT1 to AT3, which might be due to a (perceived) lower tension and a less dominant effect of single formants, as is the case in AT1. Nonetheless, if one looks only at the median, the different jitter measurement methods appear as fairly similar. Observing the distribution over the individual singers, several show especially prominent median values [OX (T); ST (H), SI (T), SU (M), ZU (H)], but singer SU seems to have not only a high median, but also a fairly wide upper range. One highly characteristic feature of SU's singing is his strikingly elaborate vibrato (dynamic and pitch variation), so that at least a period variation component had to be assumed acoustically also for the other singers. After repeated listening and re-inspection of the samples, this indeed appears to be a reasonable assumption (cf. Figure 4.14).

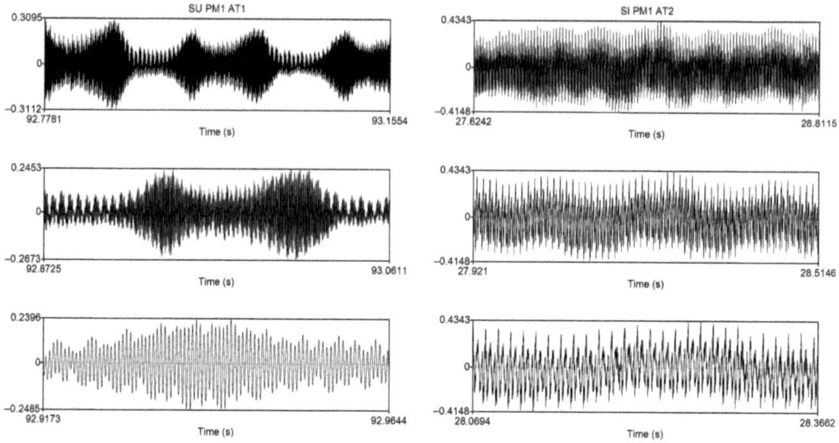

Figure 4.14: Waveforms of examples from singers with high RAP values: SU (M) with an 'extreme' elaborate dynamic vibrato and singer SI (T) with a more pitch-determined vibrato

In order to carry out a test of variance between groups the obtained measures (jitter Loc, Jitter RAP, Jitter pp5) were tested for normal distribution, both within area groups and articulation type groups. The tests applied were those of Kolmogorov-Smirnov (Massey, 1951) and Shapiro-Wilk (Shapiro and Wilk, 1965), the latter in cases of smaller numbers (< 50). Jitter values in PM1 all showed a significant deviation from a normal distribution ($p < 0.05$), not only within the area groups but also within articulation type groups.

Over the entire group of singers as a whole no specific grouping or clustering regarding singers' provenience is immediately evident (see Figure 4.16 for RAP). Nevertheless the comparison of median values (e.g. Figure 4.15) shows a slight tendency toward group differences. These differences were tested using the non-parametric test of Kruskal and Wallis (1952), also known as the H-test. This test is usually used as an extension of the Mann-Whitney U-test in cases where there are

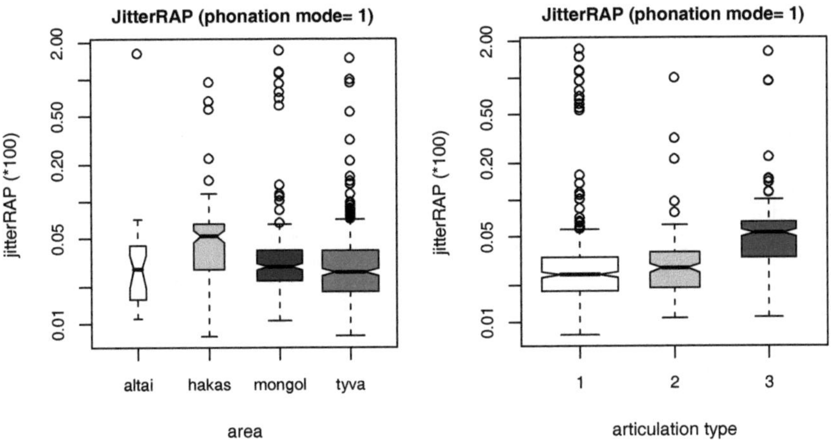

Figure 4.15: Jitter RAP values in phonation mode 1 grouped by area (left) and articulation type (right)

more than two groups of independent sets (Mann and Whitney, 1947). During the test all values are ranked irrespective of the group they belong to. If all groups end up having the same average rank the null-hypothesis is taken to be true. The results of the H-test for the two groupings show significant differences ($p < 0.05$) for both area type and articulation type in all tested parameters (jitterLoc, jitterRAP, and jitterPPQ5).

Vx Jitter in Phonation Mode 2 For PM2 the jitter parameters appear to be 'doubled' compared to the values of PM1. In this way the results may certainly give reason for PM2 to be evaluated as rough or harsh. But the relatively higher jitter value of PM2 (vs. PM1) is also not unexpected, since the nature of such two-cycle oscillation clearly inheres in an intermittent change of the period (see 4.2.3).

The parameters investigated (jitterLoc, jitterRAP and jitterppq5) overlap in their ranges; note that even a smoothing over five periods does not appear to achieve an overlap with the mean value of the jitter factor (local jitter).

The extreme outliers in the Tuvan group, AM with 0,029 ppq3 (RAP) and OB, AS, and SO (Figure 4.18), can be relativized by taking into consideration the whole

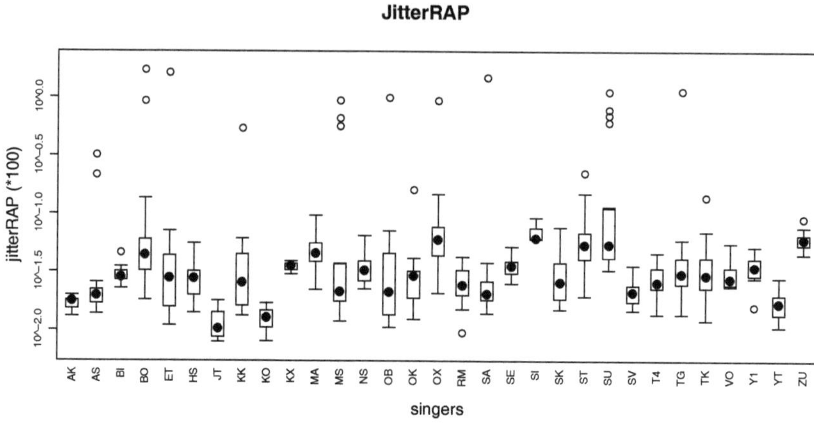

Figure 4.16: Depiction of RAP values per singer in the production of PM1

	N	Range	Minimum	Maximum	Mean	Std. Dev.
jitterLoc	881	.058108	.000988	.059096	.004439	.0043518
jitterRAP	881	.029490	.000214	.029704	.001412	.0020893
jitterppq5	881	.040184	.000001	.040184	.002735	.0036607

Table 4.5: Descriptive statistics of jitter values in PM2

distribution of jitter values over the set of singers. Here only DB shows a high median, which expresses his extraordinary 'timbre' that is reminiscent of a voice tremor. Median groupings again reveal only slight differences. So it needs to be investigated if the null-hypothesis regarding the values of certain measures within one phonation mode could be rejected for jitter (RAP, PPQ5, and local jitter). Therefore the Kruskal-Wallis test (or H-test) was applied since a test of normality had revealed that PM2 values within area groups and articulation groups do not have a normal distribution (see Appendix A.1.2.1 Table A.11). The result of the H-test shows that for all jitter values (loc, RAP, ppq5) the internal differences within the two groups are significant ($p<0.05$; see Appendix A.1.3.1 Table A.25). On the other hand it must be considered that an equal distribution of cases would possibly have lowered the median of the subgroups AT3 and Tuvan, since this

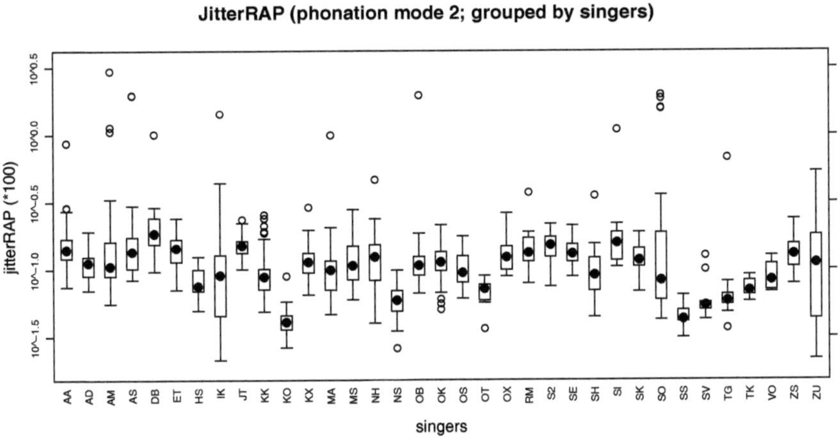

Figure 4.17: Depiction of RAP values per singer in the production of PM2

	N	Range	Minimum	Maximum	Mean	Std. Dev.
shimmerLoc	701	.260535	.011992	.272527	.067846	.0402672
shimmerapq3	701	.132601	.003783	.136384	.028415	.0209218
shimmerapq5	701	.156278	.007874	.164152	.042727	.0284164
shimmerapq11	701	.235099	.000001	.235099	.072293	.0406574

Table 4.6: Descriptive statistics of Vx shimmer values; phonation mode 1

combination (i.e. AT3 for Tuvan) makes up the majority group within PM2.

4.1.3.3 Vx Shimmer Measures

More so than with jitter, shimmer has been identified with the auditory evaluation of roughness or harshness of a given signal (Deal and Emanuel, 1978) and hence has been suggested as an index for acoustic correlates of pathological voices (e.g. Takahashi and Koike, 1976).

Vx Shimmer Phonation Mode 1 Local shimmer, apq5 and apq11 show a clear tendency towards increasing median values within the area groups, proceeding from Hakas with the lowest median value to Altai to Tuvan to Mongolian with

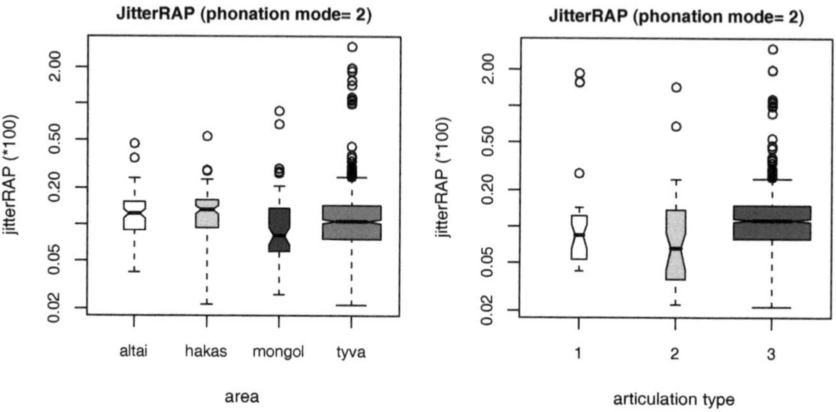

Figure 4.18: RAP values in phonation mode 2 grouped by area (left) and atype (right); y-axis has been scaled logarithmically

	N	Range	Minimum	Maximum	Mean	SD
shimmerLoc	881	.353307	.009641	.362948	.082431	.0446902
shimmerapq3	881	.183302	.004498	.187800	.038577	.0227472
shimmerapq5	881	.232836	.000001	.232836	.053950	.0298217
shimmerapq11	881	.331191	.000001	.331191	.083194	.0488907

Table 4.7: Descriptive statistics of Vx shimmer values; phonation mode 2

the highest median value, and also within the group of articulation types, going from AT3 to AT2 and to AT1 with the highest values. The prominent positions of the Mongolian singers BI, BO, SU, and TG are again presumably explicable by a distinctive strong vibrato that emerges particularly clearly in AT1 (cf. Figure 4.14).

Vx Shimmer Phonation Mode 2 Local shimmer was examined separately considered regarding a possible bias of different VPTs, in particular AEF-VF vs. VTF-VF phonation. Here, in preliminary auditory evaluations during pre-analysis, the Tuvan singers OX and TK have been presumed to be using AEF-VF phonation in PM2. Over the whole group of singers, especially the singers TK and OX in particular were found to be right in the mean area. The measures of the Tuvan

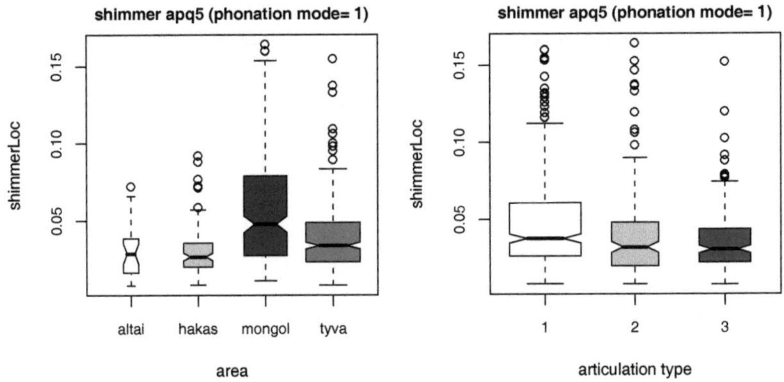

Figure 4.19: Shimmer apq5 of PM1 separately grouped into area and articulation types

singers IK, OK, and KX and the Mongolian singers AA and SH may be interpreted as being in the upper range. Here again, as in the investigation of jitter, the impact of vibrato features may be suggested as a likely interpretation. The Kruskal-Wallis test shows for PM2 that there is no significant difference ($p > .05$) between the shimmer parameters apq3 and apq5. Within these two shimmer parameters a general tendency emerges such that, aside from a slight dissimilarity for the Hakas subgroup, the areas appear as homogeneous, and among the articulation types only AT1 stands out (see Figure 4.23).

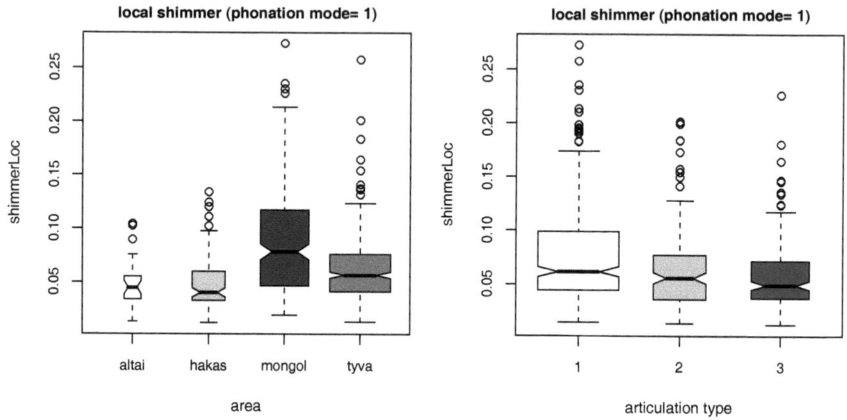

Figure 4.20: Local shimmer (left) and apq11 (right) values marked according to articulation types and clustered by area groups; the y-axis has been scaled exponentially

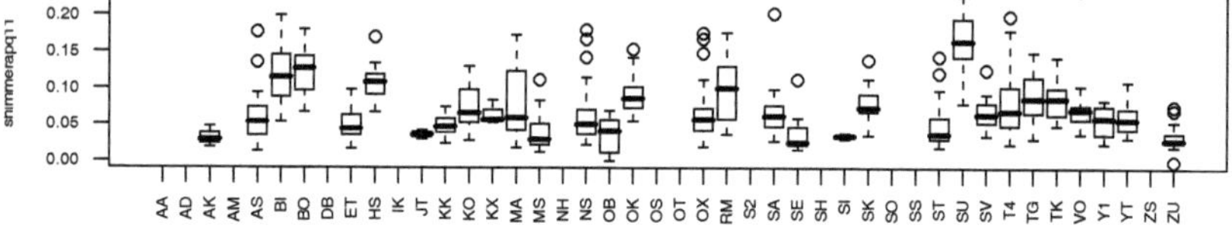

Figure 4.21: local shimmer and apq11 values for the individual singers

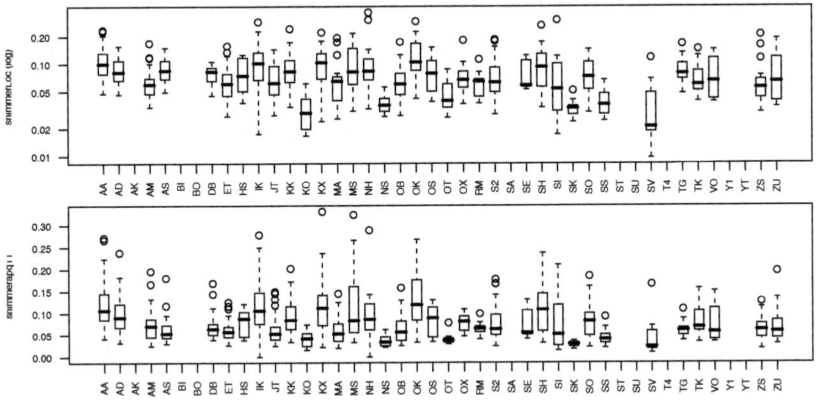

Figure 4.22: Local shimmer and shimmer apq11 measures for the individual singers; phonation mode 2

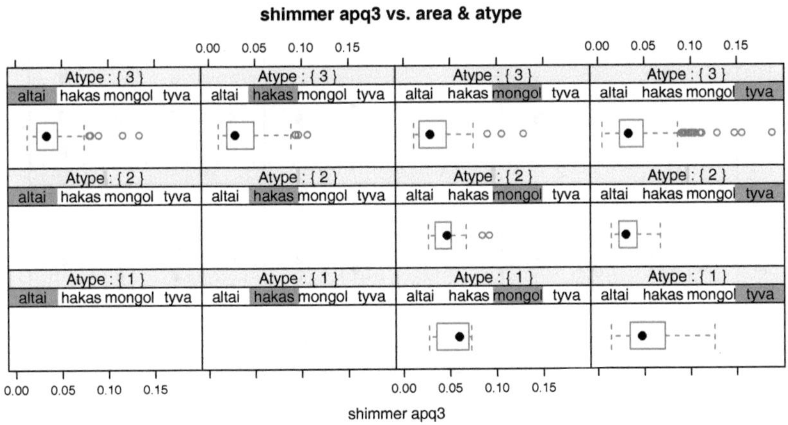

Figure 4.23: Shimmer apq3 measures grouped by area (lower panel) and articulation type (upper panel); phonation mode 2

4.1.3.4 Analysis Findings in Harmonics-to-Noise Ratio

Harmonics-to-Noise Ratio (HNR or H/N) as a measure of acoustic periodicity has been shown to correlate with such VQs as roughness and breathiness. Compared with studies of normal (non-pathological) voices the mean HNR values appear to be slightly enhanced for PM2 and in particular for PM1; the PM1 enhancement emphasizes the superposition of periodic (harmonic) components in the signal.

PM1	N	Range	Min	Max	Mean	SD	Variance
HNRmn	701	25.6	4.5	30.2	16.4	4.3	18.9
PM2	N	Range	Min	Max	Mean	SD	Variance
HNRmn	881	22.0	2.1	24.2	12.9	3.6	12.6

Table 4.8: Descriptive statistics for HNR in PM1 (upper part) and PM2 (lower part)

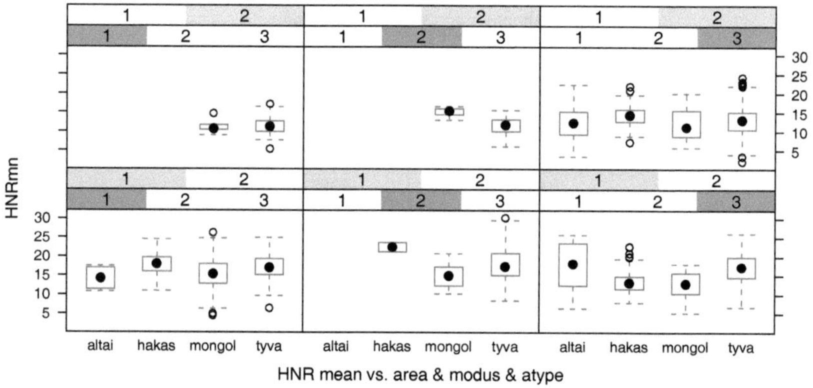

Figure 4.24: HNR values within PM1 (upper panel left) and PM2 (upper panel right) marked according to articulation types (lower panel 1-3) and clustered by area groups (styles)

In summary a grouping of mean values into AT values would result in an increasing of HNR parallel to the increasing articulatory opening (AT1 < AT2 < AT3). In PM1 those singers who stood out in jitter and shimmer measurements (BI, BO, HS, SU) now show low HNR values, indicating a higher portion of aperiodic components.

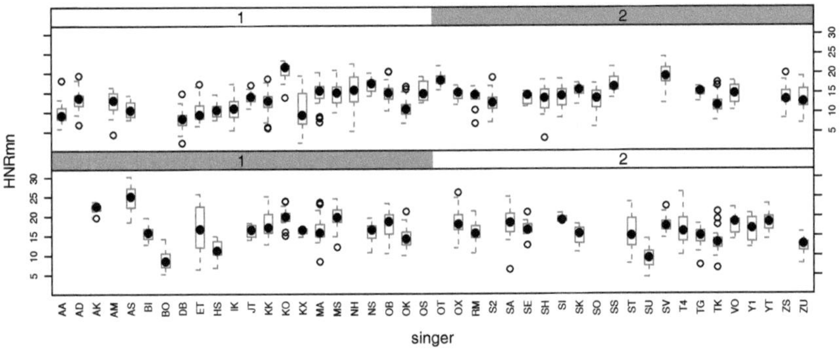

Figure 4.25: Mean HNR for Vx of PM1 and PM2 grouped by singer

The Kruskal-Wallis H-test for PM1 confirms the assumed dissimilarity between AT subgroups and gives the same ranking (A3 > AT2 > AT1), indicating a higher aperiodicity aligning with degree of jaw (mouth) closing, which seems quite surprising. Hakas and Mongolian PM1 samples are ranked on the same level, and are followed on a higher niveau by Altai and then Tuvan samples (H = M < A < T). For PM2 the Kurskall-Wallis test indicates a higher rank of Hakas samples vis-a-vìs fairly similar Tuvan, Mongolian and Altai ones. Almost inversely to PM1, for PM2 the lowest HNR is observed for AT1, followed by AT2 and then AT3.

4.1.4 Formants, Bandwidths and Reinforced Harmonics

4.1.4.1 Formant and Bandwidth Measures

The formant measures applied in PRAAT are based on LPC algorithms which have the difficulty that in the case of two formants being very close to each other (in the perspective of the LPC analysis) both formants are merged into one. This effect might be compensated for by narrowing the window and increasing the coefficients but such compensation could not prevent the missing of a damped F1. Another possible solution might be an additional specific pre-analysis of the individual overtone articulation type and a subsequently adapted formant measurement algorithm (especially regarding LPC coefficient, formant frequency bands, and exact F0). Nonetheless the results already reveal specific tendencies, which in turn lead to further detailed analysis. Nonetheless, the merging of F2, F3, F4, and F5 (see Figure 4.26), can be also observed in the individual spectrograms. And the circumstances under which such merging effects appear (labial constriction plus 'palatal' constriction plus AES) make an interpretation by the quantal theory (cf. Stevens, 1989) plausible.

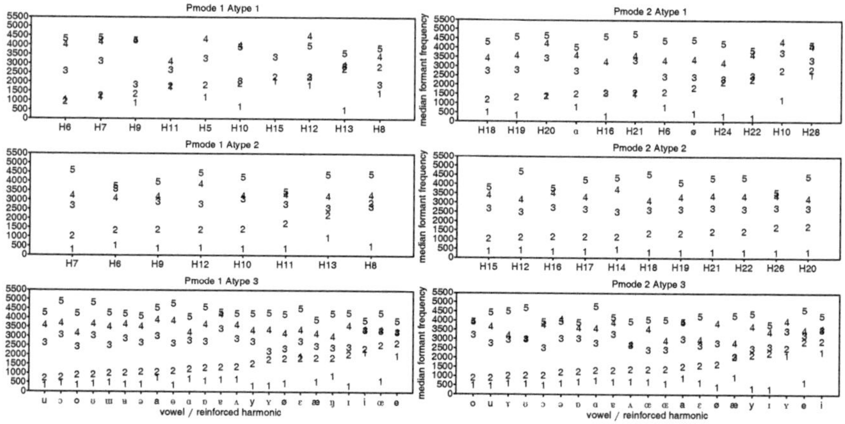

Figure 4.26: Mean values of median formant measures over all singers the samples grouped by phonation mode (PM1 left and PM2 right) and articulation type (upper, middle and lower row); note the areas of 'formant confusion' in the formant frequency measurement; the order of the vowels and reinforced on the x-axis according to F2 height

One of the clearest and most outstanding features is the selective manipulation of F2 as 'carrier' of the reinforced harmonic that creates the melody. In this way the reinforced harmonics align with tongue height or constriction of the cor-

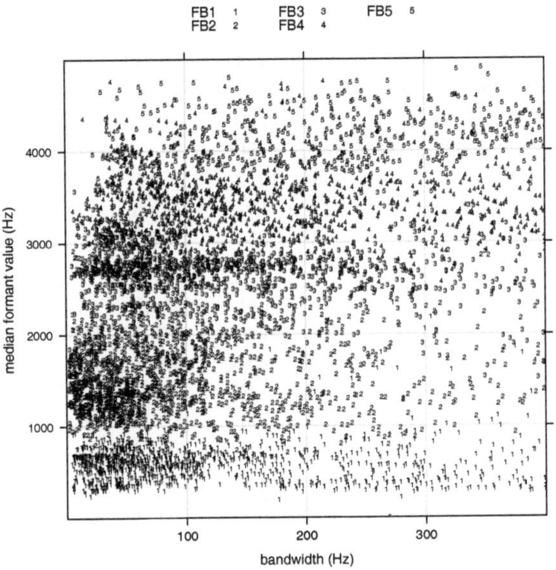

Figure 4.27: Scatterplot of formants (1-5) in the y-axis versus the corresponding bandwidths (x-axis); note that this plot explores unfiltered 'raw' values

responding articulation strategy. H5 to H13 are the harmonics used in AT1 and AT2 for PM1, and analogously H14 to H28 are used in AT1 and AT2 for PM2 (see Figure 4.27). In AT3 the F2 height determines the choice of the vowel quality, so e.g. an ascending scale could be built up by the row [u. o. ø. y. i]. This order would then be used to create the musical scale which the actual melodies are based on.

When we examine the descriptive statistics (Table 4.9) the measured formant and bandwidth values turn out to be highly variable. By scattering formant and bandwidth values one can also see that especially F1 and F2 with a very broad bandwidth overlap with the domain of the next higher formant. The picture becomes clearer, however, if the three articulation types are scattered separately (Figure 4.28). Given the relative small number of cases for AT2 and the greater number for AT1, one can also see in Figure 4.28 the relatively small bandwidth range of AT1 and AT2 vis-à-vis AT3. Nonetheless, the fairly diffuse appearance of F1, but also F2, in AT1 is probably only explicable by taking into account that bandwidths of merged or miscounted formants are often involved here (see as example Figure 4.29).

Pmode		N	Range	Min	Max	Mean	SD	Med
1	F1md	735	2139	176	2316	724	491.4	495
	F2md	735	2341	728	3070	1647	432.4	1629
	F3md	735	2229	1462	3692	2702	429.3	2735
	F4md	735	2157	2639	4796	3509	212.1	3415
	B1	735	6385	1.6	6386	422	555.6	273
	B2	735	8280	1.5	8281	150	420.5	49
	B3	735	5127	2.8	5130	352	583.6	122
	B4	735	3781	6.2	3787	374	210.1	206
2	F1md	881	2322	223	2546	661	264.7	642
	F2md	881	2360	646	3007	1529	438.4	1403
	F3md	881	2636	1533	4170	2670	302.6	2671
	F4md	881	2177	2568	4745	3418	253.0	3433
	B1	881	3265	5.5	3271	164	277.3	79
	B2	881	3294	3.9	3297	177	260.4	95
	B3	881	4124	7.2	4131	330	461.2	155
	B4	881	4400	15.0	4415	395	252.4	221

Table 4.9: Descriptive statistics of median formant and mean bandwidth values

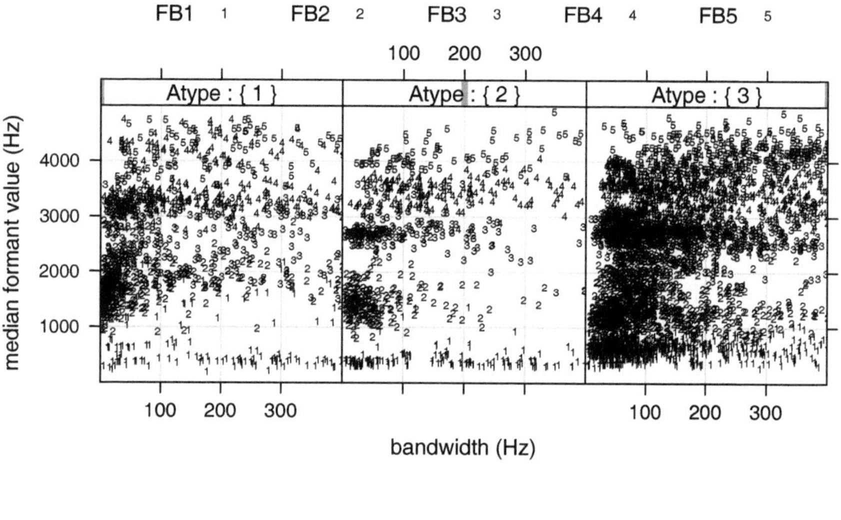

Figure 4.28: Scatterplot of formants (1-5) on the y-axis versus the corresponding bandwidths (x-axis) for each articulation type separately; note that this plot explores unfiltered 'raw' values

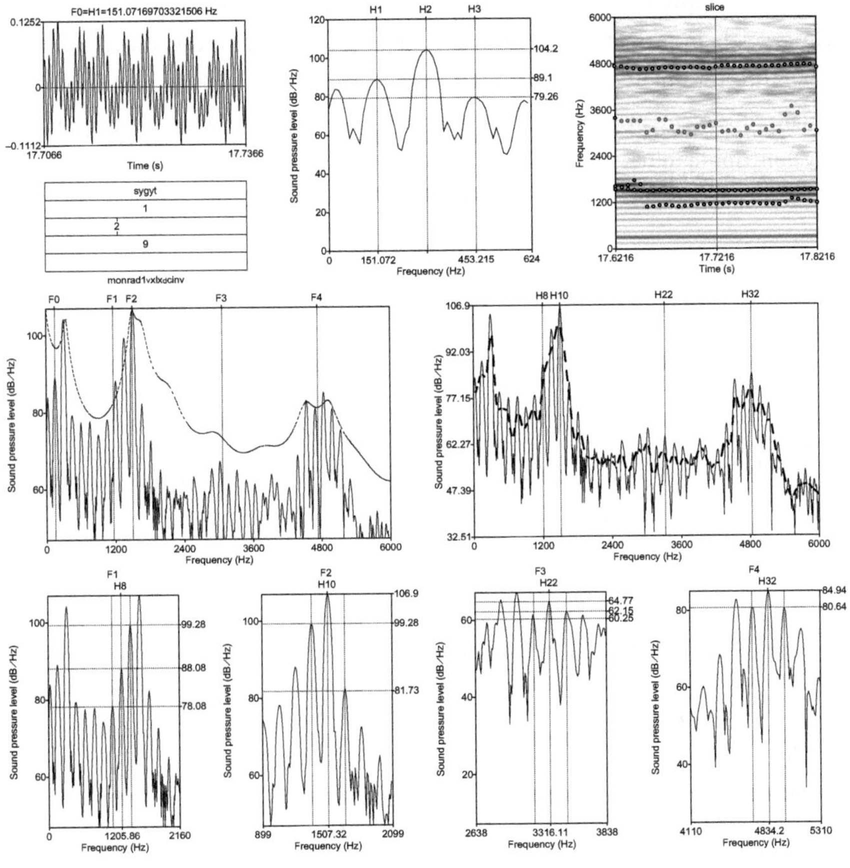

Figure 4.29: Example of a probable formant and bandwidth mismatch: F1 is damped, and so the lower margins in the tails of the F2 area are 'encountered' as F1 since they are still within the measurement frame for F1; F3, which is actually merged with F2, is expected to be higher and therefore also 'recognized' in an area of low energy

4.1.4.2 Formant Structure and Reinforced Harmonics

Formant structure analysis refers to the amplitudes of the 3 prominent harmonics which comprise the center of the formant. Especially for F2, which plays the primary role in providing the 'melody harmonic', the amplitude differences between the prominent harmonic and its adjacent neighbours give a measure of the actual reinforcement and focus (bandwidth narrowing), of which both presumably contribute in most instances to the perceptual prominence of the reinforced harmonic.

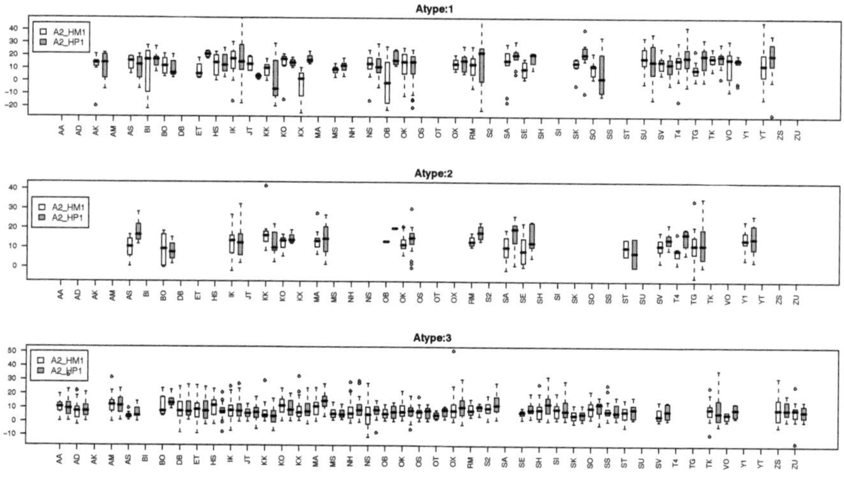

Figure 4.30: Boxplots of harmonic amplitude difference in AT1, AT2 and AT3 of PM1 and PM2 per singer; center harmonic to next-lower harmonic (Hm1; white) amplitude difference; center harmonic to next-higher harmonic (Hp1; grey) amplitude difference

Since articulation types and their underlying strategies are assumed to be the same for PM1 and PM2, it was expected to find very similar results for these two groups. In fact we find parallel tendencies: For F2 and F3 one can observe the highest mean values in AT3, whereas F1 is lower than in AT2 and AT3 (see Figure 4.31). Another overall tendency is count that we find no clear preference of greater lower-harmonic-to-center-harmonic difference vs. higher-harmonic-to-center-

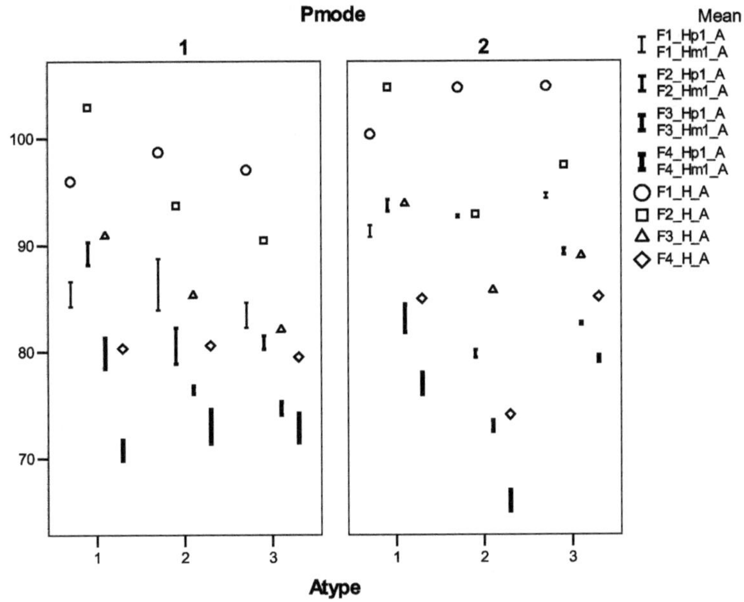

Figure 4.31: Mean difference of adjacent harmonic amplitudes (H minus 1; H; H plus 1) within a particular formant in PM1 (left) and PM2 (right)

harmonic difference. Although, the mean values in Table 4.10 could indicate that there is a slightly bigger difference of the higher-harmonic-to-center-harmonic difference reflecting simply the spectral slope. Still, differences in AT2, compared to AT1, seem to be smaller but also more compact in their range (see Figure 4.30 (top and middle) but also Table 4.10). AT3, as expected, shows an even smaller range and also lower median values (see Figure 4.30(bottom)). However, a detailed investigation of the 'overtone tuning', i.e. fine adjustment of reinforcement and bandwidth narrowing, may also need to adjust the determination method of harmonic amplitudes with respect to the individual AT.

Atype	Pmode		N	Range	Min	Max	Mean	SD
1	1	A2_Hml	367	71.91	-25.05	46.86	12.64	10.26
		A2_Hpl	367	84.86	-25.59	59.27	14.81	11.84
	2	A2_Hml	34	39.86	-15.78	24.08	11.64	8.42
		A2_Hpl	34	63.01	-11.62	51.39	10.56	14.09
2	1	A2_Hml	181	47.05	-5.36	41.69	11.46	6.13
		A2_Hpl	181	35.51	-.17	35.34	14.81	6.97
	2	A2_Hml	35	32.11	2.09	34.20	13.44	6.86
		A2_Hpl	35	31.80	.43	32.23	12.73	7.96
3	1	A2_Hml	187	62.23	-11.09	51.14	8.94	6.96
		A2_Hpl	187	38.42	-7.70	30.72	10.19	6.37
	2	A2_Hml	812	47.48	-14.80	32.68	7.88	6.14
		A2_Hpl	812	43.74	-6.70	37.04	8.43	6.59

Table 4.10: Descriptive statistics amplitude differences of F2-center harmonic and next-lower harmonic (A2-Hml) and next-higher harmonic (A2-Hpl)

4.1.5 Glottal Characteristics in the spectra (H1-H2, H1-A1, H1-A3 etc.)

4.1.5.1 Glottal characteristics of Phonation Mode 1

Additionally the measures of H1-H3 and H1-A2 have been included on the basis of preliminary observations (cf. section 3.3.2.4). In fact it turns out that for PM1 there is a clearly visible 'linear positive relationship' of H1-H2 and H1-A1 in AT1 and in AT2, which becomes more ambiguous in AT3 (see Figure 4.32). Because of the paucity of cases in AT1 and AT2 for PM2, such a relationship is only plainly noticeable for the large group of AT3. Since H1-A1 is a relative measure of the first formant bandwidth these findings become explicable by the fact, that in AT and AT2 B1 stays in a smaller range, but goes outside this range in AT3. B1 of course corresponds to the particular vowel.

4.1.5.2 Glottal Characteristics of Phonation Mode 2

The scattergrams of H1-H2 vs. H1-A1, as pointed out above, describe for AT3 positive relations; the scatters of the other difference (H1-A2) seem to follow the same tendency, but the plot loses shape and the slope becomes less clear in the relationship of H1-H2 and H1-A3.

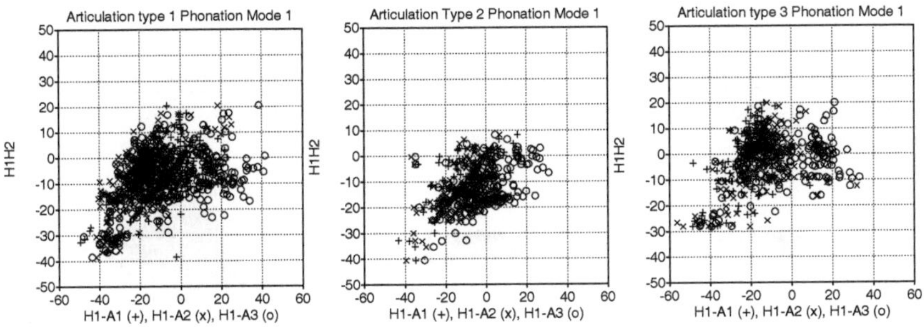

Figure 4.32: H1-H2 scattered versus H1-A1 (+), versus H1-A2 (x), and versus H1-A3 (o); the y-axis refers to H1-H2; PM1

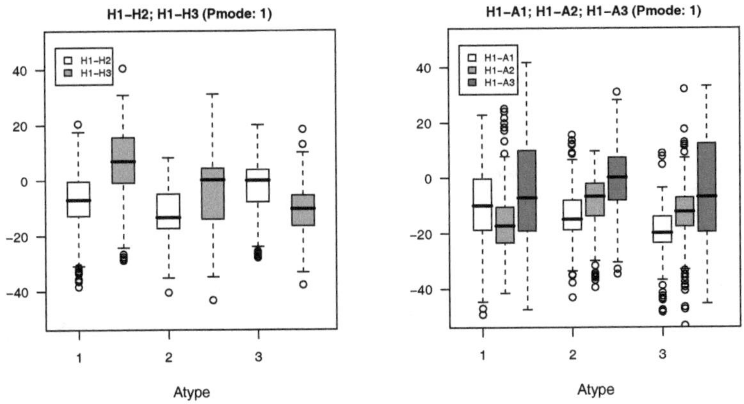

Figure 4.33: for PM1: H1-H2 and H1-H3 boxplotted in groups of articulation types (left); articulation-type-grouped boxplots of H1-A1, H1-A2, and H1-A3 (right)

In Figure 4.35 the cases for AT1 and AT2 would be completely covered by those of AT3, since here due to the variability of formant configuration the range extremely varies.

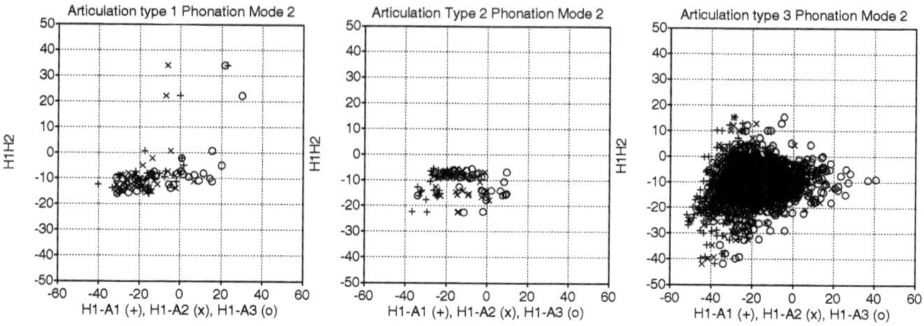

Figure 4.34: H1-H2 scattered versus H1-A1 (+), versus H1-A2 (x, and versus H1-A3 (o); Phonation Mode 2

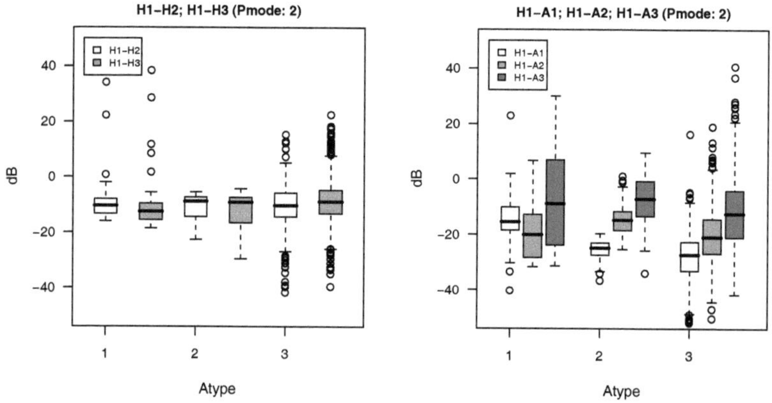

Figure 4.35: For PM2: H1-H2 and H1-H3 boxplotted in groups of articulation types (left); articulation-type-grouped boxplots of H1-A1, H1-A2, and H1-A3 (right)

4.1.6 Average Spectral Characteristics

4.1.6.1 Analysis and Findings of Noise-to-Harmonics Ratio

Since Noise-to-Harmonics Ratio (NHR) according to the MDVP manual describes more globally the noise in the signal (including jitter, shimmer, turbulence noise, subharmonic components, and voice breaks) but only between 70Hz and 4.5kHz (see section 3.3.2.3), it can be interpreted here only as general tendency.

PM1	N	Range	Min	Max	Mean	SD	Variance
NHRmn	701	0.40330	0.001114	0.4044	0.05119	0.05682	0.003
PM2	**N**	**Range**	**Min**	**Max**	**Mean**	**SD**	**Variance**
NHRmn	881	0.79653	0.00520	0.8017	0.10241	0.09060	0.008

Table 4.11: Descriptive statistics of NHR values for PM1 and PM2

NHR Phonation Mode 1 The median values of the area groups also display their ranking: Altai and Tuvan values are on a lower level, and Mongolian and Hakas on a higher level ($T \leq A < M \leq H$). Articulation type groups do not differ that much and, interestingly, AT1 and AT3 are closer to each other than to AT2 (Figure 4.36). The latter note is consistent with observations of a smaller dynamic overtone ambitus in AT2.

NHR Phonation Mode 2 Consequently NHR for PM2 was also observed regarding the proportion of Atypes (Figure 4.36). It turns out that only for the Tuvan and the Mongolian subgroup were enough values obtained to be analyzed. Nonetheless, all grouped value differences were tested statistically (see Appendix A.1.3.2) and found to be significant ($p < 0.05$). But with regard to the individual *kargyraa* strategies, i.e. PM2 production types by means of VTF and AEF, it makes more sense to look at the values for individual singers (Figure 4.37). There is no apparent way for normalizing the values. However, higher NHR values would indicate higher non-harmonic portions in high-frequency bands. These could again be an indication of AEF involvement since the additional laryngeal constriction serves presumably as turbulence source (see also 4.1.6.2).

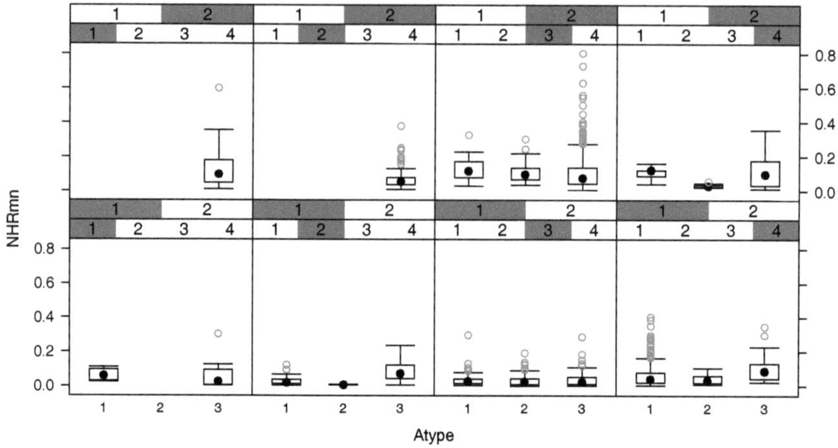

Figure 4.36: Noise-to-Harmonics Ratio (NHR) values in PM1 and PM2 (upper panel) grouped by area (lower panel) and subgrouped articulation type (x-axis); empty slots are due to paucity of data

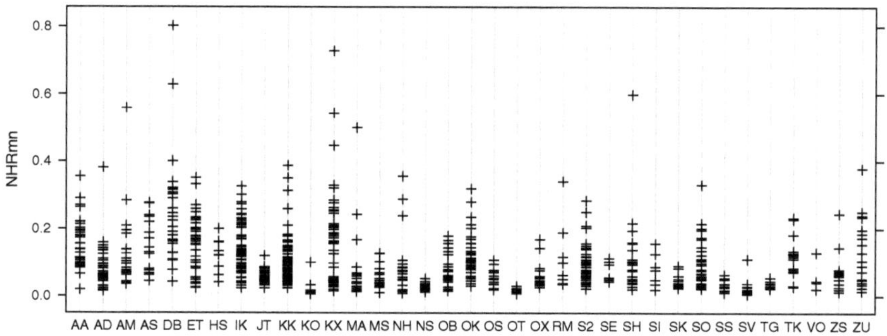

Figure 4.37: NHR values per individual singer in PM2

4.1.6.2 Band Energy Differences and Slope

BED Phonation Mode 1 The band energy differences (BED) show for both groups a clear tendency that shows for the Tuvan after the Mongolian subgroup higher differences in all selected frequency bands than in Altaian and Hakas ThS in PM1. Focusing on the median values, this could be expressed more simply as:

BED 0-2 kHz H < A < T < M AT3 <AT2 < AT1
BED 2-5 kHz H ≤ A < T < M AT3 ≥ AT2 < AT1
BED 5-8 kHz H < A < T < M AT3 < AT2 < AT1

The derived spectral slopes follow these trends.

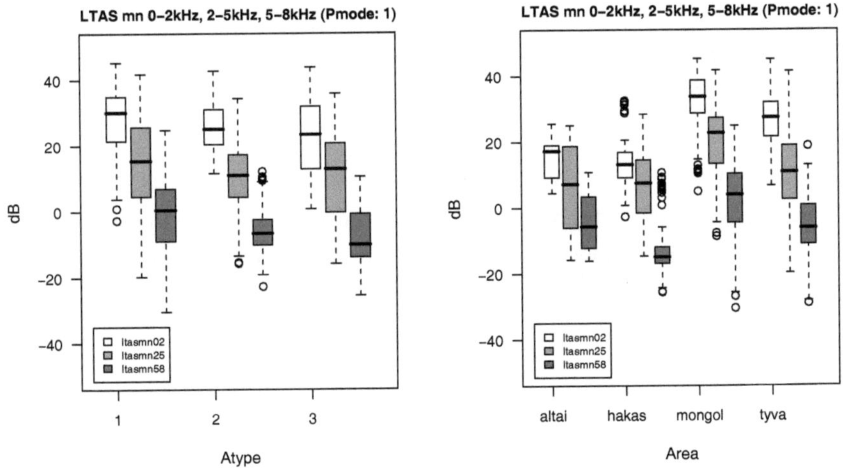

Figure 4.38: Three mean energy-band differences (derived from 'short-term LTAS') grouped into area (left) and articulation type (right) in PM1; the y-axis gives the energy differences in dB

BED Phonation Mode 2 For PM2 the tendency of high energy components in the 0-2KHz band for the Mongolian subgroup is followed by the Altai and Tuvan

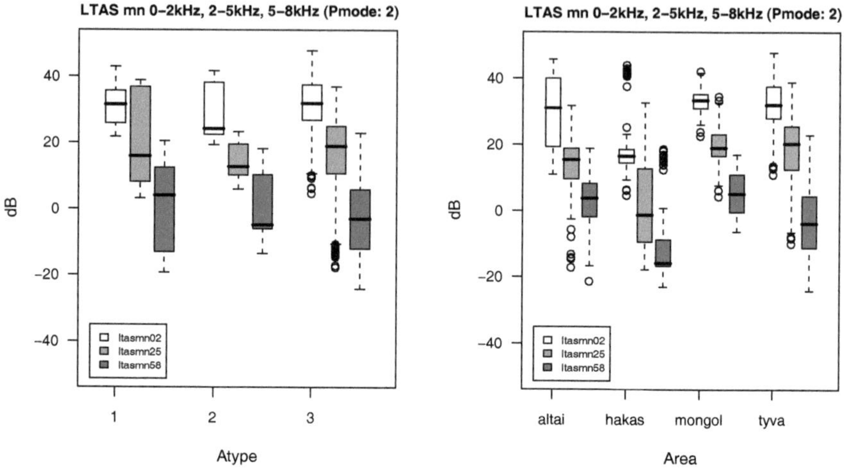

Figure 4.39: Mean energy band differences (derived from short term LTAS) grouped into area (left) and articulation type (right) in PM2; the y-axis gives the energy differences in dB

subgroup. Whereas for Hakas this band shows strikingly low values, this also indicates an overall tendency of lower values for the other bands. In the observation of articulation type groups (only) Hakas singers emerge as lower outliers for BED 0-2kHz and 2-5 kHz in AT3.

BED	0-2 kHz	H < A < T < M	AT3 > AT2 < AT1
BED	2-5 kHz	H ≤ A < T < M	AT3 > AT1 > AT2
BED	5-8 kHz	H < A < T < M	AT1 > AT3 > AT2

It is of course questionable if such an areal grouping makes sense without differentiation of articulation types. But for instance something like the very low energy in the third band (5-8 kHz) of the Hakas samples may serve as an anchor for further investigation.

Observations on LTAS A more discrete analysis of spectral features specifical on individual frequency bands can be provided by long-term-average spectra (LTAS). Here the fact must also be considered (as also expressed by Nawka et al., 1997) that frequency bands beyond the usual 5kHz may also contain valuable information about voice production characteristics of the individual subject (Figure 4.40). Although the analysis of the individual LTAS measures for each pre-defined measure point also remains for further investigation, a spot check of Tuvan PM2AT3 samples may serve as an illustration of possible tendencies, as given in Figure 4.41. It can certainly not be ruled out that the recording context (e.g. room acoustics) may bias the results. But if the focus lies for example on different ATs of one individual singer within one session, such influence of recording context may be fairly minimal.

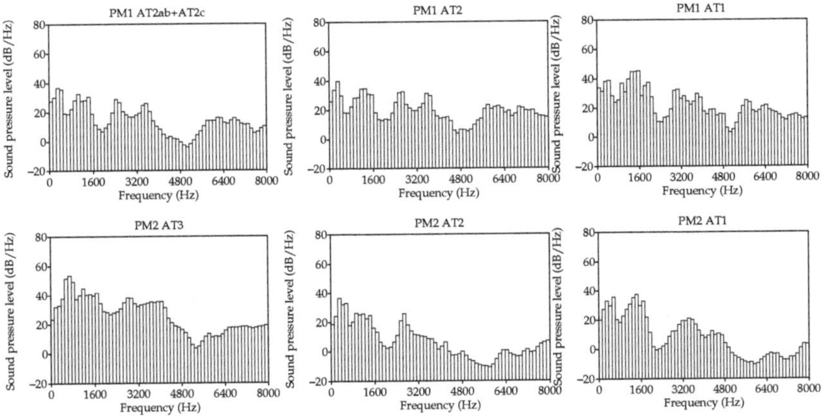

Figure 4.40: LTAS (Bandwidth 90Hz) applied on approx. 25-30 sec of different PMxATx samples of singer IK (T); y-axis gives the sound pressure level (dB/Hz)

Another observation of the PM2 sample with the most frequent articulation type AT3, illustrated in Figure 4.41, reveals a peak at around 3000-3200Hz. Another somewhat higher peak around 4800Hz is also very often present (cf. 2.4.2).

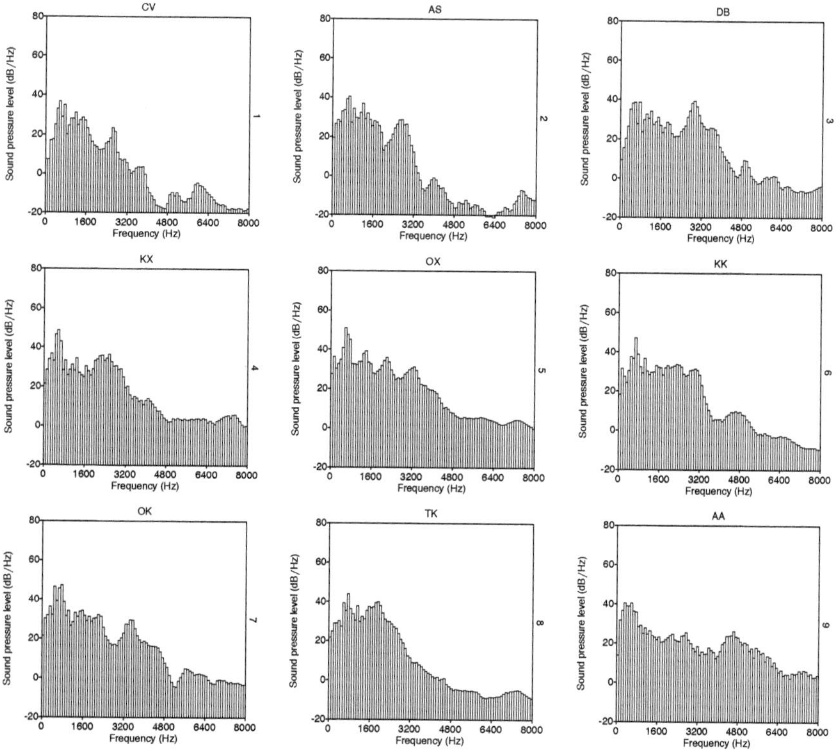

Figure 4.41: LTAS (Bandwidth 90Hz) applied on approx. 80-100sec of 9 PM2AT3 samples; singer 1-8 are Tuvan; singer 9 is Mongolian; singer 8 uses presumably AEF-VF phonation (instead of VFT-VF); y-axis gives the sound pressure level (dB/Hz)

4.1.7 Findings in Inverse Filtering Curves

As stated above, an automatically obtained inverse-filtered glottal flow and its derivative could only provide a very rough estimation due to the problems of antiresonance filter adjustment. By means of the BoGA inverse filtering program some examples could be processed. Generally the observations were based on the glottal flow curves processed in PRAAT.

Inverse Filtering of Phonation Mode 1

The instant of glottal flow abruption in the example in Figure 4.43 does not appear within the contacting phase, as might be expected. Considering also the systematic delay in Vx due to the time the microphone signal needs to travel, the inverse filtered signal still seems fairly late which would point to a possible effect on Lx. This alone illustrates the potential benefits of examining the glottal flow signal, since in this case the Vx waveform is heavily influenced by higher formant frequencies, resulting in supraperiodic behaviour.

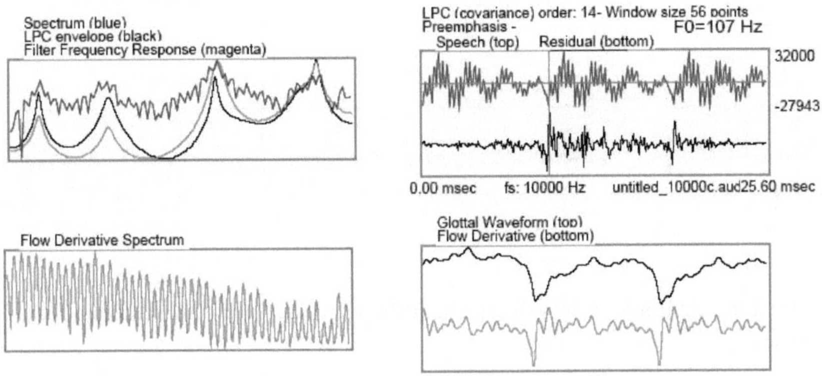

Figure 4.42: Inverse filtering (glottal flow) as provided by BoGA software; singer SK (H) PM1AT2

Figure 4.42 illustrates the qualitative difference in inverse filtering between non-manually corrected and manually corrected glottal flow curves. The glottal flow negative peak and the following phase of minimal glottal flow would then not appear as sharp dip since high-frequency noise has been filtered out. However, glottal flow curve reveals a fairly long open phase with long plateau and sharp decline at the closure instant.

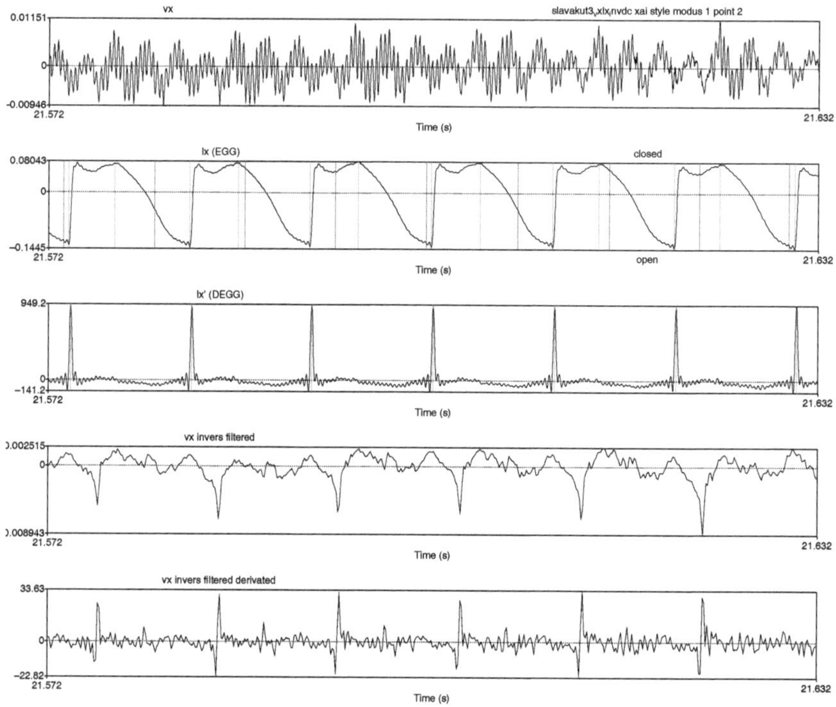

Figure 4.43: Example of waveforms including inverse-filtered Vx; singer SK (H) PM1AT2

Inverse Filtering of Phonation Mode 2

In the example in Figure 4.44 the major excitation instant (air flow abruption) seems strictly to follow the glottal instant as indicated by Vx and Lx, whereas Lx aligns within a double-cycle period at the lower peak, which would usually be interpreted as the joint VTF-VF contact phase.

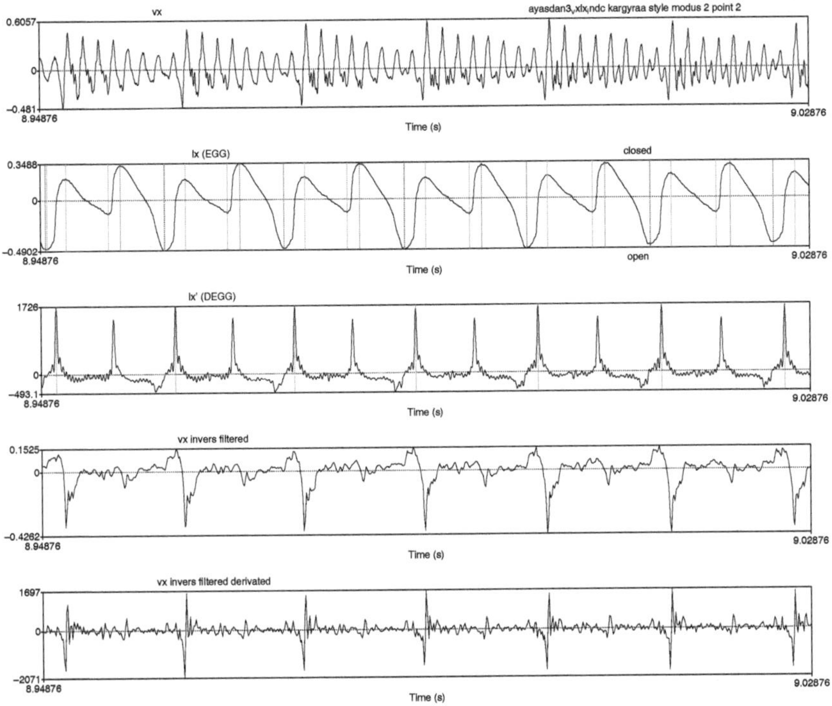

Figure 4.44: Phonation mode 2 (Tuva, *kargyraa*, AD), voice audio time signal (Vx), inverse filtered glottal flow and derived glottal flow

The other possible explanation is that the joint closure of VTF and VF serves as the real glottal instant. The second, intermittent closure implying a stop in glottal flow is either diffused or it may be incomplete.

Additionally a PM2 sample was investigated by means of the BoGA software. Here the glottal flow curve clearly reveals that there is no second air flow drop within the entire period length.

It might be very promising to look specifically in further research, at the normalized amplitude quotient (NAQ) (Alku et al., 2002), which had been successfully positively correlated to CQ in so-called "throaty" voice. Since the derivative glottal flow curve is highly dependent on low-frequency response, the recording

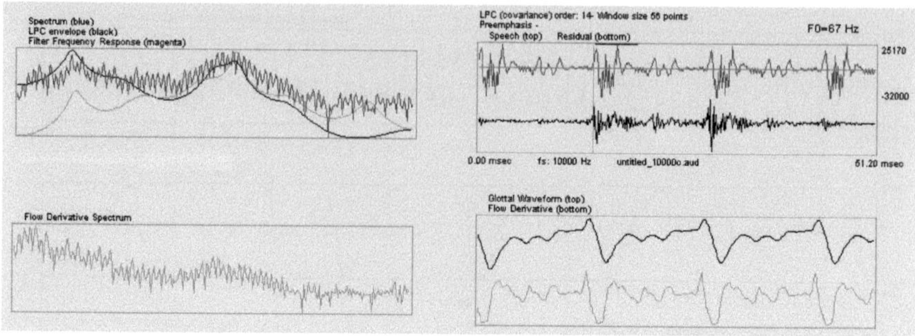

Figure 4.45: Inverse-filtered PM2 example; inverse filtering (glottal flow) as provided by BoGA software; singer AD (T) PM2AT4

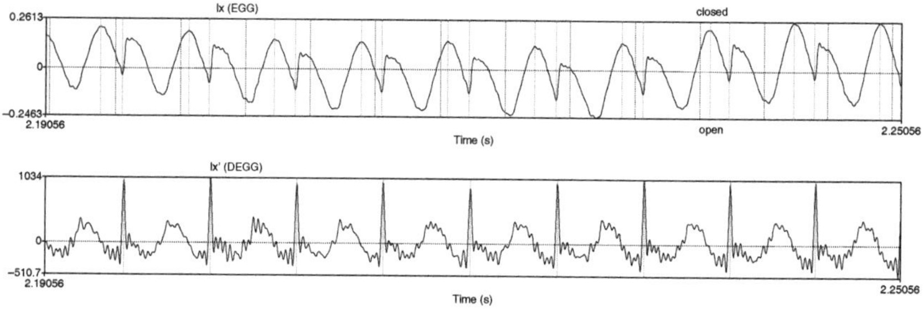

Figure 4.46: Example of PM2; singer AM (T); Vx, Lx, dLx, inverse-filtered Vx

requirements in terms of microphone choice and situative set up but also material and singing tasks might need to be reconsidered.

4.2 Analysis and Findings for Lx

4.2.1 Sub-Corpus Description

For Lx measurement and analysis, the original field data corpus was used (Corpus 1; see Table 3.2) containing 60 tracks of 1 Altai, 6 Hakas, and 9 Tuvan throat singers (in total). For singer ST no parameters of PM2 were analysed, and for singers AN and SK no PM1 values.

4.2.2 Findings in EGG and DEGG Wave Shapes (incl. Gx)

4.2.2.1 Lx and dLx Shapes:

For all measure points a time slice consisting of the following 60 milliseconds was chosen which has been selected for purposes of depiction and visual inspection (more examples are given in the Appendix A.2.3).

It should probably emphasized again, that the terms *open* and *decontacting* as well as closed and maximal contact and also *closing* and *contacting* are used here synonymous. Even though these terms remain just descriptive in sense of usual conventions. The actual contact areas in terms of ventricular-fold motion or aryepiglottic-fold motion and vocal-fold vibration remain hidden. Thus any interpretations regarding involved tissue movement are purely speculative.

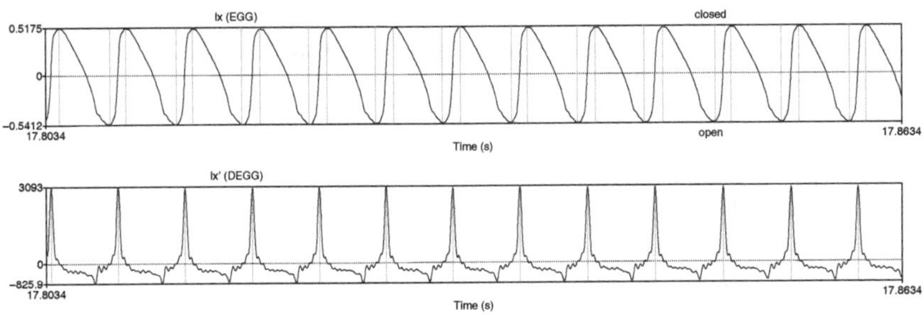

Figure 4.47: “ideal” shaped Lx and dLx curves of a trained tensed voice, Hakas singer ZU, ZU4 pt1

Lx and dLx shapes in Phonation Mode 1 Usually PM1 Lx signals show a very short closing phase followed by a short contact phase and mostly convex (positively bulged) decontacting phase. A plateau in decontacting, which as often found in modal voice, is mostly absent for ThS PM1 and indicates a short 'open phase'.

Some samples show a very sharp peak, i.e. narrow peak angle, and a skirt bulging which can also become the end point of a plateau. This plateau can be interpreted as a prolonged contacting phase, pointing to tensed or pressed phonation, and it may be the base for a negative dip.

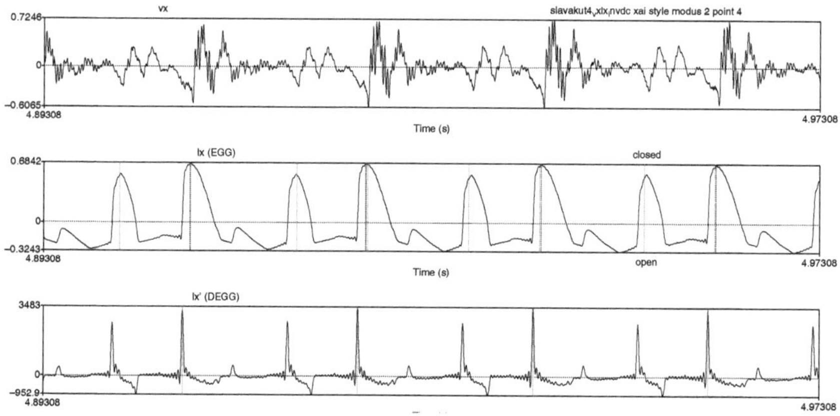

Figure 4.48: Lx and dLx shapes of a sample from Hakas singer SK; PM1; SK4 pt3SK6 pt1

Unexpectedly also in PM1 the EGG showed patterns which resemble those of PM2 or must be interpreted as double cycle patterns (e.g. Figures 4.54 and 4.53). For the example in Figure 4.49 it remains unclear where a potential second contact area actually comes into play. On the one hand the already-approximated VTFs could be involved; on the other hand, parts of the aryepiglottic sphincter may also serve as an oscillator. In either case the two oscillators seem to be out of phase. Additionally the fairly long closure time of the first half of the cycle is notable, and so it is not surprising that according to Vx, and glottal flow, it is actually the small steep rising part of the negative 'incisure' that serves as the instant of excitation. The resulting 'rough, diplophone' voice quality of the sample for Figure 4.49 was also judged by the singer as not appropriate or not "pretty enough", so that the recording at his request was repeated on another day.

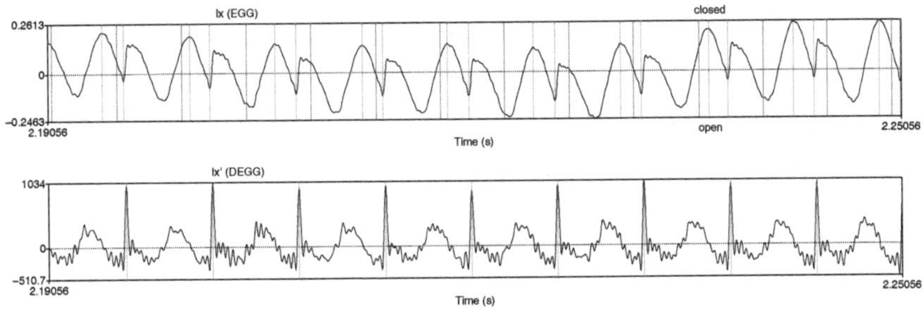

Figure 4.49: Singer AM (T) (andmon vxlx ptl)

Another example of such double cycle was provided by singer KX (T); but here the voice quality was completely 'unsuspicious'. As one explanation a second contact area may be 'bulging' right into the counter phase of the opening sequence of the glottal folds. But it must be assumed that here a more complex interference of different overlapping tissue movements is superimposed on the waveform.

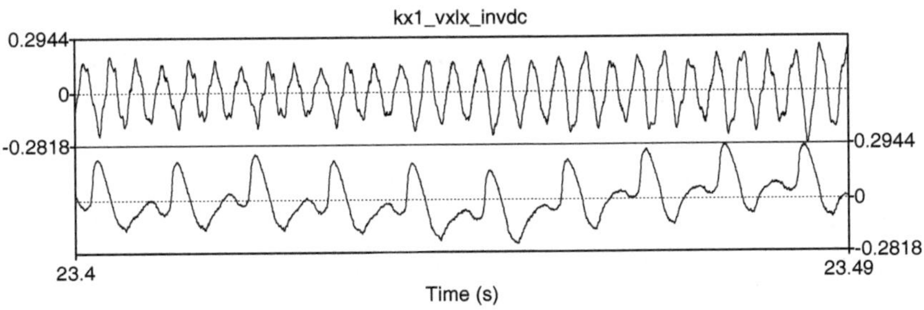

Figure 4.50: Singer KX (T) example of Lx in PM1

Lx and dLx shapes in Phonation Mode 2 The double cycle pattern usually comprises an alternation between peaks of two different relative heights, positive and negative. The positive peaks tend to be mostly sharper, while the negative peaks are mostly broader and rounder (i.e. ramping). Typically there is also a sequence of decontacting on a higher level before the lower peak. The decontacting phase before the lower peak in some cases is 'filled' with an additional positive dent which can change into a third peak (yielding a triplet-pattern). Although the two peak amplitudes in some cases are fairly close to each other, the two cycle lengths do not need to be equal (see Figure 4.52).

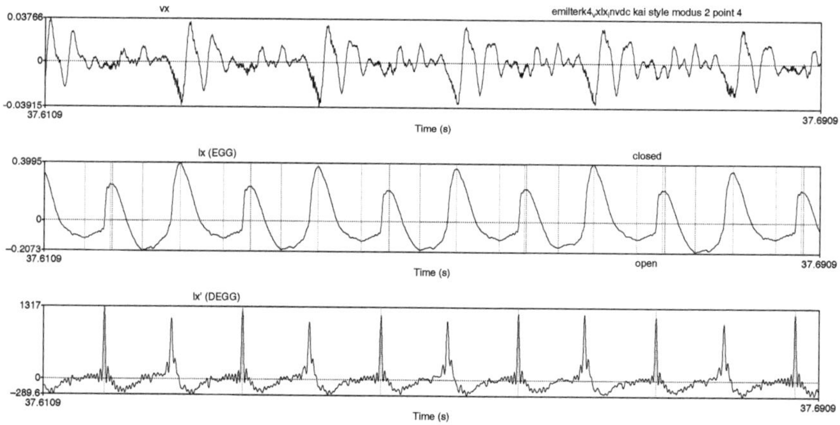

Figure 4.51: Vx, Lx and dLx waveform of PM2 of an Altai singer (ET) [emilterk4vxlxinvdc kai style modus 2 point 5]

Decontacting phases also show differences in duration and shape (skew), which leads in sample of Figure 4.53 to the assumption that in the case of slower decontacting two asynchronous masses are moving apart.

A sensible interpretation of the contact area signal can only be made in connection with Vx and glottal flow signal. Generally there seem to be two ways to achieve VTF and VF coupling. The more frequent variant is shown in Figure 4.54. Here the lower peak is interpreted as the joint VFT-VF contacting where the impedance fall, due to the remaining chinks, is lower followed by a maximal

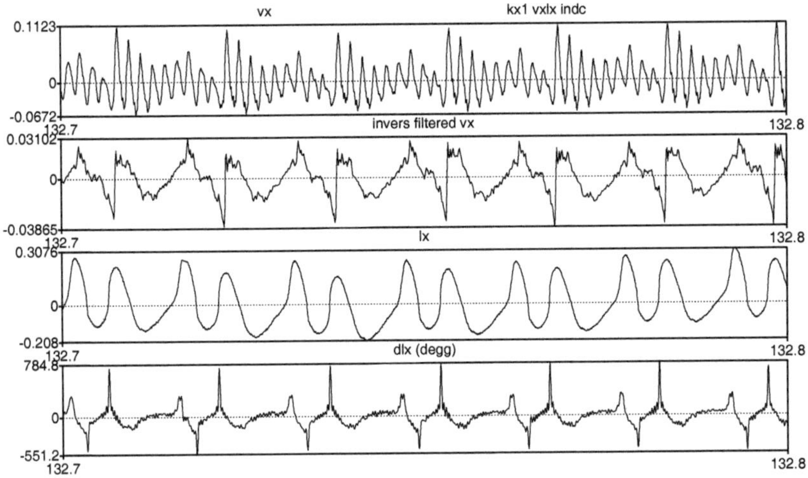

Figure 4.52: Singer KX (Tuva) Lx signal example for PM2

decontacting. After this a maximal contacting of the VFs follows which serves as the instant of excitation, as seen in the Vx (see also Figure 4.84). The adjacent decontacting phase is already influenced by an additional (surface) current.

But there are also a few examples of very roughly defined contacting phases (see Figure 4.55), which may indicate very unstable contact and which thus appear as unequal peaks. Finally, also the already predicted triple pattern (see section 3.3.2.6) can be found in some samples, whereas the origin of the third smaller peak stays questionable. Presumably here as in other cases of an in-bulging peak an asynchronicity of VTF oscillation causes a skewed contact of a singular VTF with periepiglottal tissue (or elsewhere).

By looking again at a similar example to that in section 4.1.2.6 (PM2 AT3) and also adding the Vx waveform also here the higher peak can be identified as the one accompanied by the moment of period initiation. In Figure 4.56, right before this instant, already during the initial sound pressure decline clearly an additive noise is apparent, which may be related to the glottal chink observed in endoscopy (cf. Lindestad et al., 2001).

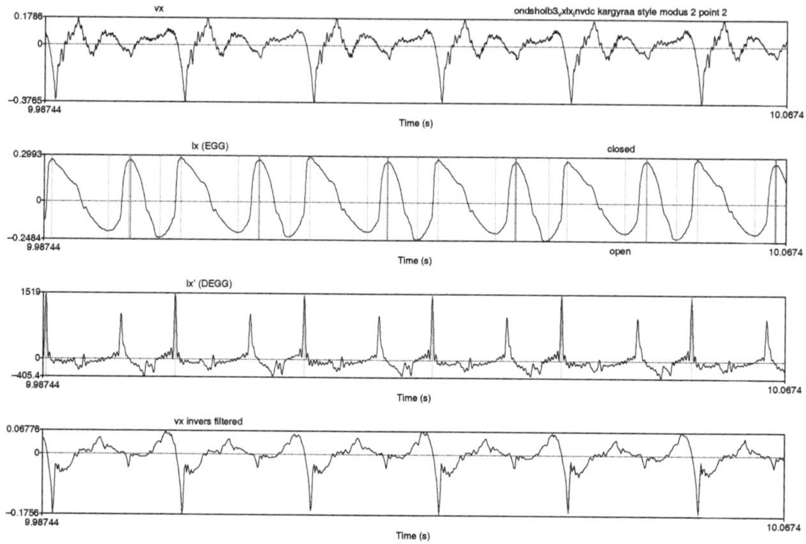

Figure 4.53: Lx and dLx of PM2 (*kargyraa*) of singer OS (T)(ondsholb 3 p2)

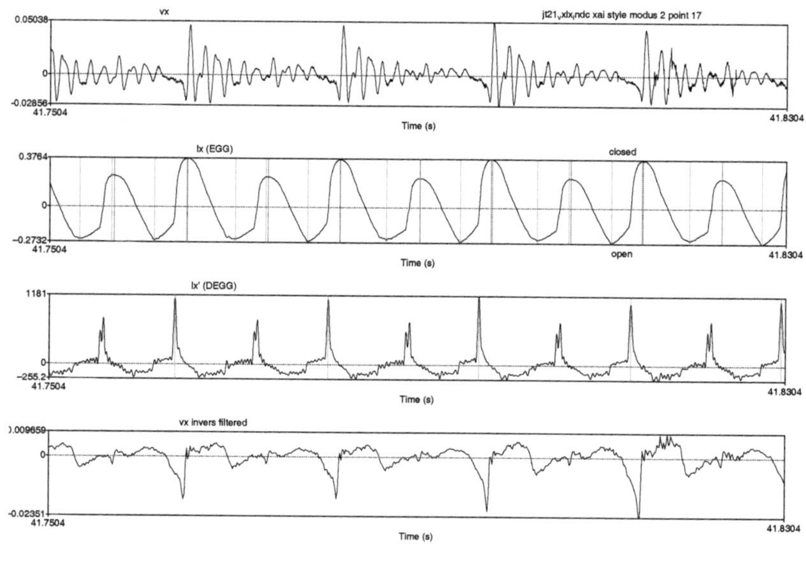

Figure 4.54: Lx and dLx shapes in JT (H) jt21 pt17 PM2 AT3

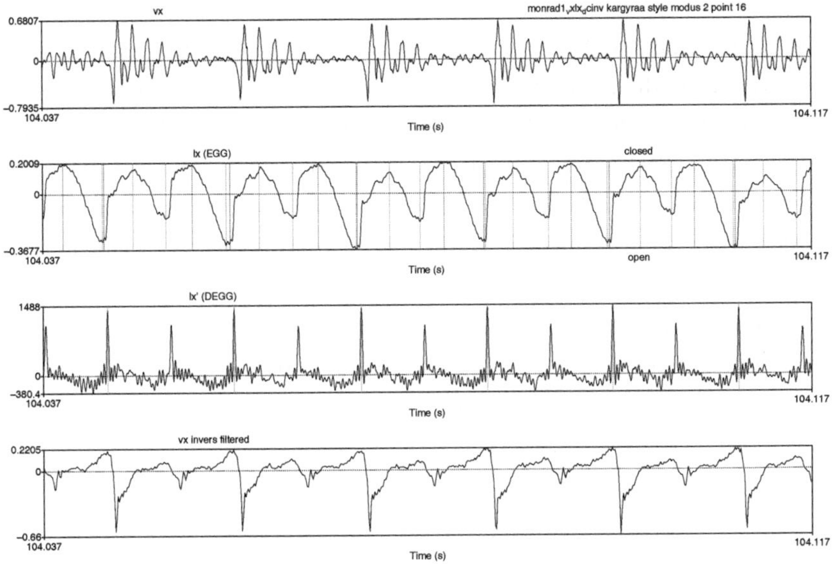

Figure 4.55: Example of Lx and dLx of *kargyraa*, singer RM (T) (file: RM4 pt 16)

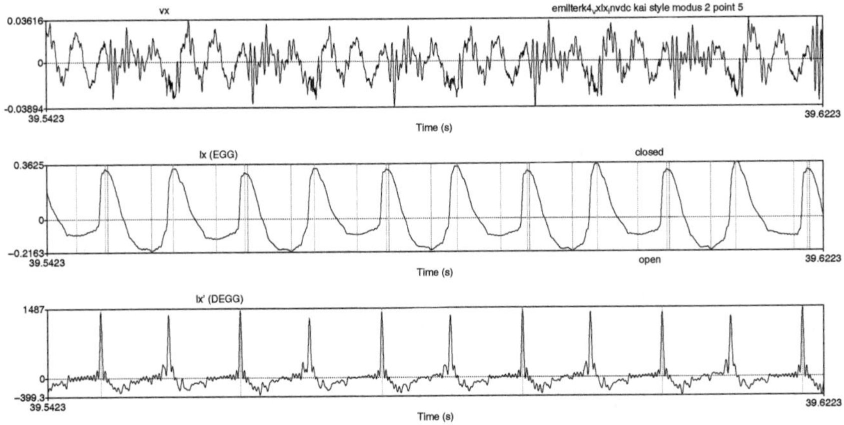

Figure 4.56: Lx and dLx singer ET (A) emilterk4_vxlx_invdc pt 5

4.2.2.2 Gx - Global Movement of the EGG-signal

Gx as the movement of the Vx baseline typically shows a very homogeneous and flat curve during the main phase of the phonatory passage. In the majority of samples of PM1 production (Fig4.57), Gx at the phrase onset rises briefly and then falls again. The same happens at the offset, while in between only a slight Gx movement is observed. This would allow us to speculate that the larynx height is fairly fixed and the smaller deviations are caused by distortions in the muscle tension of the external larynx muscles. The small movement would then result from a laryngeal movement during the the beginning of the AES constriction.

Exceptions within the corpus are found in the samples of singer (ZS). Here the Gx movement is strikingly vigorous and needs to be explained by further analysis.

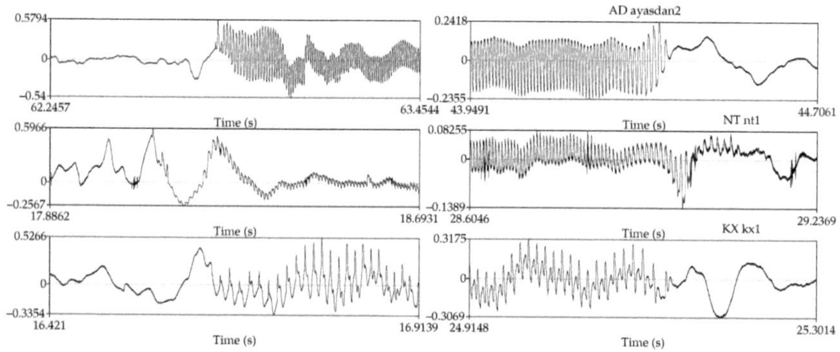

Figure 4.57: Examples from three Tuvan singers (AD, NT, KX) for Gx movement in PM1

But for examples of PM2 production (see Figure 4.58) the Gx-movement at the onset phase seems not as apparent. This fact contributes to the other observations and expectation regarding involved (supra-)laryngeal constriction mechanisms. Since a medial compression (for VTF-VF) would be presumably not demand much vertical larynx movement, for the samples lacking such onset-rise of Gx a VTF-VF phonation seems to be more plausible.

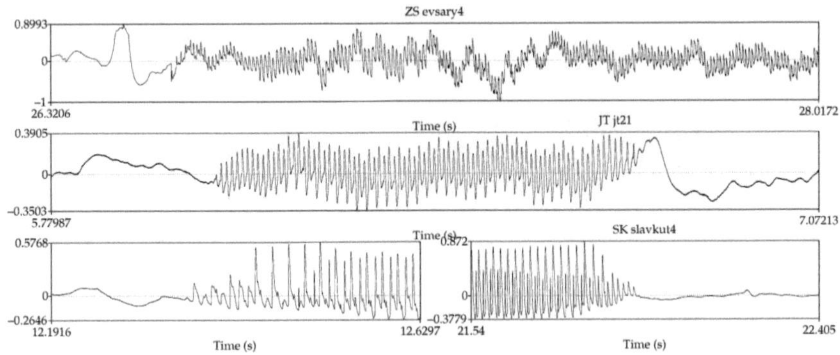

Figure 4.58: Examples from three singers [ZS(T), JT (H), SK(H)] for Gx movement in PM2

4.2.3 Periods Obtained by Lx Measurement

Usually Lx serves as a more reliable source for pitch detection since shimmer measures are hardly dependent on point definition (amplitude definition) for the PRAAT PointProcess which is again dependent on pitch (or better on signal periodicity): here the clear definition of maxima or minima. For signals with a double cycle pattern as in the ThS styles *kai*, *xai* or *kargyraa*, F0 or period length measurement was processed on the basis of two different pitch detections, resulting in two different PRAAT PointProcesses, according to the estimated pitch range (see 4.1.3.1) in phonation modes 1 and 2. The relation of period length1 to period length2, or better cycle length1 to cycle length2, is not always a pure 1:2 relation, since 1) pitch detection procedure is (as explained above) dependent on minima or maxima detection or is 2) dependent on the cross-correlation algorithm, which may find supraperiodic constants 'more attractive' and 3) also VTF-VF coordination may not always be precisely in phase, so that a change of Lx shape would also be the expected result.

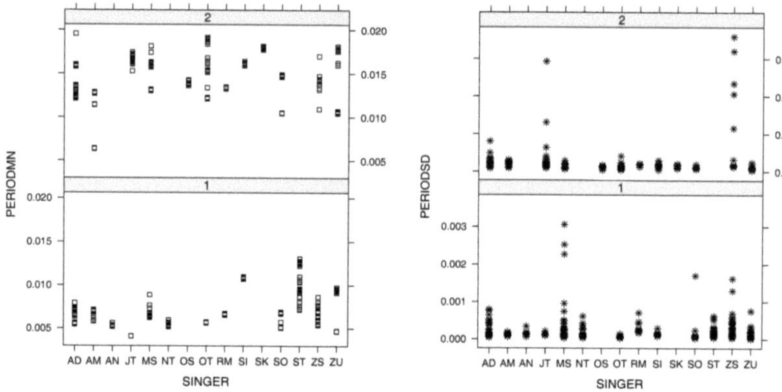

Figure 4.59: Mean period values (left) and standard deviations (right) of single cycle (1) and double cycle (2) period length

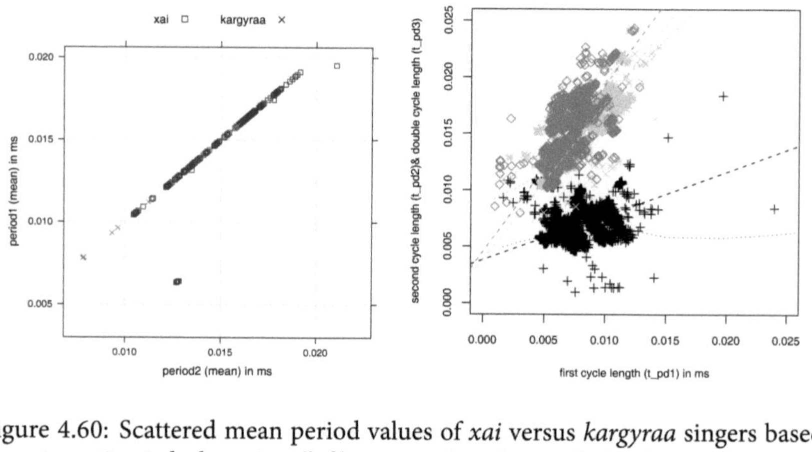

Figure 4.60: Scattered mean period values of *xai* versus *kargyraa* singers based on automatic pitch detection (left); scatterplot of period1 (cycle 1) and period2 (cycle 2) (y-axis) versus period3 (total period length) based on single value of direct measures for quotient analysis (right)

4.2.4 Jitter of the Lx Signal

Lx served as the source for perturbation measurement, since here the glottal (area) function is supposed to be more directly mapped on. Jitter measurement is also potentially interesting with respect to an investigation of inner period and period-to-period perturbation of Lx. Therefore the jitter analysis was adapted so that either the normal jitter (cycle-to-cycle) or the cycle-to-next-plus-one-cycle (period-to-period) jitter is measured. The last method is labeled with a -2 suffix.

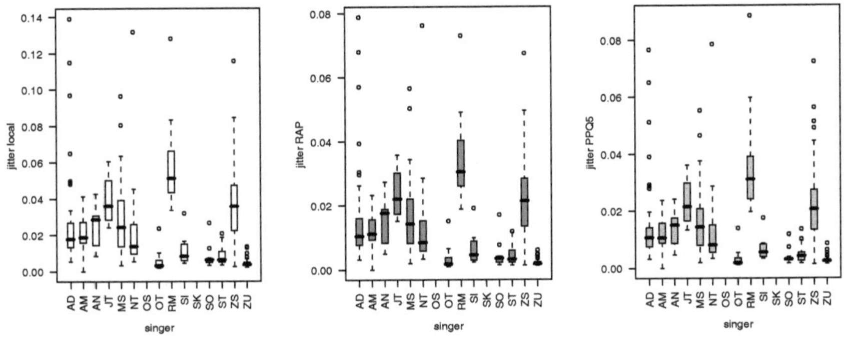

Figure 4.61: Lx jitter Loc, RAP, ppq5 for each singer of PM1

As seen in Figure 4.62 the difference between the two methods also varies from singer to singer; it can be very small, as seen for AM and SI, or quite large, as seen for MS, OT, and SK. Since especially the period-to-period measures all seem to be located in a small range, the differences observed between the cycle-to-cycle and the period-to-period jitter measures might give a specific hint regarding the period1 to period2 relationship. The perturbation 'profile' for each of the singers stays stable and does only slightly decreases by including more periods (in RAP). Interestingly, there are fairly large differences in the range of the two different measurement methods (Loc and Loc2; RAP and RAP2). However, the Mann-Whitney U-test shows significant differences between *xai* and *kargyraa* for all jitter values obtained.

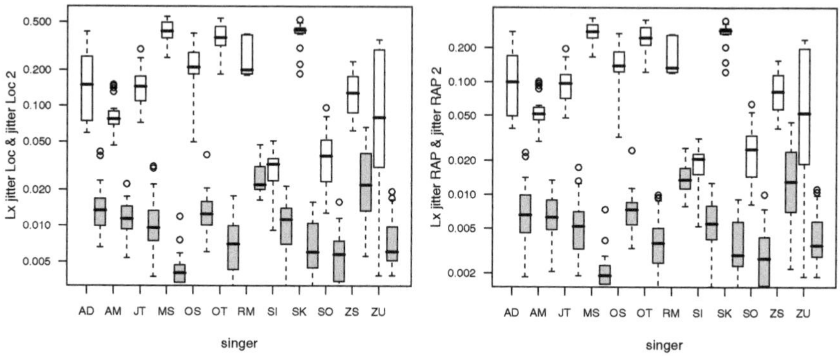

Figure 4.62: Lx jitter Loc and jitter RAP for cycle-to-cycle (white) and period-to-period (grey) measures of each singer of PM2

4.2.5 Shimmer of the Lx Signal

Here PM2 in particular stands in the focus of interest, since (especially for local shimmer) a more direct measure of the relative amplitude difference between the first and second cycle of the double cycle period is expected. As with jitter measures, this would partially reveal the inner characteristics of a period - its shape and perturbation.

	N	Minimum	Maximum	Mean	Std. Deviation
shimmerLoc	284	.000000	.854075	.34968699	.208440280
shimmerLocdB	284	.000000	7.499495	3.08816216	1.894854119
shimmerapq3	284	.000000	.568705	.22282069	.141036067
shimmerapq5	284	.000000	.412381	.12467482	.084413194
shimmerapq11	284	.000000	.514800	.19860469	.124261480
shimmerLoc2	284	.006327	.269782	.04872729	.047926420
shimmerLocdB2	284	.054932	2.304960	.42533166	.421429731
shimmerapq32	284	.003397	.148126	.02753230	.026835638
shimmerapq52	284	.004126	.192370	.03099355	.032673778
shimmerapq112	284	.004775	.194247	.03412846	.033036019

Table 4.12: Descriptive analysis table of Lx shimmer values in PM2

The comparison of different shimmer values (see Figure 4.63) reveals an interesting effect caused by the calculation method of shimmer. Whereas one can

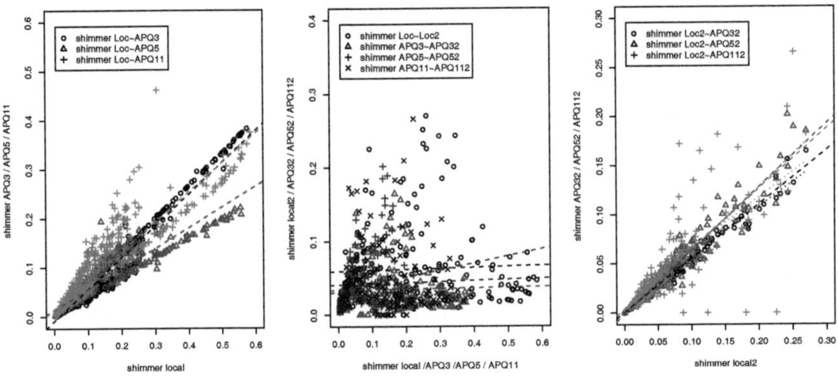

Figure 4.63: Comparison of various shimmer measure methods applied to Lx signal of PM2; each method contrasts values obtained by measures either on every cycle (left) or every second cycle

observe a decreasing of values from local shimmer over apq3 to apq5, in apq11 the shimmer value is again higher than in apq5 measures. This might be explicable due to a smoothing by the mean values of an increasing cycle number, since APQs are calculated that way. This smoothing effect seems to be lost with a higher number of compared amplitudes (apq11) and it may imply a kind of threshold for the period number chosen for shimmer measurement and for this sort of double cycle material.

By taking only the mean values (as in Table 4.12), a tendency seems to emerge for a greater cycle-to-cyle difference between adjacent amplitudes in *xai*, and a slight tendency for a greater difference between cycles of over-next neighbours in Tuvan *kargyraa*. In order to explore the outliers of local shimmer (Figure 4.65) and apq5 shimmer (Figure 4.66), values are given for all singers in PM1 and PM2. Clearly the Lx shimmer values are quite inhomogeneous, but a grouping in PM2 becomes apparent upon second inspection: there is a higher range or niveau of median values > 0.2 and a lower range of values <= 0.10.

The very high value of local shimmer for the Tuvan singer SI contradicts the auditory evaluation of his singing as very 'soft and smooth'. Nonetheless he is counted as belonging to a group of higher local shimmer values, together with

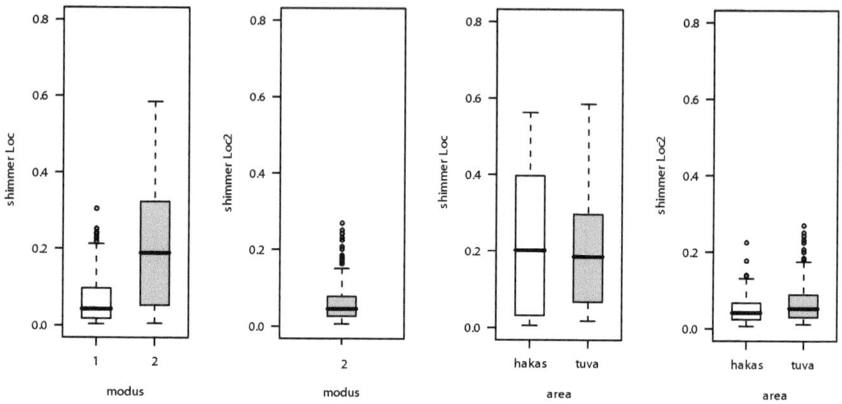

Figure 4.64: Local shimmer differences of Lx between area groups in PM2

JT (H), ZS (T), RM (T), and SO (T), which show a median value that stands out against the others [AD(T), AM(T), MS (H), OS (T), OT (H), SK (H), and ZU (H)] and which can be re-identified as the outliers in both groups of local shimmer (shimmerLoc2, Figure 4.64, most right). Considering here the higher variance in the group of Tuvan singers (*kargyraa*) it would mean the opposite to the results obtained from a group comparison based on the whole set of measures per group. When three more periods are added into the calculation (ppq5), the tendency within PM1 remains stable and seems to become more clearly defined or 'more compact' within PM2.

Within PM2 most of the cycle-to-cycle jitter values show a wide range and a fairly great distance of median values to the median of period-to-period jitter. Two singers, RM and ZS, appear exceptional so that for apq5 the median values of the two shimmer methods behaves reverse (compared to the other singers), whereas also the variance (range) seems to be very compact. Such a smaller range, i.e. homogeneity, of shimmer 2 values seems to be more typical (cf. jitter period-to-period values). The observations of the median led to a reinspection of Lx patterns and shapes for both groups in a spot check (Figure 4.67). Whereas the cycle-to-cycle differences seem to be similar to each other, in the group of higher shimmer loc values a higher variability in the difference of amplitudes of

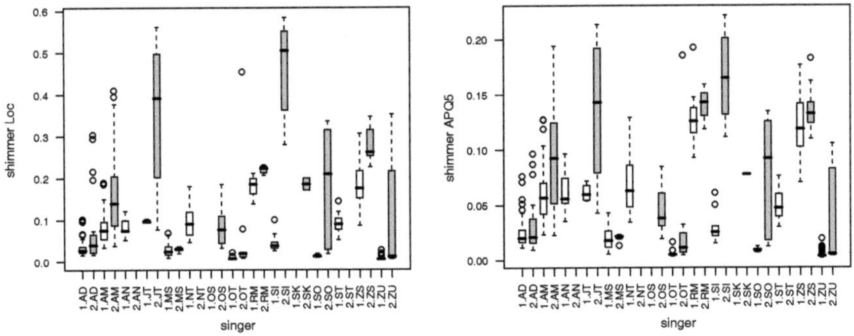

Figure 4.65: Local shimmer (left) and APQ5 (right) values of Lx over the whole group of singers in PM1 (white) and PM2 (grey); phonation modes are also indicated by "1" or "2" preceding the singer's ID; note the different ranges in the y-axis

next-plus-one neighbours with higher minimum peak and a greater remaining Gx greater variability of negative peaks was recognized.

The Mann-Whitney U-test shows that group differences are significant for all values except shimmer apq11 A.1.3.3.

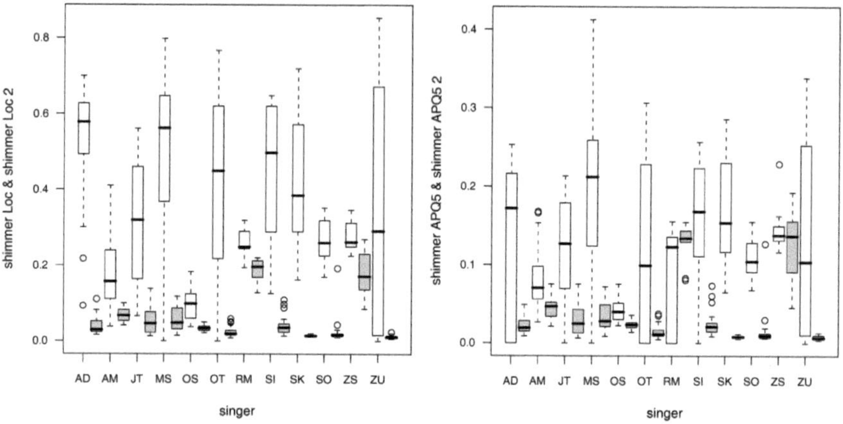

Figure 4.66: Local shimmer (left) and shimmer apq5 (right) values for single-cycle (white) and double-cycle (2; grey) measures over the whole group of singers in PM2

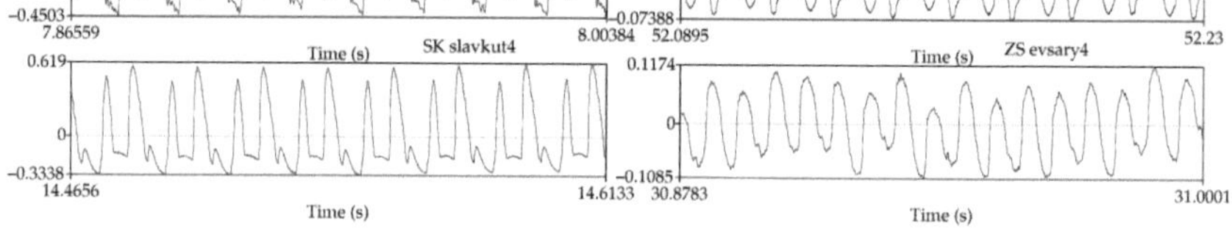

Figure 4.67: Spot check of Lx samples of singers with a low median local shimmer (left) and a high median local shimmer (right)

4.2.6 EGG Quotients – Analysis and Findings

Whereas for the above mentioned parameters each value stood for the whole measurement interval, for the Lx quotient analysis have been included all values (25-30 for PM1; 45-55 for PM2) within the measurement interval were included. A wide range of individual differences between singers may pass for an overall tendency in quotient measurement. Although the styles (area groups) show a small divergence this cannot be taken as a strong tendency, since they encompass a large range of divergent singers (see Appendix Table A.5).

4.2.6.1 Single-Cycle Source Mode (PM1)

	N	Min	Max	Mean	Std. Dev.
t3mtl/tpd_CiQ1	19537	.017009	.616785	.18794462	.102940827
t2amta2/tpd_CiQ2	19537	.001573	.954316	.12362510	.095860097
t6mt4/tpd_QOQ	19537	.018034	.973937	.50473070	.185813912
t5amt3/t3mtl_SQ	19537	.132779	51.733700	4.54537431	4.277368293
CPmOP/CPpOP_CIa	19537	-.975118	.700389	-.55418317	.309974063

Table 4.13: Descriptive statistics of Lx quotients in PM1

The measures show a very short closing phase of about 15-20% of the whole period, so that one would expect a tendency of the contact index to tend towards -1. Outliers greater than 0.6 can probably be identified as measurement errors which may be based on false closing phase detection. It seems that especially the closing phase definition for CiQ2 is susceptible to such errors. Otherwise the two methods indicate divergent tendencies for the two groups, where CiQ1 actually comprises a wider range of contacting whose end point is dependent on the highest positive peak point. Given a peak ramping the two phases could really be found different. A difference between CiQ1 and CiQ2 could then describe the characteristic of the contacting-phase-to-contact-phase transition, hence the results would point towards sharp peaks in *xai* and a more rounded left peak-half in *xöömej*.

The quasi-open quotient reveals an almost exactly equal proportion of quasi-contact or quasi-closed (positive curve half) to quasi-open or minimal-contact

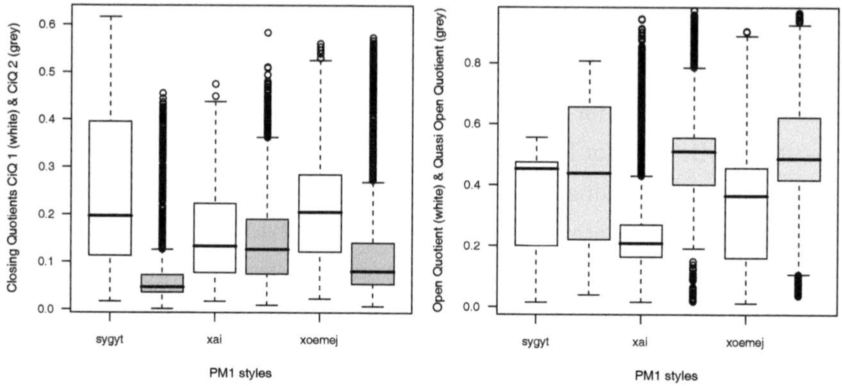

Figure 4.68: Lx quotient plots of two closing quotients [CiQ1 (white) and CiQ2 (grey)] on the left side, and open quotient (white) and quasi-open quotient (grey) on the right side; grouping by area, resp. styles (xai=Hakas, sygyt & xoemej=Tuva)

(negative curve half) for the two styles (see Figure 4.68). As indicated by the CiQs the contact index for both *xai* and *xöömej* shows median values below -0.5 (-0.73 for *xai*, -0.53 for *xöömej*), indicating a very short contacting phase. The tendency towards a smaller contacting phases for *xai* is supported by a greater median value of the speed quotient (SQ) for the Hakas group. Nevertheless for both symmetry measures the same outliers appear: ST, MS and ZU in the Hakas group and AM and NT in the Tuvan (see Figure 4.69). The Mann-Whitney U-test shows that the two groups differ significantly in all values.

Orlikoff et al. (1997) has found a CI range of -0.6 to -0.4 for men and woman "under normal vocal circumstances" so that the present results could be judged as completely abnormal. Edgerton et al. (2003), using stroboscopic evaluation for reinforced harmonics production, obtained the opening phase as 45% of the period, while the closing phase was 55%. It is difficult to say how this aligns with the obtained measures in the present study, since none of the various methods are readily comparable. But the two symmetry indices (SQ and CI) at least point in the same direction.

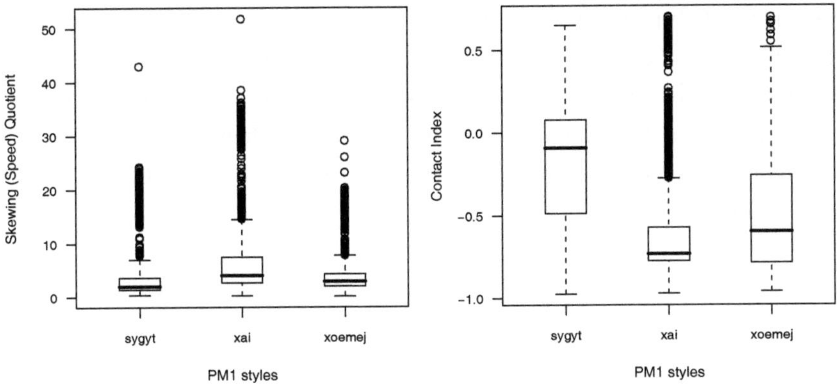

Figure 4.69: Lx quotient plots of skew (speed) quotient measurements (left) and contact index (right); grouping by area (styles: xai=Hakas, xoemej=Tuva)

4.2.6.2 Double-Cycle Source Mode (PM2)

Here the method of quotient obtainment had to be adapted, so that for every double cycle investigated each individual cycle was measured separately (see chapter 3.3.2.6), since in the case of a double cycle there were observed differing shapes, periods and amplitudes, which also point to differing quotients. In fact the quotients of the two cycles show unequal values for the closing quotient and open quotient measurement, with the same (or similar) tendency in evidence in both in *xai* and *kargyraa*, Hakas and Tuvan PM2 ThS. Starting from the observations of waveform shapes it is not surprising to find slightly longer closing phases for the second cycle[3]. This cycle-to-cycle difference is strongest in the Hakas group for CiQ1, measuring here the contacting phase from peak to peak (negative to positive) (see Figure 4.70 left). The negative half of the second cycle seems to be only very slightly shorter (QOQ md 0.524 < 0.542) than in the first cycle of *kargyraa*, but slightly longer (QOQmd 0.636 > 0.588) than in the first cycle of *xai* (see Figure 4.70). However, all QOQ md measures indicate a longer negative

[3]The cycle with the stronger positive peak in terms of amplitude height (supposedly caused by simultaneous VF and VTF contact) is defined as the first cycle, consequently the following cycle, with a weaker amplitude, is defined as the second cycle (supposedly caused by contact of the VFs only).

half (quasi-open phase) than positive half of the two cycles, whereas the 'true' open quotient (OQ), as a more closely defined measurement of the minimal contact phase, would further support this finding. OQ measurement shows for both styles a greater minimal contact phase in the first cycle than in the second, while the differences between styles are fairly small (T 0.315 > 0.277; H 0.379 > 0.338) (see Figure 4.70).

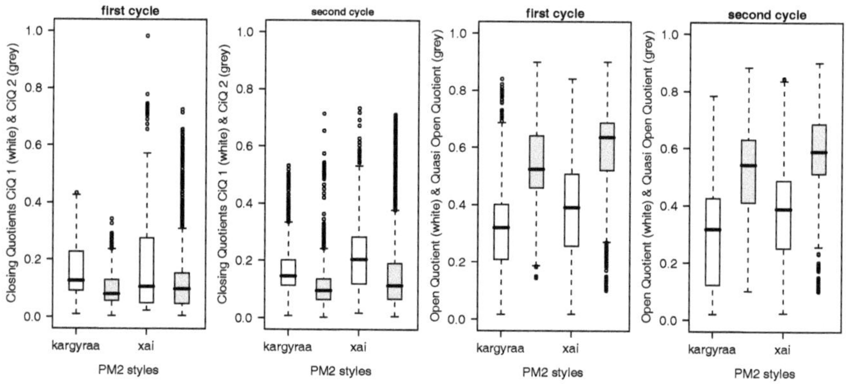

Figure 4.70: Boxplotted values of two closing quotient methods (left) and two open quotient methods (right); PM2; grouping according to style; each group contains the boxplot for CiQ method1 (white) and CiQ method2 (grey) for the first cycle and CiQ1 (white) and CiQ2 (grey) outliers are labeled by singer; Note for the open quotient diagram (right) that the boxplots in the lower range and the ones in the upper range both belong to the same method.

The symmetry indicators (SQ and CI) show the same tendencies for both styles, *xai* and *kargyraa*: the contacting phase in the first cycle is shorter than in the second cycle (Figure 4.71). SQ and CI also show that only the second cycle contacting phase differs slightly between Hakas and Tuvan PM2 styles (for SQ in T 4.07 > 3.74, and in H 3.73 > 2.48; for CI in T -0.616 < -0.558, and in H -0.616 < -0.499), so that for *kargyraa* the closing phase of cycle 2 tends to be shorter than in *xai*. In fact, the Mann-Whitney test shows that the quotient values all differ significantly between *kargyraa* and *xai*, with only one exception: the contact index for the first cycle (CIa).

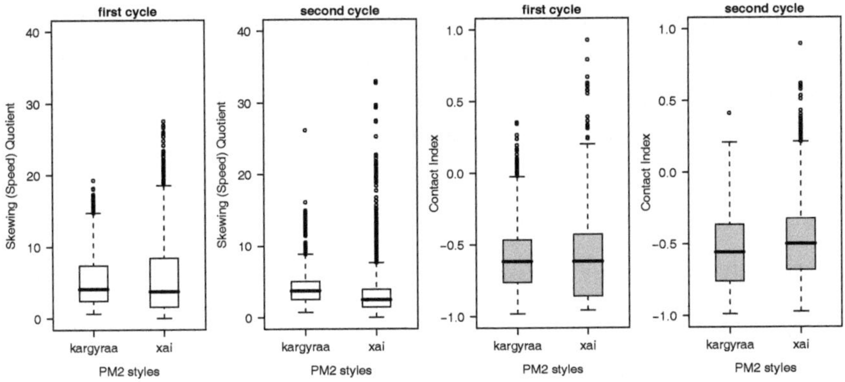

Figure 4.71: Boxplotted values of speed quotient (left) and contact index (right) grouped by styles with a separate plot for each part of the period: cycle 1 (1st & 3rd bpl.) and cycle 2 (2nd & 4th bpl.)

4.3 Analysis and Findings for the Subglottal Pressure Wave Signal (Sx)

4.3.1 Sub-Corpus Description

As already mentioned in chapter 3.2.6, due to signal distortion (clipping) and inadequate channel separation, most field recordings of Sx were lost. The available subcorpus thus contains only 10 recordings of 10 Tuvan singers which are available for analysis. Therefore in the present study only a first description of findings and general tendencies can be made.

4.3.2 Coordination of Vx, Lx and Sx

Only one complete recording including all three channels (Vx, Lx, Sx) was successfully acquired. It is the recording of singer SI (T). Of course in particular the discrete analysis of time-related events in sub- and supraglottal tract makes it necessary to synchronize the signals precisely. Here the glottal instant again serves preferably as marker for the synchronisation of signal Vx, which of course needs to be adjusted for each signal (see Figure 4.73). Depending on air temperature, VT tract length, and microphone distance as the basic factors, a delay of approximately 0.8-1.0 milliseconds should be expected (see Figure 4.72), yielding a mismatch of the Vx signal to the other two.

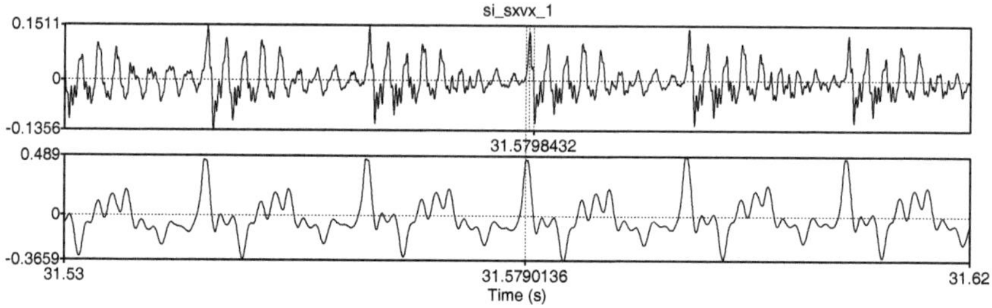

Figure 4.72: 0.0008sec skew of Vx to Sx; example from SI PM2

Neumann et al. (2003) additionally pointed out that the jugular microphone wave also reacts slower than the actual internal pressure wave. Therefore the first positive peak also lies 0.1-0.2ms behind the assumed instant of closure.

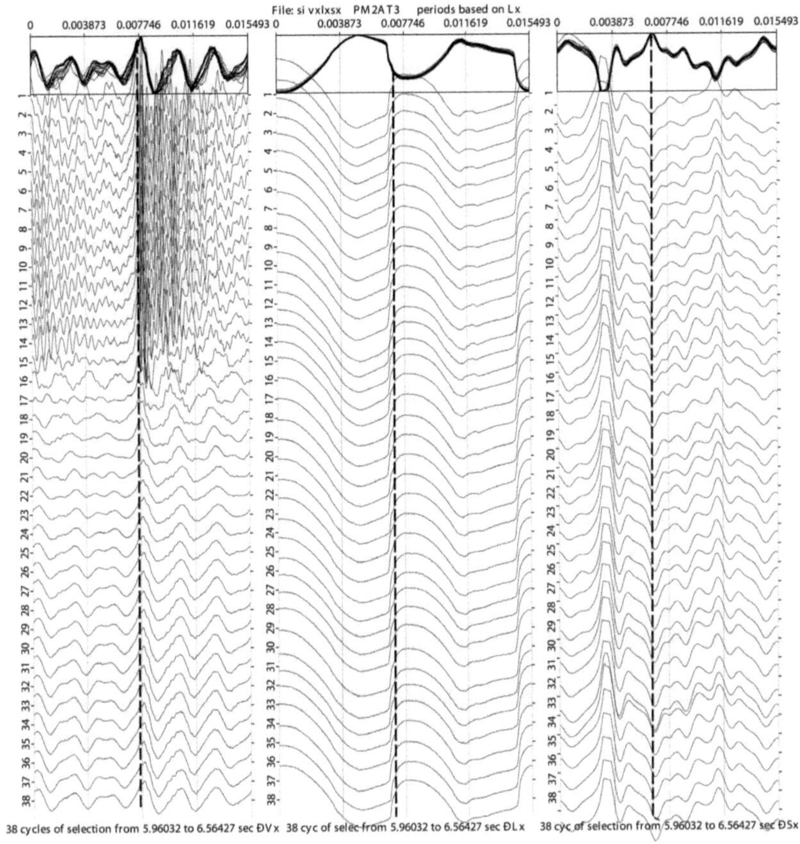

Figure 4.73: Synchronization of Vx (left), Lx (mid), and Sx (right); the vertical bold dashed lines determine the approximate position of the 'glottal' closure instant; the boxes in the upper part contain the entire cohort of curve segments drawn in the same window

4.3.3 Sx vs. Vx Waveform Comparison

The analysis of Sx (vs. Vx) was carried out primarily by waveform inspection. Especially the methods of comparison by Neumann, Gall and Schutte (2003) suggested a need to be adapted for larger corpora. Though the waterfall plot seems to be appropriate for Sx analysis, a more linear waveform display was also chosen. Additional examples of Sx are given in the Appendix (A.2.3).

4.3.3.1 Sx-Vx-Waveform Comparison in PM1

The signal of the jugular microphone appears not just as a smoothed and phase-reversed Vx, since the higher VT resonances are much less dominant while the subglottal resonances show a much stronger impact. Hence especially in cases of supraperiodic waveforms, Sx can serve as a more clearly structured waveform for period segmentation – although this cannot really substitute for Lx as a glottal closure instant indicator unless one could assume a skew or parallel offset which stays constant.

Both waveforms are dominated by F1; in Sx F1 turns into a noticeably strong and steep peak at the beginning of the period.

4.3.3.2 Sx-Vx-Waveform Comparison in PM2

In PM2 Sx and Vx show more similarities; this may be interpreted as a narrow coupling since here also the excitation of the subglottal cavity is expected to be very high.

4.3.4 Spectral Analysis of Sx

Another approach to the analysis and comparison of Vx and Sx is the investigation of spectral components. Here a LTAS with a 125Hz bandwidth was carried out on the sequences (approx. 50-60 periods) for waveform comparison. Due to the relatively fixed subglottal resonance tract a preference for certain resonance frequencies is expected. These frequencies have been discussed in the literature, and even for the first subglottal formant a whole range of values have been found

[Van den Berg: F1 =300Hz; Ishizaka et al. , Fant: F1=640Hz Boves: F1=475Hz (Boves, 1984; Fant et al., 1972; Ishizaka et al., 1976; van den Berg, 1960).

4.3.4.1 Spectral Analysis of Sx in PM1

Generally Sx shows a prominent H2 (in FFT) which as the octave of H1 refers to the VF frequency and specifies the first subglottal formant. The subglottal spectral tilt often has in the lower frequency range (0-3kHz) almost the same slope as the supraglottal spectra. In Figure 4.76 the formant values for F1, F2, F3, and F4 in both signals correspond to each other in amplitude and frequency. Only the subglottal first formant bandwidth (F1 at about 300-400Hz) appears to be higher than in Vx. F5 is finally damped in Sx, marking the end of the slope.

4.3.4.2 Spectral Analysis of Sx in PM2

The subglottal resonance spectrum in Figure 4.77 as an example for PM2 shows a very similar behaviour to the Vx spectrum. Only the peaks between 2.5-4 kHz are somewhat rounder and lower, and in comparison to Vx the spectral tilt seems to drop beyond 3000Hz. The strong formant peaks of subglottal F2 and F3 corroborate the observations of F2 and F3 as superimposed on Sx waveforms. As seen in PM1, also in this sample of PM2 a very high H2-amplitude is observed. H2 corresponds here to the VF vibration frequency one octave above F0.

It is clear that these observations and findings still have a very tentative and preliminary character and must demand a more systematic analysis.

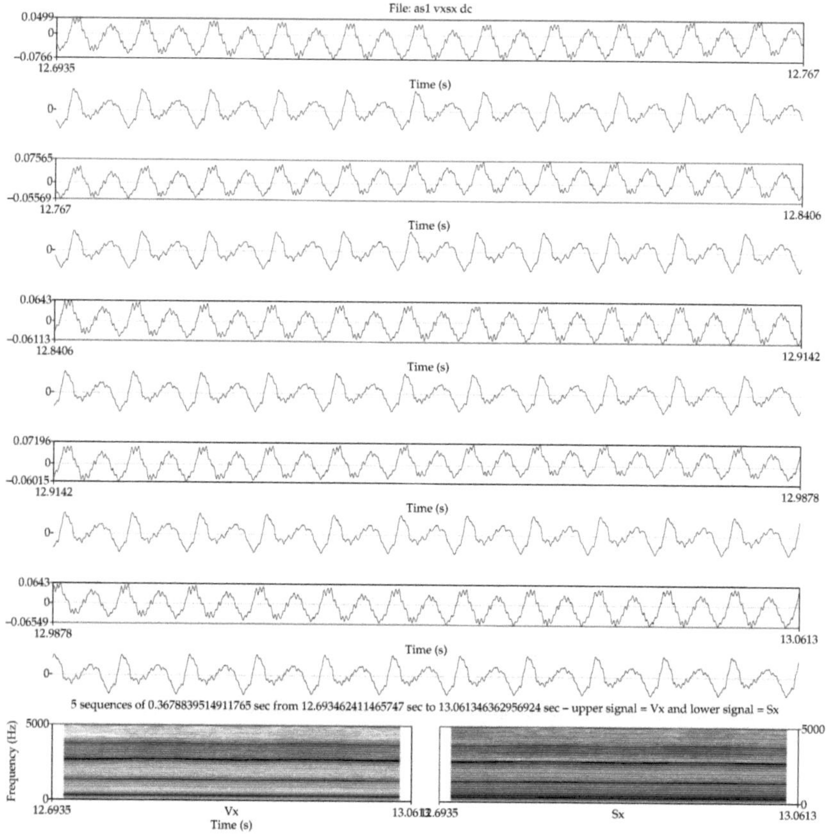

Figure 4.74: Example of singer AS for PM1AT2, linear waveform comparison of Vx and Sx; uncorrected delay and inversed phase in Vx

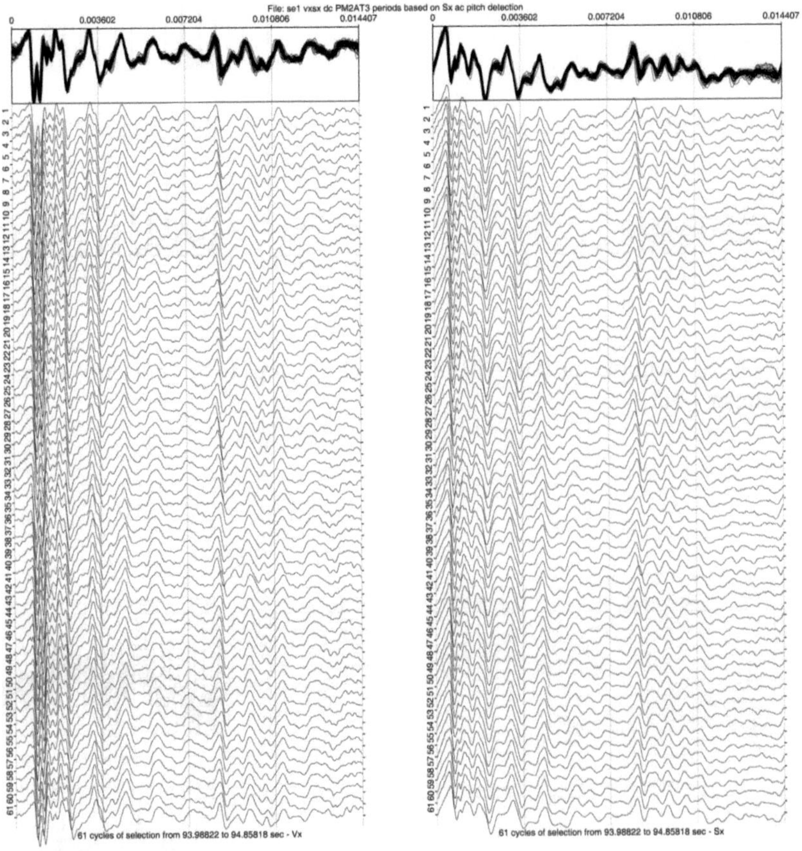

Figure 4.75: Cascaded signals of Vx (left) and Sx (right) of PM2; both waveforms are depicted with the same phases after Sx (i.e. phase inversion of Vx is uncorrected)

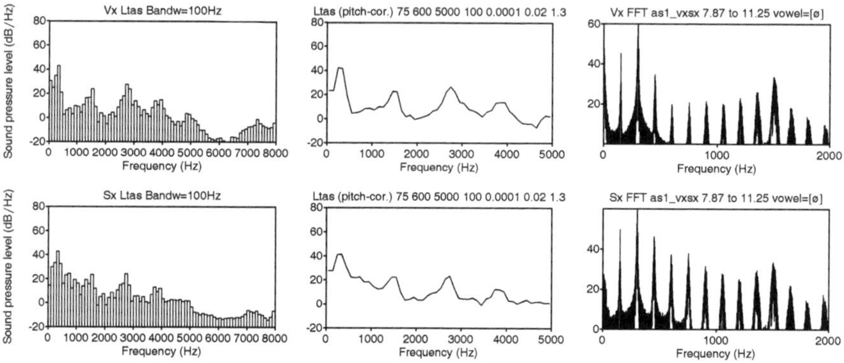

Figure 4.76: Example for PM1AT3 of spectral Vx (top) to Sx (bottom) comparison; singer AS(T)

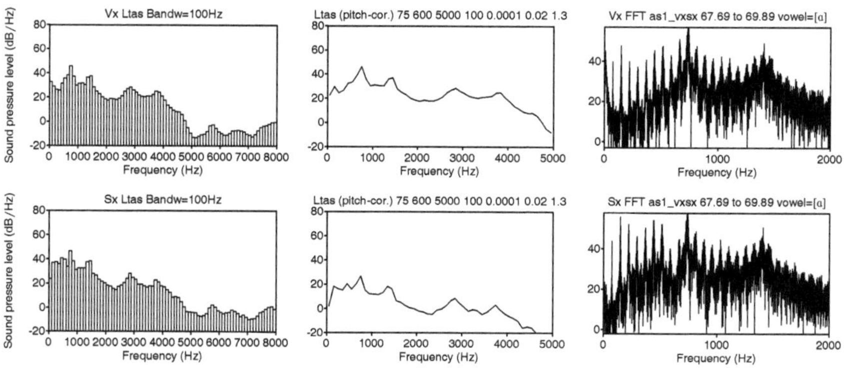

Figure 4.77: Example for PM2AT3 of spectral Vx (top) to Sx (bottom) comparison; singer AS (T)

4.4 Additional Observations

4.4.1 Air Flow in Different VPT

An additional experiment was carried out at ZAS (Zentrum für Allgemeine Sprachwissenschaft) Berlin as a lab investigation of the air flow (rate) by means of PC-QUIRER X16 system (SCICON RD.) comprising a synchronous recording of Vx, Lx, and Ux . The experiment, carried out in August 2004, was performed with the assistance of Dipl.-Ing. Jörg Dreyer. The apparatus was calibrated beforehand and the mask was additionally sealed with tape in order to avoid any leakage. While the subject pressed the mask against his face (enclosing mouth and nose) and performed the phonation tasks, voice Vx, laryngographic signal Lx, and mean airflow Ux (air flow rate) had been recorded simultaneously. According to PC-QUIRER X16 system specifications, this was carried out at a sample rate of 4kHz for the airflow measurement while the other channel (Vx, Lx) was sampled at 44.1 kHz. Four different voice production types (modal voice, AES-VF phonation, pulse register phonation and AEF-VF phonation) were produced by one subject (the author). Each VPT was applied to the three vowels (/a/, /i/, and /u/) with 3 repetitions per vowel. Air flow values were obtained as the mean values of a phonatory (voiced) sequence.

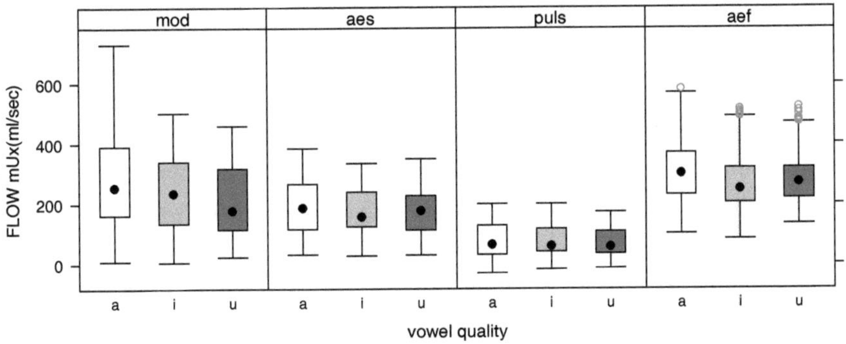

Figure 4.78: Boxplot of mean airflow values (mUx) during production of three vowels for four phonation types in one subject (SG); y-axis refers to mean air flow in ml/sec

The VPT groups (modal, AES-VF, pulse, AEF-VF) were treated as independent variables and were tested regarding difference (and ranking) (Kruskall-Wallis H-test and Mann-Whitney U-test). The results showed a significant difference between all grouped values; whereas AEF-VF phonation showed the highest median value, followed by modal voice and then AES-VF phonation. Pulse register phonation showed the lowest air flow but was also lowest in loudness. This corresponds to the results obtained by Blomgren et al. (1998). The difference between modal and AES-VF phonation is especially interesting since the low air flow fits well with the observations of extremely long sung passages in PM1. The results for AEF-VF fit well with the observation of short sung passages in (presumably) AEF-VF phonation in the different ThS varieties (incl. *umŋqokolo*) of PM2. It emerges clearly that subglottal pressure is not correlated with mean air flow since in particular for AES-VF one would then have expected higher mUx values (see also Table A.7).

4.4.2 Aryepiglottic Sphincter Constriction (MV → AESV) in Lx

In addition to the above observations the corpus was analysed in a simple experimental setting aimed at answering the question: How does aryepiglottic sphincter formation modify the associated waveform parameters? Within the corpus most voice onset phases start immediately with the sphinctered voice or show a rapid adjustment phase. Therefore in several repetitions involving various pitches and time frames a transition from modal voice into AES-VF was performed. In Lx the constriction typically results in a steeper contacting phase, whereas in Vx the upper formants (F2, F3) emerge clearly. In experimental settings there is sometimes also a pitch rising phenomenon associated with the constriction which shows that the lower the starting pitch is in modal voice, the stronger the signal is affected. Here, of course, the larynx elevation and the corresponding increase of tension and decrease of contact area come into play. Endoscopic findings and videofluoroscopy, however, reveal that these tendencies are not always this extreme, as demonstrated in section 2.3.1.3 and 2.3.2.

The Lx in Figure 4.79 also reveals a phenomenon that could be interpreted as an in-bulging of an additional contact area. At least during the initial constric-

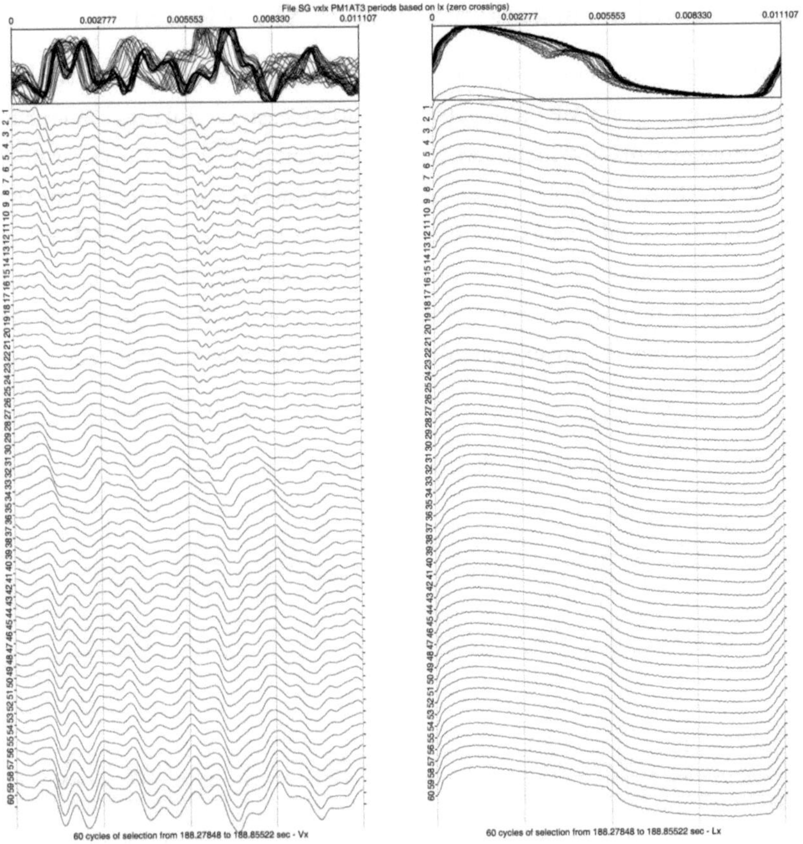

Figure 4.79: Transition of modal to AES-VF phonation; corrected (equalized) period length

tion phase, during decontacting (opening of the vocal contact area = increasing impedance), a short impedance 'dent' appears which then is 'integrated' into a lower impedance level, presumably because the VFCA has been diminished by the compression.

4.4.3 Variations in *kargyraa* (VTF-V, AEF-VF, etc.)

One of the hypotheses tested was the assumption of the co-existence of two ways of producing *kargyraa* VP: in the Tuvan group, at least, several observations had previously been made which lead to a confrontation of VTF-VF vs. AEF-VF (AEF-VTF-VF) as possible types. Additionally, the author received a positive evaluation by several singers and singing teachers for his own AEF-VF VP as a possible way of *kargyraa* production. Only by examining the alignment of Lx and the glottal flow signal will it be visible that also in AEF-VF phonation, too, the cycle 'carrying' the lower peak in Lx serves as the cycle of major excitation.

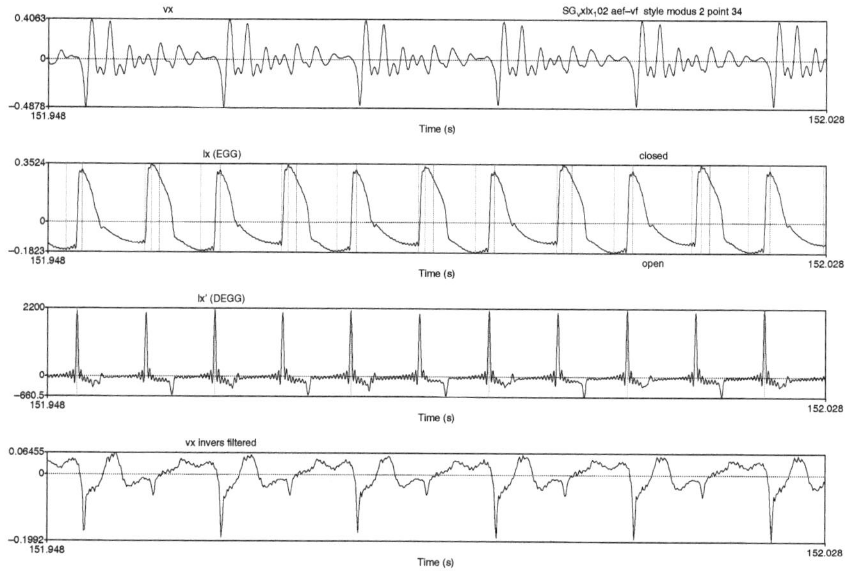

Figure 4.80: Demonstration of AEF-VF phonation (subject SG, the author): voice signal, EGG-signal, inverse filtered Vx signal and derived inverse filtered signal;

On the basis of perceptual judgments and of the indications delivered by LTAS and spectrograms, the sample of the Tuvan singer TK was evaluated as the only true sample of AEF-VF within the corpus. This sample belongs to the extended corpus (Corpus 2) and has no additional Lx or Sx channel. Although the inverse filtered Vx (glottal flow) signal shows similar features to the signal produced by the author, the assignment of singer TK's production to the AEF-VF phonation type is of course not unambiguous. Consequently the definitive identification of specific AEF-VF features and and of necessary acoustic or electrophysiological parameters must remain for further research in a laryngoscopically controlled setting. Here for example the observations on Gx-movement in the onset of a phonation phase (see 4.2.2.2) could already give a hint.

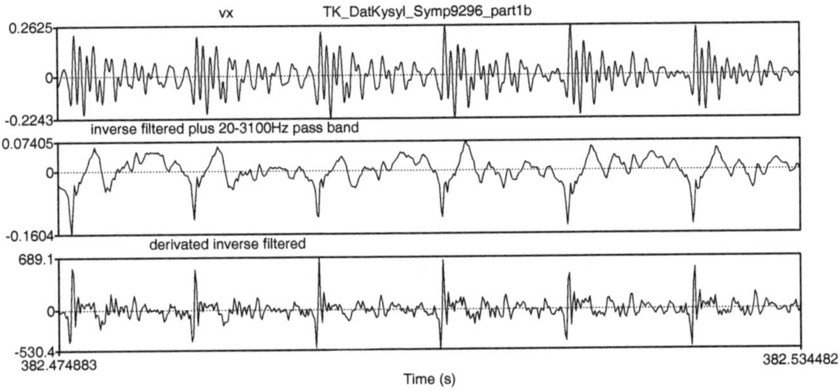

Figure 4.81: (supposed) AEF-VF VPT usage in PM2 of singer TK (T): voice signal, (inv. filt.) glottal flow, and derivated glottal flow

Additional observations point again (see LTAS) to higher inharmonic portions in a band of 7kHz to 12kHz in 'AEF-phonation' as well as to a stronger prominence of the first harmonic (F0).

VTF-VF to VF modus transition While exercising and practicing the *kargyraa* style or *xai* it quite often happens that in an instable phase a kind of switching effect appears: F0 switches to F0/2 and back again, caused by VTF involvement. And indeed this phenomenon is found in the corpus (e.g. AM(T) AM25 or MA(T) MA1). Singers apparently try to compensate for this effect mostly by increasing tension and breath support, which would involve medial compression and subglottal pressure.

On the other hand, singer SI(T), for example, exhibits such a transition from VTF-VF (or better VF-VTF) into VF-(AES) as very smooth and controlled, although it should be noted that his AES-VF production appears to be very soft and modal, which could be caused by a looser constriction of AES. The latter point could be demonstrated by the corresponding values for H1-H2 or CiQ. A very clear transition (or better switch) is depicted in Figure 4.82. In the majority of cases the switch-over to VTF-VF occurs rapidly from one cycle to the next and can be clearly observed in the waveform as an increase of amplitude, whereas the periodlength simply doubles (see Figure 4.84).

However, some cases show a smoother transition (see Figure 4.83), probably depending on a gentle medial compression and oscillatory masses involved, which have to coordinate and synchronize in their closure. In the sample of singer SI(T) the VTFs cause a bulging effect during the minimal contact phase, indicating an asynchronous vibration pattern which ultimately (i.e. only after eight cycles) stabilizes and follows every second VF cycle.

In the demonstration by the author (Figure 4.84) the impact of the VTFs becomes clearly evident, even though the sudden appearance of noise during the VF cycle needs to be investigated. For the time being it may be explained by an incomplete closure of the VFs which is caused by anterior medial compression of the VTFs.

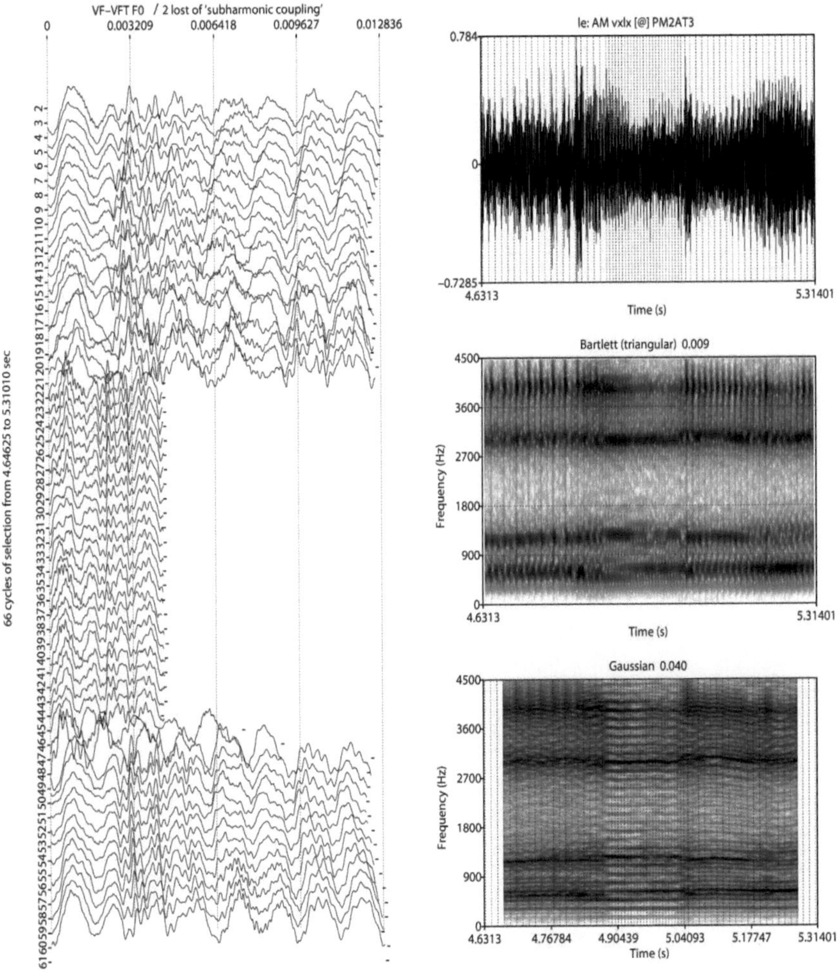

Figure 4.82: Typical intermittent effect of 'switching VTFs on and off' during phonation; subject AM(T)

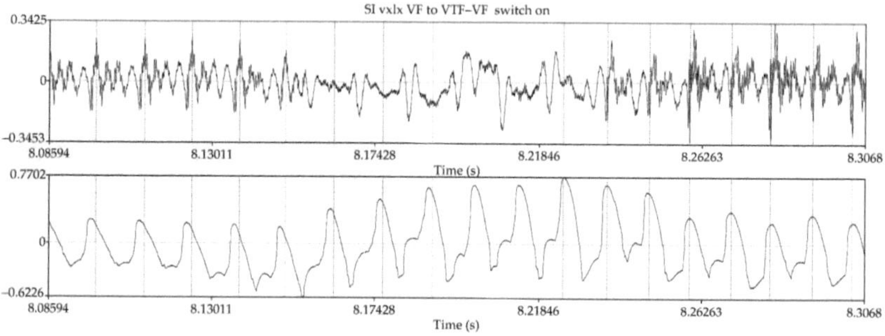

Figure 4.83: VF-VTF-VF transition; singer SI (T); Vx (top) and Lx (bottom); 1ms delay uncorrected; vertical lines in Lx are taken from the pitch detection in Vx

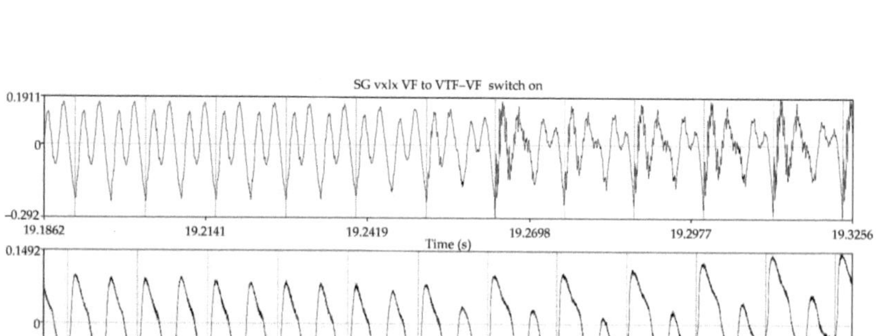

Figure 4.84: VF to VTF-VF mode transition; SG (author); vertical lines in Lx refer to the period points in Vx

4.5 DISCUSSION

4.5.1 Interrelations and Correlations Between Measures

Correlations have been investigated as bivariate correlations between individual perturbation values, wherein periodlength was included in order to investigate whether perturbation is already effected by F0 (within a phonation mode). The dependence on a phonation mode makes sense for spectral components but was not investigated for the time being. For the other measures such relationship to phonation mode seems to be as evident. The statistic correlations were investigated by means of the nonparametric Spearman rho correlation, which is also based on ranks (see for detailed results Appendix A.1.3). Period standard deviation and local jitter and shimmer show of course a correlation within the PPQ as well as within APQ parameters.

One of the more interesting questions which may also have greater implications is: Are AES, VTF, VTF-VF, VF-VF registers VPTs characterized by specific acoustic parameters? The present results do not clearly indicate specific relations but there are certainly a number of findings pointing to a combination e.g. of certain perturbation values (local Lx jitter, loc Lx shimmer) and spectral values.

Dependence on Atype - articulation type Overtone articulation strategies (ATs) should indicate certain spectral properties: NHR and articulation type for example show a positive correlation in the way that with an increasing articulatory closure tendency (AT3 → AT1) higher values of NHR are obtained. This could be presumably explained by the prominence of the particular narrow banded formant in terms of the reinforced harmonic

Throughout the data exploration it became clear that there is a 'dependence' on area but apparently also on individual singers. Could it be that singers of different areas (stylistic backgrounds) group together regarding specific parameters? Or, how consistent (homogeneous) are the groups defined by style (area)? How (acoustically) different interpret singers their styles? How restrict do the singers follow the 'norms' and standards provided by the role models of their area? (see above correlation to VPT). The relationships of such individual characteristics may need to be re-investigated regarding such internal corpus clusters.

4.5.2 Possible Voice Production Types

The basic voice production types involved in ThS can be described as follows: There is on the one hand the sphinctered (A-P compression) voice, called AES-VF phonation (PM1). The aryepiglottic sphincter contributes to the narrowing of the epilaryngeal space and may sometimes be constricted very tightly, just leaving a small jet-like orifice.

On the other hand there is a rough, growling, 'subharmonic' phonation (PM2). In some cases the AES (or AEFs) can act as coupled mass and vibrate in PM1 or PM2, but VTF-VF phonation, as double-cycle oscillation of a joint VTF-VF cycle and a single VF cycle, serves presumably as the major phonation type in PM2. Therefore the corpus provides primarily information about variability and group-specific characteristics of this variety of PM2. In light of the empirical findings, AEF-VF phonation has to be revised as not significantly frequent enough to be considered a common phonatory variant; nonetheless, AEF-VF voice cannot be completely ruled out. It may occur as an individual or personal style feature. Likewise, the so-called asymmetrical VF diplophonation (cf. Edgerton et al., 2003) may serve as an individual interpretation of PM2.

PM1	PM2		
AES-VF	AEF-VF	VTF-VF	VF-VTF
xöömej, sygyt, xoomij, xail, kail	kargyraa2 (xos-kargyraa, tespeŋ kargyraa) example: TK(T)	kargyraa1 xöömej-kargyraa xarxiraa, xai2, kai2 examples: IK(T), SK(H)	kargyraa3 (ün-kargyraa) examples: SI(T), DB(T)

Table 4.14: Hypothetical VPT in ThS

There are 'artefacts' of 'real' *xöömej kargyraazy*, meaning AES-VF-VTF phonation, which either appear as *xöömej* with a strong medial compression (see corpus mal_vxsx or andmon1_vxlx) or *kargyraa* with a high VF proportion (singer SI, see Figure 4.73). The are referred to as *ün-kargyraa* ('voice kargyraa') as a third category (kargyraa3) and therefore the opposite end of PM2 voice production types (Table 4.14).

At present there appears to be no clear justification for adding an 'asymmetrical double source' VPT (VF1-VF2) to the VPTs used in south-Siberian ThS, despite the fact that Edgerton et al. (2003) have described this VPT as an 'alternative choice' in the realisation of PM2. This asymmetry would then refer to the "11 [oscillation] mode" as described by Titze (1994a: 97-99) (see also Edgerton, 2005: 18-19; 86-87). Sveč (1996) has found such behaviour in modal voice and characterized it as subharmonic vibratory pattern. A style differentiation of *xai* vs. *kai* vs. *karygraa* vs. *xarxiraa* may then proceed by means of such VPT varieties as medial and A-P compression, tissue involvement, breath support (air flow rate, subglottal pressure), VT coupling, and nasal coupling. Nonetheless does the Tuvan material demonstrate a high variability on the level of singers, which rather suggests a 'continuum', which would employ different structures of medial and A-P compression along the gradation of constriction.

4.5.3 Similarities to Other Pathological and Non-pathological Voice Patterns

A comparison of the author's data on voice parameters with other phonetic data as given by MDVP or as provided by investigations in the field of voice pathology and singing pedagogics will be useful in order to provide a context and background for the obtained measurements of ThS in the present study. On the one hand a context is already implicit in the various descriptions of ThS styles and phonation types (see Table 2.5); on the other hand the physiological difference between the various phonaton types already difficulties in achieving any basis for comparison. Regarding a *tertium comparationis* it must be stated that the lack of comparable 'normal voice data' potentially diminishes the informational value of the results of this study. Although during some recording sessions in the field such normal-voice data was in fact acquired for 6 singers, these data have not been included in the present results. Analogies to other laryngeal modes, such as inspiratory, creaky voice, or pulse register, can also be drawn on the basis of similarity waveform shapes and patterns.

According to Blomgren et al. (1998) waveforms in vocal fry show a long decontacting phase followed by either a small short pulse (contacting peak) or a doublet or triplet of closely connected pulses. Here the data on perturbation values of vocal fry phonation obtained by Blomgren et al. (1998) should serve well for comparison, since the authors were investigating especially subjects who were capable of producing long sustained passages of vocal fry or pulse register voice. Blomgren et al.'s results of 8.8 - 14.9 % for jitter factor and 1.38 - 1.41dB for (absolute) shimmer in vocal fry point to higher jitter and higher shimmer values compared to the acoustic jitter and shimmer values of PM2 phonation in the present corpus. If indeed the acoustic measurements across phonation types are comparable and the values appear to be as similar, the question may arise as to whether EGG and acoustic perturbation values may be used interchangeably - which, according to Vieira et al. (1997, 2002), is clearly not advisable.

Chen et al. (2002) carried out a parametrization of multiple phases within one vibratory period of vocal fry, defining multiple opening and closing times with respect to this parameterization. But since they used only a very rough determination (see 2.1.1) which does not even resemble that of the quasi-open-quotient their results can hardly be compared with the parameters used in the present study. Lindestad et al. (2004) have contrasted ventricular dysphonia and ventricular voice and found for both types cases of high period-to-period variation (approx. 20%) and of roughness in cases of desynchronized vibrations. They concluded that only the degree in vibrational amplitude magnitude (VTF closure) and regularity (symmetry) of VTF co-vibration in relation to the glottal level determines the vocal outcome.

In her study of Vx and Lx patterns of pathological voices (organic disordered voices) Stelzig (1996) pointed out waveforms of voice after recurrent nerve paresis which strikingly resemble the double-cycle pattern of PM2. Regarding acoustic and physiological correlates of voice qualities similar to PM1 the so-called ringing voice quality has been already mentioned. This voice quality refers to a "ringing" 3kHz marker and has also been identified as so-called singing or singers formant, since this characteristic is typical for operatic voices. Yanagisawa et al. (1989) had detected the contribution of AES to this characteristic, which has been also described in contrast to other "Voice modes" by Colton and Estill (1981). Colton and Estill had described components of "negative airflow (airflow in an inspiratory direction) during closed phase" for ring and twang phonations (Colton and Estill, 1981: 383-385). Such phenomena can also be found in PM1 examples in the present corpus (see Appendix A.2.1), whereas also the peak between 2,800 and 4,300Hz can be described for samples in the two ThS phonation modes. Since this is not met all over the corpus it may just indicate also a component of brilliance and brightness which contribute to a higher penetrance power of those voices. Nonetheless, the impressionistic evaluations of ThS voice based on observation by various individual researchers need to be proven in terms of perceptional experiments with a larger group of listeners. Such listeners could be drawn either from the community of throat singers or in that of clinical voice specialists or phoneticians.

Chapter 5

SUMMARY

5.1 Macrostructure and Microstructure of ThS – Summary Hypotheses

Regarding the articulation types and phonation modes found in the course of this study, it has to be stated that neither the usage of VTF-VF type/mode nor the usage of AES-VF type/mode is unique to ThS. Endoscopic findings strengthen a theory of structures of the *aditus laryngis* as sphincter (AES), source and articulator. A comparison with descriptions of similar phonatory phenomena reveals that the usage of VTF-VF and AES-VF, or the involvement of the laryngeal sphincter, is probably more common than clinicians and phoneticians would usually expect. Nonetheless, phonation modes exploiting AES-VF and VTF-VF are specific within ThS as basic voices defining styles and style groups. AES setting is adjusted for overtone enhancement; the VTF-VF mode is adjusted for sustained oscillation in longer passages (including pitch shifting). But phonation mode 2 demands new specific categories for VQ in (throat) singing, and due to its deviant vibrational pattern it demands an adjusted parameterization too. While certain phenomena, such as longer decontacting phases in samples of experienced singers or the adaptation of voice source in OtS (Grawunder, 2003a), point to a 'continuum' between OtS and ThS regarding VP; nevertheless ThS is significantly different from the kind of VP which is characteristic of OtS. The acquired data support a theory of reinforcement or enhancement of harmonics by means of:

(1) voice source variation (closing phase, excitation strength, or intermediate cycle);

(2) increased subglottal pressure, while air flow remains constant or even lower than in modal voice (for PM1);

(3) (for AT1/AT2) formant melting of F2, F3 and F4 due to multiple vocal tract constrictions (this refers to quantal theory,(cf. Stevens, 2000: 145));

(4) coupling of source to the adjacent epilaryngeal tube of 1/6 VT for a resonant voice (Titze and Story, 1997);

(5) concatenated vocal tract (resonator) coupling at 1/6 VT (Stevens, 2000: 143-44);

(6) bandwidth tuning; adjustment of lip radiation (cf. Edgerton et al., 2003);

(7) probably also certain nasal coupling in order to damp F4 and F5.

Microstructure

The findings of the present study reveal primarily differences between groups of singers. Groupings are based on area (Altai, Hakassia, Tuva, Mongolia), (overtone) formant articulation type, and sometimes on the individual singer. Area and articulation type group differences have been tested by means of nonparametric tests and must therefore also be interpreted as differences regarding the central tendencies of all values reflecting a rank.

1. for PM1 and PM2 significant area group differences have been detected in

    (a) Vx Jitter
    (PM1: jLoc T<H<M<A; jRAP A<T<M<H; jPPQ5 A=T<A<H)
    (PM2: jLoc M<H<T<A; jRAP M<T<A<H; jPPQ5 M<T<H<A)

   (b) Vx Shimmer
   (PM1: sLoc H<A<T<M; sAPQ3 A<T<H<M; sAPQ5&11 H<A<T<M)
   (PM2: sLoc H<M<A=T; sAPQ3 H<A<T<M; sAPQ5&11 H<M<A<T)

   (c) Vx HNR
   (PM1: HNR M=H<A<T; PM2: HNR A<M<T<H)

   (d) Vx NHR
   (PM1: NHR A<H<M<T; PM2: NHR H<M<T<A)

   (e) Lx jitter
   (PM2: jLoc T<H; jRAP T<H; jLoc2 H<T; jRAP2 H<T)

   (f) Lx shimmer
   (PM2: sLoc T<H; sAPQ5 T<H; sLoc2 H<T; sAPQ52 H<T)

   (g) Lx quotients
   (PM1: CiQ1 H<T; CiQ2 T<H, QOQ H<T, SQ T<H, CI H<T)
   (PM2: CiQ1 H<T, CiQ2 T<H, OQ[1] T<H, QOQ T<H, SQ H<T, CI H=T CiQ1b T<H, CiQ2b T<H, OQb T<H, QOQb T<H, SQb H<T, CIb T<H)

2. significant articulation type differences have been found for example in

   (a) Vx Jitter
   (PM1: jLoc AT2<AT1<AT3; PM2: jLoc AT2<AT1<AT3)

   (b) Vx Shimmer
   (PM1: sLoc AT3<AT2<AT1; PM2: sLoc AT3<AT2<AT1)

   (c) Vx HNR
   (PM1: AT3<AT1<AT2; PM2: AT1<AT2<AT3)

   (d) Vx NHR
   (PM1: AT2<AT1<AT3; PM2: AT2=AT3<AT1)

3. PM1 (phonation modus 1), i.e. AES-VF phonation, typically results in a

   (a) steep contacting phase, very short minimal contact phase in Lx;

[1] Only for PM2.

   (b) barely predictable glottal flow for AT1 because of supraperiodical features in Vx;
   (c) mean Ux (air flow rate) lower than in modal phonation.

4. PM2 (phonation modus 2)
   (a) primarily uses a VTF-VF phonation type in which a joint VTF-VF closure alternates with a glottal (VF) closure. The latter serves in most of the cases as a / the source of VT excitation;
   (b) produced by a switch-on or engaging of VTF's co-vibration results in an octave (down) shift and an emerging of subharmonic components (perception of roughness);typically exhibits a double- or triple-cycle pattern, in which peak shape and amplitude height do not unambiguously point to the underlying contact area structures (VTF-VF or VF);
5. Subject-dependent differences appear sometimes as very strong in such parameters as Lx quotients, local Vx jitter and local Vx shimmer. But perturbation and source parameters do also potentially restrain possible types or VPModes which point to tension, breath support, VT adaptation and voice source adjustment.

5.2 Are Throat Singers High-Risk Vocal Performers?

Phonation modes similar to throat singing are also found in musical genres of world-wide pop cultures. There is, for example, in reggae the so-called "toasting" voice, or in jazz the Armstrong-like voice, which appear very similar to kargyraa-type phonation (cf. Sakakibara et al., 2004a). In addition, new musical compositions contain voices which demand going beyond the 'usual' phonation types (cf. Edgerton, 2005; Sakakibara et al., 2004a). Hoffmann-Ruddy et al. (2001) refer to performers employing these techniques as high-risk performers. Hence, by analogy to other vocal performers using such 'rough' voice techniques, it makes sense to look into possible risks for throat singers too. Regarding the aryepiglottic constriction which has been discussed in connection with the so called "ringing" voice quality in certain (personal) singing techniques, Yanagisawa et al. (1989) had already cast doubt on the belief "that laryngeal constriction inevitably results in voice deterioration" (342). And the studies of other researchers Koufman et al. (1996); Stager et al. (2000) cannot prove that such constrictions unavoidably damage the voice, even in case of longer practise. But a potential risk (in particular for younger adepts) regarding deterioration of laryngeal tissue is of course not ruled out completely, especially when such extreme voice usage in performance situations coincides with psychological and physical stress, dehydration, or voice fatigue. But there is apparently not enough laryngoscopic data of ThSingers (just four singers provided by Edgerton et al. 2003 plus one singer by Esling 2002a) that could either support a hypothesis of precisely controlled aryepiglottic and ventricular constriction (A-P and medial compression) or, directly speaking, support the proof of harmlessness of ThS practise over the long term. However, the corpus analysed for this study does also contain examples of suboptimal voice usage in ThS, but it can also comprise a number of core features which from an acoustic standpoint does not necessarily indicate a pathological deviation.

5.3 Perspectives

The chosen method clearly needs to be developed further and specifically redesigned with a real time monitoring device. An adaptation of a multichannel EGG setting, as suggested by Rothenberg (1992), may offer better estimations of laryngeal height and could possibly help evaluate the movements of the larynx during phonation onset. With respect to vocology research on voices in other styles should be discussed such issues like penetrance power. Hence also the dependence or relation of performance practice (hall, rooms vs. outside countryside, amplification) and adaptation of the voice source characteristics may be investigated. This is especially appropriate for ThS since traditionally ThS was performed mainly outside (in the steppe or forest). As addressed in chapter 2.5.1, structural similarities of certain sounds in Yi, Bai, !Xóõ and other languages are quite striking. It needs to be investigated whether these observations can hold in a larger corpus of subjects, but also whether such phonation type appearing as voice quality markers are perhaps more frequent in the languages of the world. However, the occurrence of ventricular and aryepiglottic voice in other traditional (singing) context (see chapter 1) and in vocal communication of infants points to a not complete negligibility of such phonation types. Within this framework also a comparison of human voice and voice in animal communication (e.g. grunts among primates) may be a reasonable task, since usage of AES (AEFs and VTFs) may not be limited to humans, which also could shed more light on the function and potentially also the phylogenesis of AES structures. Regarding the articulation of rHs in terms of articulatory strategies also movement, i.e. dynamics of individual articulators, need to be further observed. Therefore an articulatory investigation of simultaneous acoustical change during the small definite modifications in the constricted VT (in particular AT1). Due to a certain limit in time and space the author had to give up the undertaking of a chapter on perception. This would also have shifted the focus quite strongly. Nevertheless the perception of reinforced harmonics and formant clusters etc., as well the perception of subharmonic and supraperiodic sound, are subjects not to be missed. Considering other similar difficulties in the evaluation of VQ and phonatory types, it would probably be reasonable to look at phenomena such as the differenciation of double and triple rhythms regarding JNDs in temporal and rhythmic structures. In this way potential correlations of acoustic analysis parameters to perception (inclusively VQ evaluations) may become evident. For such experiments should be considered ThSingers and voice pathology experts as well. Possible findings may provide insights into ...

- 'unusual' voice type identifications
- distinction articulatory characteristics in the lower VT
- distinction of glottal cycle patterns (roughness of low frequency vibration)
- perception of supraperiodical phenomena (in particular pitch perception during shifting of the fundamental of a supraperiodic sound)
- perception of subharmonics (Omori, 1997).

Another focus may be brought on the discrimination of close OTs within a formant cluster (masking effects) (cf. Hartmann, 1997: 124-129), also regarding bandwidths of formants and associated clarity brilliance (Bloothooft et al., 1992).

Appendix A

TABLES, DIAGRAMs & SCRIPTS

A.1 Tables

A.1.1 Descriptive Statistics

A.1.1.1 Vx perturbation measures (descriptive statistics)

	Range	Minimum	Maximum	Mean	SD
periodmn	.013123	.003837	.016960	.00659328	.001738267
periodsd	.004269	.000003	.004272	.00010972	.000342477
pitchmn	201.66	58.96	260.62	1.603	3.499248
jitterLoc	.047604	.000327	.047931	.00241460	.003820007
jitterRAP	.017116	.000079	.017195	.00056056	.001500586
jitterppq5	.041571	.000195	.041766	.00121431	.002951036
shimmerLoc	.260535	.011992	.272527	.06784614	.040267243
shimmerapq3	.132601	.003783	.136384	.02841545	.020921867
shimmerapq5	.156278	.007874	.164152	.04272778	.028416422
shimmerapq11	.235099	.000000	.235099	.07229387	.040657423
HNRmn	25.672	4.513	30.185	1.638144	4.353732
NHRmn	.403304	.001114	.404418	.05119385	.056820668

Table A.1: Perturbation values, phonation modus 1, ungrouped, N=701

	Range	Minimum	Maximum	Mean	SD
periodmn	0.019081	0.003529	0.02261	0.013465	0.0023069
periodsd	0.003613	0.00003	0.003643	0.000193	0.0003421
pitchmn	239.14	44.23	283.37	77.07	18.45245
jitterLoc	0.058108	0.000988	0.059096	0.004439	0.0043518
jitterRAP	0.02949	0.000214	0.029704	0.001412	0.0020893
jitterppq5	0.040184	0	0.040184	0.002735	0.0036607
shimmerLoc	0.353307	0.009641	0.362948	0.082431	0.0446902
shimmerapq3	0.183302	0.004498	0.1878	0.038577	0.0227472
shimmerapq5	0.232836	0	0.232836	0.053950	0.0298217
shimmerapq11	0.331191	0	0.331191	0.08319	0.0488907
HNRmn	22.063	2.143	24.206	12.95556	3.551493
NHRmn	0.796533	0.005209	0.801742	0.10241827	0.090605

Table A.2: Perturbation values, phonation modus 2, ungrouped, N=881

A.1.1.2 Lx perturbation measures and quotients (descriptive)

	N	Range	Min	Max	Mean	SD
periodmnl	394	0.013072	0	0.013072	0.00717087	0.002005225
periodsdl	394	0.003059	0	0.003059	0.00018726	0.000285408
jitterLoc	394	0.139123	0	0.139123	0.02071745	0.021010562
jitterRAP	394	0.07885	0	0.07885	0.0121783	0.0124203
jitterppq5	394	0.088588	0	0.088588	0.01215679	0.012644372
shimmerLoc	394	0.305884	0	0.305884	0.06492917	0.061062166
shimmerapq3	394	0.126459	0	0.126459	0.02990156	0.027902604
shimmerapq5	394	0.192795	0	0.192795	0.04391284	0.040777557
shimmerapq11	394	0.462182	0	0.462182	0.05929435	0.061054286

Table A.3: Lx perturbation measures; modus = 1; ungrouped

	N	Range	Min	Max	Mean	SD
periodmn1	236	0.019544	0	0.019544	0.01448543	0.003211171
periodsd1	236	0.00356	0.000036	0.003596	0.00022657	0.000414134
periodmn2	236	0.0115	0.0104	0.0219	0.015042	0.0023288
periodsd2	236	0.0036	0	0.0036	0.000221	0.0004143
jitterLoc	236	0.087279	0.001255	0.088534	0.00837153	0.014905512
jitterRAP	236	0.05893	0.00044	0.05937	0.0042377	0.01005494
jitterppq5	236	0.035654	0.000806	0.03646	0.00442916	0.005866337
shimmerLoc	236	0.584441	0	0.584441	0.1539727	0.175519444
shimmerapq3	236	0.383018	0	0.383018	0.09614587	0.114592574
shimmerapq5	236	0.22182	0	0.22182	0.05688575	0.06594807
shimmerapq11	236	0.375321	0	0.375321	0.08591995	0.104478514
jitterLoc2	236	0.02865	0.001255	0.029905	0.00553759	0.003444728
jitterRAP2	236	0.009777	0.000436	0.010213	0.00229834	0.001559344
jitterppq52	236	0.017526	0.000806	0.018332	0.00336286	0.001859908
shimmerLoc2	236	0.263908	0.006259	0.270167	0.059698	0.05060347
shimmerapq32	236	0.161211	0.003389	0.1646	0.03359781	0.028135342
shimmerapq52	236	0.197601	0.004151	0.201752	0.03748549	0.033919992
shimmerapq112	236	0.265785	0	0.265785	0.04218108	0.039128184

Table A.4: Lx perturbation measures; modus = 2; ungrouped

	N	Mean	SD	Min	Max	Percentiles		
						25th	50th	75th
t3mt1/tpd_CiQ1	19537	0.1879	0.1029	0.01701	0.6167	0.1027	0.1698	0.2613
t2amta2/tpd_CiQ2	19537	0.1236	0.0958	0.00157	0.9543	0.0569	0.0973	0.1628
t6mt4/tpd_QOQ	19537	0.5047	0.1858	0.01803	0.9739	0.4054	0.5060	0.6015
t5amt3/t3mt1_SQ	19537	4.54	4.27	0.13	51.73	2.17	3.17	5.22
CPmOP/CPpOP_CIa	19537	-0.554	0.309	-0.975	0.700	-0.777	-0.683	-0.351

Table A.5: Descriptive statistics of EGG-quotients: closing quotient (CiQ), quasi-open quotient (QOQ), speed quotient (SQ), and contact index (CI); single cycle mode

	N	Mean	SD	Min	Max	Percentiles 25th	50th	75th
t3mt1/tpd_CiQ1	7055	0.1617	0.12064	0.01	2.28	0.0586	0.1244	0.237
t2amta2/tpd_CiQ2	7055	0.1076	0.08017	0	0.73	0.0519	0.0885	0.1405
t5bmt5a/tpd_OQ	7055	0.3249	0.16328	0	0.84	0.2147	0.3378	0.4322
t6mt4/tpd_QOQ	7055	0.5724	0.13535	0.1	0.9	0.4727	0.5862	0.6788
t5amt3/t3mt1_SQ	7055	5.4787	4.34885	0.03	58.93	2.0463	3.9938	7.9194
CPmOP/CPpOP_CIa	7055	-0.5981	0.26038	-0.98	0.93	-0.8513	-0.6164	-0.4486
t7mt5b/tpd2_CiQ1	7055	0.1942	0.12833	0.01	3.6	0.1138	0.1752	0.2534
t6amta6/tpd2_CiQ2	7055	0.1297	0.10529	0	0.71	0.065	0.1033	0.162
t9bmt9a/tpd2_OQ1	7055	0.2804	0.20075	-3.74	0.85	0.0945	0.3172	0.4415
t10mt8/tpd2_QOQ	7055	0.5494	0.15749	0.1	0.9	0.4473	0.5727	0.6539
t9amt7/t7mt5b_SQ	7055	3.882	3.13847	0.01	69.83	1.9654	3.0363	4.7725
CPmOP/CPpOP_CIb	7055	-0.5069	0.58472	-0.99	31.73	-0.7221	-0.5354	-0.3453

Table A.6: Descriptive statistics of EGG-quotients: closing quotient (CiQ), open quotient (OQ), quasi-open quotient (QOQ), speed quotient (SQ), and contact index (CI); double cycle mode

A.1.1.3 oral flow (Ux) (descriptive)

	MODUS											
	mod			aes			puls			aef		
	VOWEL			VOWEL			vowel			VOWEL		
	a	i	u	a	i	u	a	i	u	a	i	u
Ux Mean	283	240	211	193	179	172	76	76	68	302	264	274

Table A.7: Mean oral flow (Ux) values per mode and vowel

A.1.2 Normal Distribution Tests

A.1.2.1 Normal Distribution of Vx Perturbation Measures

	AType	N
For all values in PM1	1	367
	2	154
	3	180

Table A.8: Vx pertub Atype cases PM1

	area	N
For all values in PM1	altai	28
	hakas	101
	tyva	350
	mongol	222

Table A.9: Vx pertub area cases PM1

	Atype	Kolmogorov-Smirnov			Shapiro-Wilk		
		Statistic	df	Sig.	Statistic	df	Sig.
Period sd	1	0.437	367	0	0.219	367	0
	2	0.352	154	0	0.22	154	0
	3	0.347	180	0	0.258	180	0
Jitter Loc	1	0.32	367	0	0.316	367	0
	2	0.278	154	0	0.388	154	0
	3	0.251	180	0	0.366	180	0
Jitter RAP	1	0.436	367	0	0.222	367	0
	2	0.373	154	0	0.191	154	0
	3	0.363	180	0	0.204	180	0
Jitter ppq5	1	0.43	367	0	0.216	367	0
	2	0.339	154	0	0.217	154	0
	3	0.352	180	0	0.211	180	0
Shimmer Loc	1	0.124	367	0	0.883	367	0
	2	0.131	154	0	0.854	154	0
	3	0.127	180	0	0.899	180	0
Shimmer apq3	1	0.142	367	0	0.819	367	0
	2	0.173	154	0	0.765	154	0
	3	0.129	180	0	0.882	180	0
Shimmer apq5	1	0.143	367	0	0.872	367	0
	2	0.151	154	0	0.79	154	0
	3	0.131	180	0	0.889	180	0
Shimmer apq11	1	0.101	367	0	0.937	367	0
	2	0.091	154	0.003	0.938	154	0
	3	0.124	180	0	0.876	180	0
HNR mn	1	0.059	367	0.004	0.983	367	0
	2	0.097	154	0.001	0.96	154	0
	3	0.09	180	0.001	0.971	180	0.001

Table A.10: Normal distribution tests Vx perturbation measures Atype grouped; Lilliefors Significance Correction; phonation modus = 1

area	area	Kolmogorov-Smirnov Statistic	df	Sig.	Shapiro-Wilk Statistic	df	Sig.
Period sd	altai	0.376	28	0	0.299	28	0
	hakas	0.377	101	0	0.272	101	0
	tyva	0.404	350	0	0.163	350	0
	mongol	0.416	222	0	0.209	222	0
Jitter Loc	altai	0.351	28	0	0.322	28	0
	hakas	0.297	101	0	0.477	101	0
	tyva	0.298	350	0	0.299	350	0
	mongol	0.317	222	0	0.341	222	0
Jitter RAP	altai	0.485	28	0	0.227	28	0
	hakas	0.388	101	0	0.339	101	0
	tyva	0.369	350	0	0.205	350	0
	mongol	0.437	222	0	0.224	222	0
Jitter ppq5	altai	0.479	28	0	0.232	28	0
	hakas	0.373	101	0	0.345	101	0
	tyva	0.333	350	0	0.26	350	0
	mongol	0.422	222	0	0.199	222	0
Shimmer Loc	altai	0.179	28	0.022	0.926	28	**0.048**
	hakas	0.161	101	0	0.896	101	0
	tyva	0.092	350	0	0.898	350	0
	mongol	0.116	222	0	0.917	222	0
Shimmer apq3	altai	0.122	28	.200(*)	0.913	28	0.023
	hakas	0.156	101	0	0.879	101	0
	tyva	0.112	350	0	0.812	350	0
	mongol	0.126	222	0	0.879	222	0
Shimmer apq5	altai	0.109	28	.200(*)	0.939	28	**0.102**
	hakas	0.139	101	0	0.853	101	0
	tyva	0.102	350	0	0.885	350	0
	mongol	0.132	222	0	0.9	222	0
Shimmer apq11	altai	0.126	28	.200(*)	0.946	28	**0.157**
	hakas	0.164	101	0	0.866	101	0
	tyva	0.087	350	0	0.936	350	0
	mongol	0.118	222	0	0.938	222	0
HNRmn	altai	0.139	28	0.179	0.924	28	**0.045**
	hakas	0.107	101	0.006	0.966	101	0.01
	tyva	0.053	350	0.019	0.987	350	0.003
	mongol	0.052	222	.200(*)	0.987	222	0.035

Table A.11: normal distribution tests Vx perturbation measures area grouped;phonation modus = 1; Lilliefors Significance Correction; *This is a lower bound of the true significance

	AType	N
Values for PM2	1	32
	2	50
	3	798

Table A.12: Vx pertub Atype cases PM2

	Area	N
For all values PM2	altai	86
	hakas	95
	tyva	623
	mongol	76

Table A.13: Vx pertub area cases PM2

	Atype	Kolmogorov-Smirnov			Shapiro-Wilk		
		Statistic	df	Sig.	Statistic	df	Sig.
periodsd	1	0.426	32	0	0.457	32	0
	2	0.456	50	0	0.265	50	0
	3	0.327	798	0	0.324	798	0
pitchmn	1	0.315	32	0	0.571	32	0
	2	0.277	50	0	0.73	50	0
	3	0.072	798	0	0.969	798	0
jitterLoc	1	0.382	32	0	0.476	32	0
	2	0.316	50	0	0.403	50	0
	3	0.224	798	0	0.439	798	0
jitterRAP	1	0.45	32	0	0.414	32	0
	2	0.318	50	0	0.411	50	0
	3	0.293	798	0	0.296	798	0
jitterppq5	1	0.466	32	0	0.391	32	0
	2	0.32	50	0	0.423	50	0
	3	0.277	798	0	0.32	798	0
shimmerLoc	1	0.081	32	.200(*)	0.971	32	0.516
	2	0.12	50	0.068	0.947	50	0.025
	3	0.111	798	0	0.89	798	0
shimmerapq3	1	0.106	32	.200(*)	0.956	32	0.211
	2	0.143	50	0.012	0.92	50	0.002
	3	0.133	798	0	0.876	798	0
shimmerapq5	1	0.088	32	.200(*)	0.971	32	0.532
	2	0.124	50	0.053	0.946	50	0.024
	3	0.101	798	0	0.903	798	0
shimmerapq11	1	0.183	32	0.008	0.942	32	0.086
	2	0.201	50	0	0.867	50	0
	3	0.112	798	0	0.894	798	0
HNRmn	1	0.126	32	.200(*)	0.982	32	0.848
	2	0.082	50	.200(*)	0.976	50	0.389
	3	0.027	798	.200(*)	0.997	798	0.093

Table A.14: Normal distribution tests Vx perturbation measures Atype grouped; Lilliefors Significance Correction; phonation modus = 2; * This is a lower bound of the true significance

	area	Kolmogorov-Smirnov			Shapiro-Wilk		
		Statistic	df	Sig.	Statistic	df	Sig.
periodsd	altai	0.311	86	0	0.438	86	0
	hakas	0.326	95	0	0.299	95	0
	tyva	0.356	623	0	0.304	623	0
	mongol	0.42	76	0	0.248	76	0
pitchmn	altai	0.154	86	0	0.879	86	0
	hakas	0.287	95	0	0.71	95	0
	tyva	0.204	623	0	0.629	623	0
	mongol	0.159	76	0	0.883	76	0
jitterLoc	altai	0.134	86	0.001	0.845	86	0
	hakas	0.137	95	0	0.711	95	0
	tyva	0.271	623	0	0.402	623	0
	mongol	0.208	76	0	0.625	76	0
jitterRAP	altai	0.138	86	0	0.83	86	0
	hakas	0.109	95	0.007	0.842	95	0
	tyva	0.326	623	0	0.296	623	0
	mongol	0.232	76	0	0.543	76	0
jitterppq5	altai	0.145	86	0	0.731	86	0
	hakas	0.09	95	0.053	0.979	95	**0.129**
	tyva	0.324	623	0	0.305	623	0
	mongol	0.253	76	0	0.492	76	0
shimmerLoc	altai	0.163	86	0	0.757	86	0
	hakas	0.17	95	0	0.866	95	0
	tyva	0.11	623	0	0.919	623	0
	mongol	0.112	76	0.02	0.904	76	0
shimmerapq3	altai	0.158	86	0	0.839	86	0
	hakas	0.162	95	0	0.871	95	0
	tyva	0.129	623	0	0.881	623	0
	mongol	0.119	76	0.01	0.897	76	0
shimmerapq5	altai	0.132	86	0.001	0.81	86	0
	hakas	0.152	95	0	0.882	95	0
	tyva	0.105	623	0	0.923	623	0
	mongol	0.126	76	0.004	0.88	76	0
shimmerapq11	altai	0.137	86	0	0.887	86	0
	hakas	0.177	95	0	0.734	95	0
	tyva	0.107	623	0	0.92	623	0
	mongol	0.129	76	0.003	0.874	76	0
HNRmn	altai	0.088	86	0.095	0.981	86	**0.235**
	hakas	0.046	95	.200(*)	0.992	95	**0.855**
	tyva	0.03	623	.200(*)	0.995	623	**0.047**
	mongol	0.114	76	0.016	0.947	76	0.003

Table A.15: Normal distribution tests Vx perturbation measures area grouped; phonation modus = 2; Lilliefors Significance Correction;* This is a lower bound of the true significance.

A.1.2.2 Normal Distribution Analysis of Vx Spectral Components Measures

	Atype	Kolmogorov-Smirnov			Shapiro-Wilk		
		Statistic	df	Sig.	Statistic	df	Sig.
NHRmn	1	0.24	367	0	0.653	367	0
	2	0.144	154	0	0.845	154	0
	3	0.146	180	0	0.858	180	0

Table A.16: NHR Atype grouped Tests of Normality, modus = 1; Lilliefors Significance Correction

	area	Kolmogorov-Smirnov			Shapiro-Wilk		
		Statistic	df	Sig.	Statistic	df	Sig.
NHRmn	altai	0.209	28	0.003	0.758	28	0
	hakas	0.13	101	0	0.886	101	0
	tyva	0.172	350	0	0.724	350	0
	mongol	0.226	222	0	0.731	222	0

Table A.17: NHR Area grouped Tests of Normality, modus = 1; Lilliefors Significance Correction

	area	Kolmogorov-Smirnov			Shapiro-Wilk		
		Statistic	df	Sig.	Statistic	df	Sig.
NHRmn	altai	0.147	86	0	0.856	86	0
	hakas	0.208	95	0	0.725	95	0
	tyva	0.146	623	0	0.78	623	0
	mongol	0.175	76	0	0.878	76	0

Table A.18: NHR Area grouped Tests of Normality, modus = 2; Lilliefors Significance Correction

	Atype	Kolmogorov-Smirnov			Shapiro-Wilk		
		Statistic	df	Sig.	Statistic	df	Sig.
NHRmn	1	0.115	32	.200(*)	0.94	32	0.076
	2	0.138	50	0.019	0.88	50	0
	3	0.155	798	0	0.785	798	0

Table A.19: NHR Atype grouped Tests of Normality, modus = 2; * This is a lower bound of the true significance; Lilliefors Significance Correction

A.1.2.3 Test of Normality of Lx Quotients

	styles	Kolmogorov-Smirnov Statistic	df	Sig.
period	xai	0.253	9065	0
	xoemej	0.269	10472	0
t3mtl/tpd_CiQ1	xai	0.13	9065	0
	xoemej	0.088	10472	0
t2amta2/tpd_CiQ2	xai	0.105	9065	0
	xoemej	0.178	10472	0
t6mt4/tpd_QOQ	xai	0.181	9065	0
	xoemej	0.061	10472	0
t5amt3/t3mtl_SQ	xai	0.175	9065	0
	xoemej	0.18	10472	0
CPmOP/CPpOP_CIa	xai	0.191	9065	0
	xoemej	0.146	10472	0

Table A.20: Test of Normality Lx qotients area PM1

A.1.3 Nonparametric Rank Test

A.1.3.1 Ranking tests of vx perturbation values

	Period mn	Period sd	Jitter Loc	Jitter RAP	Jitter ppq5
Chi-Square	98.536	20.436	13.415	40.837	28.868
df	3	3	3	3	3
Asymp. Sig.	0	0	0.004	0	0
	Shimmer Loc	**Shimmer apq3**	**Shimmer apq5**	**Shimmer apq11**	**HNR mn**
Chi-Square	76.197	47.908	69.764	96.435	60.596
df	3	3	3	3	3
Asymp. Sig.	0	0	0	0	0

Table A.21: H-Test (Kruskal Wallis Test) for grouped perturbation values of PM1; Grouping Variable: area

	Period mn	Period sd	Jitter Loc	Jitter RAP	Jitter ppq5
Chi-Square	126,935	43,102	30,016	20,163	15,377
df	3	3	3	3	3
Asymp. Sig.	0	0	0	0	0.002
	Shimmer Loc	**Shimmer apq3**	**Shimmer apq5**	**Shimmer apq11**	**HNR mn**
Chi-Square	11,294	3,395	7,303	25,220	21,232
df	3	3	3	3	3
Asymp. Sig.	0.01	**0.335**	**0.063**	0	0

Table A.22: H-Test (Kruskal-Wallis test) for grouped perturbation values of PM2; Grouping Variable: area

modus	1			2			
	area	N	Mean Rank		area	N	Mean Rank
periodmn	altai	28	365.79	periodmn	altai	86	372.88
	hakas	101	530.32		hakas	95	711.91
	tyva	350	333.01		tyva	623	419.68
	mongol	222	295.92		mongol	77	355.31
periodsd	altai	28	420	periodsd	altai	86	560.77
	hakas	101	372.58		hakas	95	429.7
	tyva	350	317.42		tyva	623	443.67
	mongol	222	385.41		mongol	77	299.55
jitterLoc	altai	28	384.27	jitterLoc	altai	86	505.37
	hakas	101	369.46		hakas	95	405.32
	tyva	350	323.26		tyva	623	453.99
	mongol	222	382.15		mongol	77	308.04
jitterRAP	altai	28	315.52	jitterRAP	altai	86	498.18
	hakas	101	466.14		hakas	95	512.85
	tyva	350	321.74		tyva	623	431.94
	mongol	222	349.22		mongol	77	361.82
jitterppq5	altai	28	323.88	jitterppq5	altai	86	503.2
	hakas	101	447.31		hakas	95	462.38
	tyva	350	325.56		tyva	623	440.24
	mongol	222	350.71		mongol	77	351.32
shimmerLoc	altai	28	253.75	shimmerLoc	altai	86	451.7
	hakas	101	243.14		hakas	95	358.45
	tyva	350	335.96		tyva	623	451.89
	mongol	222	436.05		mongol	77	442.75
shimmerapq3	altai	28	295.96	shimmerapq3	altai	86	434.15
	hakas	101	323.29		hakas	95	397.47
	tyva	350	314.29		tyva	623	446.91
	mongol	222	428.42		mongol	77	454.51
shimmerapq5	altai	28	270.29	shimmerapq5	altai	86	441.05
	hakas	101	254.47		hakas	95	378.37
	tyva	350	331.41		tyva	623	452.46
	mongol	222	435.98		mongol	77	425.51
shimmerapq11	altai	28	232.48	shimmerapq11	altai	86	450.24
	hakas	101	203.44		hakas	95	319.41
	tyva	350	353.42		tyva	623	459.51
	mongol	222	429.27		mongol	77	430.97
HNRmn	altai	28	370.2	HNRmn	altai	86	407.45
	hakas	101	287.5		hakas	95	552.86
	tyva	350	408.45		tyva	623	430.74
	mongol	222	286.9		mongol	77	423.43

Table A.23: Ranks of vx perturbation values; area grouped; phonation modus = 1; total N for all groups 701

	Jitter Loc	Jitter RAP	Jitter ppq5	Shimmer Loc	Shimmer apq3	Shimmer apq5	Shimmer apq11
Chi-Square	74,474	137,340	136,163	34,361	18,569	34,940	51,212
df	2	2	2	2	2	2	2
Asymp. Sig.	0	0	0	0	0	0	0

Table A.24: Kruskal-Wallis H-test for articulation type grouped vx perturbation values; Grouping Variable: Atype, modus = 1

	Jitter Loc	Jitter RAP	Jitter ppq5	Shimmer Loc	Shimmer apq3	Shimmer apq5	Shimmer apq11
Chi-Square	24.525	19.984	20.38	17.463	13.046	12.443	20.19
df	2	2	2	2	2	2	2
Asymp. Sig.	0	0	0	0	0.001	0.002	0

Table A.25: Kruskal-Wallis H-test for articulation type grouped vx perturbation values; Grouping Variable: Atype; phonation modus = 2

modus	PM1			PM2			
	Atype	N	Mean Rank		Atype	N	Mean Rank
Jitter Loc	1	367	325.66	Jitter Loc	1	32	367.33
	2	154	284.2		2	50	280.55
	3	180	459.81		3	798	453.46
Jitter RAP	1	367	290.18	Jitter RAP	1	32	325.09
	2	154	319.14		2	50	318.46
	3	180	502.26		3	798	452.77
Jitter ppq5	1	367	292.92	Jitter ppq5	1	32	321.02
	2	154	312.59		2	50	319.08
	3	180	502.27		3	798	452.9
Period mn	1	367	256.33	Period mn	1	32	244.13
	2	154	385.21		2	50	332.97
	3	180	514.76		3	798	455.11
Period sd	1	367	328.12	Period sd	1	32	378.53
	2	154	304.73		2	50	287.69
	3	180	437.24		3	798	452.56
Shimmer Loc	1	367	392.29	Shimmer Loc	1	32	616
	2	154	323.93		2	50	478.42
	3	180	289.97		3	798	431.09
Shimmer apq3	1	367	378.77	Shimmer apq3	1	32	599
	2	154	296.27		2	50	447.27
	3	180	341.21		3	798	433.72
Shimmer apq5	1	367	393.89	Shimmer apq5	1	32	593.53
	2	154	311.27		2	50	456.94
	3	180	297.54		3	798	433.33
Shimmer apq11	1	367	398.99	Shimmer apq11	1	32	623.78
	2	154	332.08		2	50	493.21
	3	180	269.35		3	798	429.85
HNR mn	1	367	350.36	HNR mn	1	32	319.86
	2	154	401.29		2	50	398.45
	3	180	309.28		3	798	447.97

Table A.26: Ranking for articulation type grouped vx perturbation values; PM1 (left) and PM2 (right)

A.1.3.2 Ranking test of Vx spectral components

modus		area	N	Mean Rank
1	NHRmn	altai	28	334.18
		hakas	101	419.29
		tyva	350	294.53
		mongol	222	411.09
		Total	701	
2	NHRmn	altai	86	483.7
		hakas	95	325.46
		tyva	623	456.26
		mongol	77	412.39
		Total	881	

Table A.27: NHR ranking area grouped

modus		NHRmn
1	Chi-Square	58.44
	df	3
	Asymp. Sig.	0
2	Chi-Square	25.219
	df	3
	Asymp. Sig.	0

Table A.28: NHRmn ranks; Kruskal Wallis Test; Grouping Variable: area

modus		Atype	N	Mean Rank
1	NHRmn	1	367	354.55
		2	154	289.24
		3	180	396.61
		Total	701	
2	NHRmn	1	32	552.5
		2	50	434.68
		3	799	436.93
		Total	881	

Table A.29: NHR ranking Atype grouped

modus		NHRmn
1	Chi-Square	23.567
	df	2
	Asymp. Sig.	0
2	Chi-Square	6.379
	df	2
	Asymp. Sig.	0.041

Table A.30: NHR Kruskal Wallis Test; Grouping Variable: Atype

A.1.3.3 Ranking test of Lx jitter shimmer values

	style2	N	Mean Rank	Sum of Ranks
periodsd1	kargyraa	146	101.34	14796
	xai	138	186.04	25674
periodsd2	kargyraa	146	161.86	23631
	xai	138	122.02	16839
jitterLoc	kargyraa	146	103.9	15170
	xai	138	183.33	25300
jitterRAP	kargyraa	146	103.9	15170
	xai	138	183.33	25300
jitterppq5	kargyraa	146	104.67	15282
	xai	138	182.52	25188
shimmerLoc	kargyraa	146	131.24	19161
	xai	138	154.41	21309
shimmerapq3	kargyraa	146	128.67	18786
	xai	138	157.13	21684
shimmerapq5	kargyraa	146	129.58	18918.5
	xai	138	156.17	21551.5
shimmerapq11	kargyraa	146	133.33	19466
	xai	138	152.2	21004
jitterLoc2	kargyraa	146	169.51	24749
	xai	138	113.92	15721
jitterRAP2	kargyraa	146	167.75	24491.5
	xai	138	115.79	15978.5
jitterppq52	kargyraa	146	165.94	24227
	xai	138	117.7	16243
shimmerLoc2	kargyraa	146	162.9	23783.5
	xai	138	120.92	16686.5
shimmerapq32	kargyraa	146	162.49	23723
	xai	138	121.36	16747
shimmerapq52	kargyraa	146	164.68	24043.5
	xai	138	119.03	16426.5
shimmerapq112	kargyraa	146	162.55	23733
	xai	138	121.28	16737
	Total	284		

Table A.31: Ranks Lx perturbation; area (=style) grouped

	period	jitter	jitter	jitter	shimmer	shimmer	shimmer	shimmer
	sd1	Loc	RAP	ppq5	Loc	apq3	apq5	apq11
U	4065	4439	4439	4551	8430	8055	8187.5	8735
Asymp. Sig.	0	0	0	0	0.017	0.004	0.006	0.053
	period	jitter	jitter	jitter	shimmer	shimmer	shimmer	shimmer
	sd2	Loc2	RAP2	ppq52	Loc2	apq32	apq52	apq112
U	7248	6130	6387.5	6652	7095.5	7156	6835.5	7146
Asymp. Sig.	0	0	0	0	0	0	0	0

Table A.32: Mann-Whitney U Test Lx perturbation PM2

A.1.3.4 Ranking tests of Lx quotients – Single-cycle mode (PM1)

	style	N	Mean Rank	Sum of Ranks
t3mt1/tpd_CiQ1	xai	9065	7979.25	72331866
	xoemej	10472	11318.29	118525087
t2amta2/tpd_CiQ2	xai	9065	11509.6	104334558.5
	xoemej	10472	8262.26	86522394.5
t6mt4/tpd_QOQ	xai	9065	9557.37	86637517.5
	xoemej	10472	9952.2	104219435.5
t5amt3/t3mt1_SQ	xai	9065	11609.45	105239637
	xoemej	10472	8175.83	85617316
CPmOP/CPpOP_CIa	xai	9065	8602.04	77977451
	xoemej	10472	10779.17	112879502
	Total	19537		

Table A.33: Ranks Mann-Whitney Test Lx quotients PM1

	$\frac{t3mt1}{tpd}$	$\frac{t2amta2}{tpd}$	$\frac{t6mt4}{tpd}$	$\frac{t5amt3}{t3mt1}$	$\frac{CPmOP}{CPpOP}$
Mann-Whitney U	31240221	31685766.5	45545872.5	30780688	36885806
Wilcoxon W	72331866	86522394.5	86637517.5	85617316	77977451
Z	-41.268	-40.135	-4.88	-42.437	-26.908
Asymp. Sig. (2-tailed)	0	0	0	0	0

Table A.34: Mann-Whitney Test Lx quotients PM1; Grouping Variable: area (=style)

A.1.3.5 Ranking tests of Lx quotients – Double-cycle mode (PM2)

	styles	N	Mean Rank	Sum of Ranks
t3mt1/tpd_CiQ1	xai	3628	3406.2	12357692
	kargyraa	3427	3656.94	12532348
t2amta2/tpd_CiQ2	xai	3628	3626.74	13157826
	kargyraa	3427	3423.46	11732214
t5bmt5a/tpd_OQ	xai	3628	3920.65	14224123.5
	kargyraa	3427	3112.32	10665916.5
t6mt4/tpd_QOQ	xai	3628	3986.6	14463385
	kargyraa	3427	3042.5	10426655
t5amt3/t3mt1_SQ	xai	3628	3389.64	12297628
	kargyraa	3427	3674.47	12592412
CPmOP/CPpOP_CIa	xai	3628	3508.59	12729167
	kargyraa	3427	3548.55	12160873
t7mt5b/tpd2_CiQ1	xai	3628	3971.95	14410237
	kargyraa	3427	3058.01	10479803
t6amta6/tpd2_CiQ2	xai	3628	3796.17	13772489
	kargyraa	3427	3244.11	11117551
t9bmt9a/tpd2_OQ1	xai	3628	3729.43	13530368
	kargyraa	3427	3314.76	11359672
t10mt8/tpd2_QOQ	xai	3628	3926.94	14246923
	kargyraa	3427	3105.67	10643117
t9amt7/t7mt5b_SQ	xai	3628	2946.25	10689005
	kargyraa	3427	4143.87	14201035
CPmOP/CPpOP_CIb	xai	3628	3739.15	13565623
	kargyraa	3427	3304.47	11324417
	Total	7055		

Table A.35: Ranks Mann-Whitney Test Lx quotients PM2; grouping by area (=style: *kargyraa* (Tuva), *xai* (Hakassia))

Cycle 1	$\frac{t3mt1}{tpd}$ CiQ1	$\frac{t2amta2}{tpd}$ CiQ2	$\frac{t5bmt5a}{tpd}$ OQ	$\frac{t6mt4}{tpd}$ QOQ	$\frac{t5amt3}{t3mt1}$ SQ	$\frac{CPmOP}{CPpOP}$ CIa
Mann-Whitney U	5774686	5858336	4792038.5	4552777	5714622	6146161
Asymp. Sig. (2-tailed)	0.0001	0.0001	0.0001	0.0001	0.0001	**0.41**
Cycle 2	$\frac{t7mt5b}{tpd2}$ CiQ1	$\frac{t6amta6}{tpd2}$ CiQ2	$\frac{t9bmt9a}{tpd2}$ OQ1	$\frac{t10mt8}{tpd2}$ QOQ	$\frac{t9amt7}{t7mt5b}$ SQ	$\frac{CPmOP}{CPpOP}$ CIb
Mann-Whitney U	4605925	5243673	5485794	4769239	4105999	5450539
Asymp. Sig. (2-tailed)	0.0001	0.0001	0.0001	0.0001	0.0001	0.0001

Table A.36: Mann-Whitney Test Lx quotients (doublecycle)PM2; Grouping Variable: style

A.1.3.6 MeanUx

	modus	N	Mean Rank
Ux value	mod	11205	23669.1
	aes	7699	19500.36
	puls	11356	7829.26
	aef	7671	28046.49
	Total	37931	

Table A.37: Kruskall-Wallis test for mean Ux ranks grouped by VPT (=phonation mode)

	Ux value
Chi-Square	19107.973
df	3
Asymp. Sig.	0.0001

Table A.38: Kruskal-Wallis test of mean Ux ranks; Grouping Variable: phonation modus

A.1.4 Tables of Correlation Analysis

A.1.4.1 Correlation analysis for Vx perturbation values

Spearman's rho		Period sd	Jitter Loc	Jitter RAP	Jitter ppq5	Shimmer Loc	Shimmer apq3	Shimmer apq5	Shimmer apq11	HNR mn	NHR mn
period	Corr coeff	1	.888**	.584**	.633**	.224**	.224**	.207**	.212**	-.365**	.387**
sd	Sig. 2-tail.	.	0	0	0	0	0	0	0	0	0
jitter	Corr coeff	.888**	1	.758**	.818**	.277**	.303**	.272**	.262**	-.448**	.472**
Loc	Sig. 2-tail.	0	.	0	0	0	0	0	0	0	0
jitter	Corr coeff	.584**	.758**	1	.985**	.249**	.377**	.277**	.151**	-.500**	.507**
RAP	Sig. 2-tail.	0	0	.	0	0	0	0	0	0	0
jitter	Corr coeff	.633**	.818**	.985**	1	.232**	.343**	.259**	.159**	-.479**	.492**
ppq5	Sig. 2-tail.	0	0	0	.	0	0	0	0	0	0
shimmer	Corr coeff	.224**	.277**	.249**	.232**	1	.904**	.967**	.912**	-.621**	.597**
Loc	Sig. 2-tail.	0	0	0	0	.	0	0	0	0	0
shimmer	Corr coeff	.224**	.303**	.377**	.343**	.904**	1	.926**	.712**	-.710**	.677**
apq3	Sig. 2-tail.	0	0	0	0	0	.	0	0	0	0
shimmer	Corr coeff	.207**	.272**	.277**	.259**	.967**	.926**	1	.882**	-.655**	.628**
apq5	Sig. 2-tail.	0	0	0	0	0	0	.	0	0	0
shimmer	Corr coeff	.212**	.262**	.151**	.159**	.912**	.712**	.882**	1	-.497**	.486**
apq11	Sig. 2-tail.	0	0	0	0	0	0	0	.	0	0
HNRmn	Corr coeff	-.365**	-.448**	-.500**	-.479**	-.621**	-.710**	-.655**	-.497**	1	-.980**
	Sig. 2-tail.	0	0	0	0	0	0	0	0	.	0
NHRmn	Corr coeff	.387**	.472**	.507**	.492**	.597**	.677**	.628**	.486**	-.980**	1
	Sig. 2-tail.	0	0	0	0	0	0	0	0	0	.
	N	701	701	701	701	701	701	701	701	701	701

Table A.39: Correlation analysis for Vx perturbation values; Phonation Mode 1; ** Correlation is significant at the 0.01 level (2-tailed.); NHR is clearly no perturbation value but has been included here for reasons of comparison since NHR was acquired at the same time.

Spearman's rho		period sd	Jitter Loc	Jitter RAP	Jitter ppq5	Shimmer Loc	Shimmer apq3	Shimmer apq5	Shimmer apq11	HNR mn	NHR mn
period	Corr coeff	1	.845**	.529**	.658**	.370**	.363**	.365**	.336**	-.353**	.385**
sd	Sig. 2-tail.	.	0	0	0	0	0	0	0	0	0
jitter	Corr coeff	.845**	1	.759**	.890**	.421**	.414**	.431**	.377**	-.495**	.527**
Loc	Sig. 2-tail.	0	.	0	0	0	0	0	0	0	0
jitter	Corr coeff	.529**	.759**	1	.919**	.357**	.411**	.374**	.242**	-.519**	.556**
RAP	Sig. 2-tail.	0	0	.	0	0	0	0	0	0	0
jitter	Corr coeff	.658**	.890**	.919**	1	.399**	.417**	.419**	.324**	-.497**	.527**
ppq5	Sig. 2-tail.	0	0	0	.	0	0	0	0	0	0
shimmer	Corr coeff	.370**	.421**	.357**	.399**	1	.949**	.964**	.867**	-.581**	.557**
Loc	Sig. 2-tail.	0	0	0	0	.	0	0	0	0	0
shimmer	Corr coeff	.363**	.414**	.411**	.417**	.949**	1	.920**	.736**	-.605**	.587**
apq3	Sig. 2-tail.	0	0	0	0	0	.	0	0	0	0
shimmer	Corr coeff	.365**	.431**	.374**	.419**	.964**	.920**	1	.872**	-.562**	.539**
apq5	Sig. 2-tail.	0	0	0	0	0	0	.	0	0	0
shimmer	Corr coeff	.336**	.377**	.242**	.324**	.867**	.736**	.872**	1	-.446**	.423**
apq11	Sig. 2-tail.	0	0	0	0	0	0	0	.	0	0
HNRmn	Corr coeff	-.353**	-.495**	-.519**	-.497**	-.581**	-.605**	-.562**	-.446**	1	-.967**
	Sig. 2-tail.	0	0	0	0	0	0	0	0	.	0
NHRmn	Corr coeff	.385**	.527**	.556**	.527**	.557**	.587**	.539**	.423**	-.967**	1
	Sig. 2-tail.	0	0	0	0	0	0	0	0	0	.
	N	881	881	881	881	881	881	881	881	881	881

Table A.40: Correlation analysis for Vx perturbation values; Phonation Mode 2; ** Correlation is significant at the 0.01 level (2-tailed.)

A.1.4.2 Correlation analysis for Vx spectral component analysis

	Spearman's rho	H1-H2	H1-A1	H1-A2	H1-A3	H1-H3	B1
H1-H2	CorrCoef	1	.381(**)	.306(**)	.252(**)	.246(**)	.083(*)
	Sig. (2-tail.)	.	0	0	0	0	0.024
H1-A1	CorrCoef	.381(**)	1	.282(**)	.262(**)	.640(**)	.605(**)
	Sig. (2-tail.)	0	.	0	0	0	0
H1-A2	CorrCoef	.306(**)	.282(**)	1	.553(**)	.211(**)	-.289(**)
	Sig. (2-tail.)	0	0	.	0	0	0
H1-A3	CorrCoef	.252(**)	.262(**)	.553(**)	1	.228(**)	-.220(**)
	Sig. (2-tail.)	0	0	0	.	0	0
H1-H3	CorrCoef	.246(**)	.640(**)	.211(**)	.228(**)	1	.283(**)
	Sig. (2-tail.)	0	0	0	0	.	0
B1	CorrCoef	.083(*)	.605(**)	-.289(**)	-.220(**)	.283(**)	1
	Sig. (2-tail.)	0.024	0	0	0	0	.
	N	735	735	735	735	735	735

Table A.41: Correlation analysis of Vx spectral components PM1;** Correlation is significant at the 0.01 level (2-tailed);* Correlation is significant at the 0.05 level (2-tailed).

	Spearman's rho	H1-H2	H1-A1	H1-A2	H1-A3	H1-H3	B1
H1-H2	CorrCoef	1	.245(**)	.228(**)	.152(**)	.456(**)	-0.05
	Sig. (2-tail.)	.	0	0	0	0	0.138
H1-A1	CorrCoef	.245(**)	1	.668(**)	.574(**)	.310(**)	.328(**)
	Sig. (2-tail.)	0	.	0	0	0	0
H1-A2	CorrCoef	.228(**)	.668(**)	1	.576(**)	.245(**)	-.124(**)
	Sig. (2-tail.)	0	0	.	0	0	0
H1-A3	CorrCoef	.152(**)	.574(**)	.576(**)	1	.172(**)	-.091(**)
	Sig. (2-tail.)	0	0	0	.	0	0.007
H1-H3	CorrCoef	.456(**)	.310(**)	.245(**)	.172(**)	1	-.082(*)
	Sig. (2-tail.)	0	0	0	0	.	0.015
B1	CorrCoef	-0.05	.328(**)	-.124(**)	-.091(**)	-.082(*)	1
	Sig. (2-tail.)	0.138	0	0	0.007	0.015	.
	N	881	881	881	881	881	881

Table A.42: Correlation analysis of Vx spectral components PM2; ** Correlation is significant at the 0.01 level (2-tailed);* Correlation is significant at the 0.05 level (2-tailed).

		F2_H	F2_H_F	F2_H_A	F2_Hm1	F2_Hm1_F	F2_Hm1_A	F2_Hp1	F2_Hp1_F	F2_Hp1_A	Atype	area
F2_H	CorrCoef	1	.620**	-.187**	1.000**	.671**	-.135**	1.000**	.568**	0.008	.177**	-.190**
	Sig. 2-tail.	.	0	0	.	0	0	.	0	0.827	0	0
F2_H_F	CorrCoef	.620**	1	.167**	.620**	.997**	.181**	.620**	.997**	.329**	-.300**	0.008
	Sig. 2-tail.	0	.	0	0	0	0	0	0	0	0	0.825
F2_H_A	CorrCoef	-.187**	.167**	1	-.187**	.137**	**.741****	-.187**	.198**	.681**	-.455**	.559**
	Sig. 2-tail.	0	0	.	0	0	0	0	0	0	0	0
F2_Hm1	CorrCoef	1.000**	.620**	-.187**	1	.671**	-.135**	1.000**	.568**	0.008	.177**	-.190**
	Sig. 2-tail.	.	0	0	.	0	0	.	0	0.827	0	0
F2_Hm1_F	CorrCoef	.671**	.997**	.137**	.671**	1	.157**	.671**	.989**	.305**	-.264**	-0.014
	Sig. 2-tail.	0	0	0	0	.	0	0	0	0	0	0.714
F2_Hm1_A	CorrCoef	-.135**	.181**	**.741****	-.135**	.157**	1	-.135**	.205**	.565**	-.341**	.529**
	Sig. 2-tail.	0	0	0	0	0	.	0	0	0	0	0
F2_Hp1	CorrCoef	1.000**	.620**	-.187**	1.000**	.671**	-.135**	1	.568**	0.008	.177**	-.190**
	Sig. 2-tail.	.	0	0	.	0	0	.	0	0.827	0	0
F2_Hp1_F	CorrCoef	.568**	.997**	.198**	.568**	.989**	.205**	.568**	1	.349**	-.332**	0.031
	Sig. 2-tail.	0	0	0	0	0	0	0	.	0	0	0.396
F2_Hp1_A	CorrCoef	0.008	.329**	.681**	0.008	.305**	.565**	0.008	.349**	1	-.314**	.464**
	Sig. 2-tail.	0.827	0	0	0.827	0	0	0.827	0	.	0	0
Atype	CorrCoef	.177**	-.300**	-.455**	.177**	-.264**	-.341**	.177**	-.332**	-.314**	1	-.384**
	Sig. 2-tail.	0	0	0	0	0	0	0	0	0	.	0
area	CorrCoef	-.190**	0.008	.559**	-.190**	-0.014	.529**	-.190**	0.031	.464**	-.384**	1
	Sig. 2-tail.	0	0.825	0	0	0.714	0	0	0.396	0	0	.
	N	735	735	735	735	735	735	735	735	735	735	735

Table A.43: Correlation analysis of formant structure measures PM1;** Correlation is significant at the 0.01 level (2-tailed);* Correlation is significant at the 0.05 level (2-tailed).

A.1.4.3 Correlation analysis for Lx perturbation and Lx quotient values

		period mnl	period sd1	jitter Loc	jitter RAP	jitter ppq5	shimmer Loc	shimmer apq3	shimmer apq5	shimmer apq11	style
period mnl	Cor coef	1	.179**	-.285**	-.319**	-.273**	-.202**	-.125*	-.256**	-.302**	-.358**
	Sig.	.	0	0	0	0	0	0.013	0	0	0
Period sd1	Cor coef	.179**	1	.727**	.681**	.704**	.462**	.471**	.437**	.430**	.169**
	Sig.	0	.	0	0	0	0	0	0	0	0.001
Jitter Loc	Cor coef	-.285**	.727**	1	.995**	.993**	.567**	.532**	.585**	.590**	.397**
	Sig.	0	0	.	0	0	0	0	0	0	0
Jitter RAP	Cor coef	-.319**	.681**	.995**	1	.990**	.558**	.522**	.580**	.584**	.405**
	Sig.	0	0	0	.	0	0	0	0	0	0
Jitter ppq5	Cor coef	-.273**	.704**	.993**	.990**	1	.558**	.522**	.579**	.583**	.395**
	Sig.	0	0	0	0	.	0	0	0	0	0
Shimmer Loc	Cor coef	-.202**	.462**	.567**	.558**	.558**	1	.988**	.991**	.976**	.470**
	Sig.	0	0	0	0	0	.	0	0	0	0
Shimmer apq3	Cor coef	-.125*	.471**	.532**	.522**	.522**	.988**	1	.970**	.941**	.407**
	Sig.	0.013	0	0	0	0	0	.	0	0	0
Shimmer apq5	Cor coef	-.256**	.437**	.585**	.580**	.579**	.991**	.970**	1	.985**	.521**
	Sig.	0	0	0	0	0	0	0	.	0	0
Shimmer apq11	Cor coef	-.302**	.430**	.590**	.584**	.583**	.976**	.941**	.985**	1	.530**
	Sig.	0	0	0	0	0	0	0	0	.	0
style	Cor coef	-.358**	.169**	.397**	.405**	.395**	.470**	.407**	.521**	.530**	1
	Sig.	0	0.001	0	0	0	0	0	0	0	.
	N	394	394	394	394	394	394	394	394	394	394

Table A.44: Correlation analysis for Lx perturbation values PM1

		period mn1	period sd1	period mn2	period sd2	jitter Loc	jitter RAP	shim Loc	shim apq3	jitter Loc2	jitter RAP2	shim Loc2	shim apq32	style2
period	CorCof	1	.280**	**.997****	.137*	.142*	.141*	-0.032	0.015	-0.099	-0.09	-0.084	-0.066	.470**
mn1	Sig.	.	0	0	0.021	0.017	0.017	0.588	0.801	0.095	0.132	0.159	0.265	0
period	CorCof	.280**	1	.285**	0.028	**.980****	**.978****	0.081	0.068	-0.015	-0.018	.128*	.133*	.516**
sd1	Sig.	0	.	0	0.643	0	0	0.175	0.251	**0.806**	0.757	0.031	0.025	0
period	CorCof	**.997****	.285**	1	.145*	.146*	.145*	-0.025	0.023	-0.092	-0.084	-0.084	-0.067	.466**
mn2	Sig.	0	0	.	0.014	0.014	0.014	0.679	0.699	0.124	0.159	0.157	0.262	0
Period	CorCof	.137*	0.028	.145*	1	-0.059	-0.065	0.002	-0.036	**.783****	.688**	.489**	.475**	-.243**
sd2	Sig.	0.021	0.643	0.014	.	0.319	0.277	0.972	0.55	0	0	0	0	0
Jitter	CorCof	.142*	**.980****	.146*	-0.059	1	1.000**	0.081	0.067	-0.051	-0.048	0.094	0.097	.484**
Loc	Sig.	0.017	0	0.014	0.319	.	0	0.171	0.262	0.391	0.421	0.116	0.103	0
Jitter	CorCof	.141*	**.978****	.145*	-0.065	1.000**	1	0.085	0.071	-0.055	-0.052	0.089	0.092	.484**
RAP	Sig.	0.017	0	0.014	0.277	0	.	0.152	0.234	0.353	0.382	0.136	0.122	0
shimmer	CorCof	-0.032	0.081	-0.025	0.002	0.081	0.085	1	**.918****	-0.033	-0.042	-.212**	-.205**	.141*
Loc	Sig.	0.588	0.175	0.679	0.972	0.171	0.152	.	0	0.582	0.484	0	0	0.017
shimmer	CorCof	0.015	0.068	0.023	-0.036	0.067	0.071	.918**	1	-0.069	-0.071	-.229**	-.225**	.174**
apq3	Sig.	0.801	0.251	0.699	0.55	0.262	0.234	0	.	0.244	0.231	0	0	0.003
jitter	CorCof	-0.099	-0.015	-0.092	**.783****	-0.051	-0.055	-0.033	-0.069	1	**.976****	.435**	.433**	-.339**
Loc2	Sig.	0.095	0.806	0.124	0	0.391	0.353	0.582	0.244	.	0	0	0	0
jitter	CorCof	-0.09	-0.018	-0.084	.688**	-0.048	-0.052	-0.042	-0.071	.976**	1	.383**	.388**	-.317**
RAP2	Sig.	0.132	0.757	0.159	0	0.421	0.382	0.484	0.231	0	.	0	0	0
shimmer	CorCof	-0.084	.128*	-0.084	.489**	0.094	0.089	-.212**	-.229**	.435**	.383**	1	**.991****	-.256**
Loc2	Sig.	0.159	0.031	0.157	0	0.116	0.136	0	0	0	0	.	0	0
shimmer	CorCof	-0.066	.133*	-0.067	.475**	0.097	0.092	-.205**	-.225**	.433**	.388**	.991**	1	-.251**
apq32	Sig.	0.265	0.025	0.262	0	0.103	0.122	0	0	0	0	0	.	0
style2	CorCof	.470**	.516**	.466**	-.243**	.484**	.484**	.141*	.174**	-.339**	-.317**	-.256**	-.251**	1
	Sig.	0	0	0	0	0	0	0.017	0.003	0	0	0	0	.
	N	284	284	284	284	284	284	284	284	284	284	284	284	284

Table A.45: Correlation analysis for Lx perturbation values PM2

	Spearman's rho	period	t3mt1/tpd CiQ1	t2amta2/tpd CiQ2	t6mt4/tpd QOQ	t5amt3/t3mt1 SQ	CPmOP/CPpOP CIa
period	CorrCoef	1	-.142(**)	.222(**)	0.013	.136(**)	0.003
	Sig. (2-tail.)	.	0	0	0.068	0	0.717
	N	19537	19537	19537	19537	19537	19537
t3mt1/tpd	CorrCoef	-.142(**)	1	.299(**)	-.214(**)	-.829(**)	.467(**)
CiQ1	Sig. (2-tail.)	0	.	0	0	0	0
	N	19537	19537	19537	19537	19537	19537
t2amta2/tpd	CorrCoef	.222(**)	.299(**)	1	-.167(**)	-.109(**)	.100(**)
CiQ2	Sig. (2-tail.)	0	0	.	0	0	0
	N	19537	19537	19537	19537	19537	19537
t6mt4/tpd	CorrCoef	0.013	-.214(**)	-.167(**)	1	-.153(**)	.288(**)
QOQ	Sig. (2-tail.)	0.068	0	0	.	0	0
	N	19537	19537	19537	19537	19537	19537
t5amt3/t3mt1	CorrCoef	.136(**)	-.829(**)	-.109(**)	-.153(**)	1	-.663(**)
SQ	Sig. (2-tail.)	0	0	0	0	.	0
	N	19537	19537	19537	19537	19537	19537
CPmOP/CPpOP	CorrCoef	0.003	.467(**)	.100(**)	.288(**)	-.663(**)	1
CIa	Sig. (2-tail.)	0.717	0	0	0	0	.
	N	19537	19537	19537	19537	19537	19537

Table A.46: Correlation analysis of Lx quotient values

A.2 Diagrams and Plots

A.2.1 Descriptive Plots & Diagrams

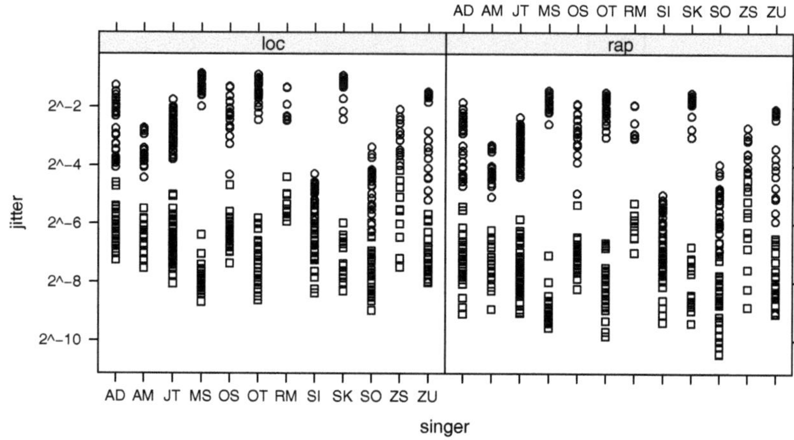

Figure A.1: Lx jitter values of local jitter and RAP jitter measures for single cycle-to-cycle (circle) and double (boxes) cycle 'mode' in PM2

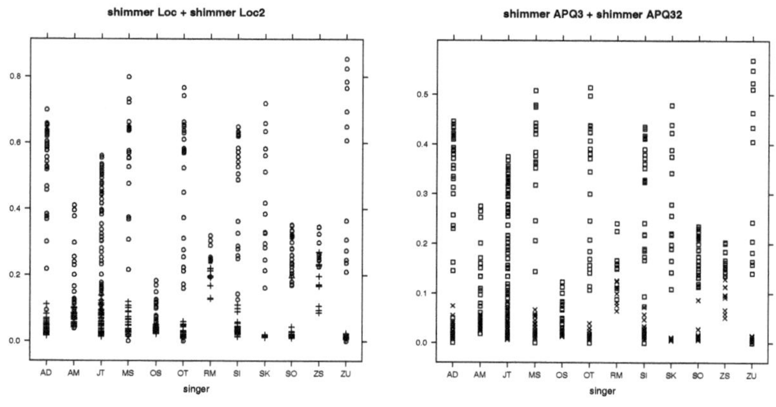

Figure A.2: Lx local shimmer and shimmer APQ3 measures grouped by singer for cycle-to-cycle (upper) and double (lower) cycle 'mode' in PM2

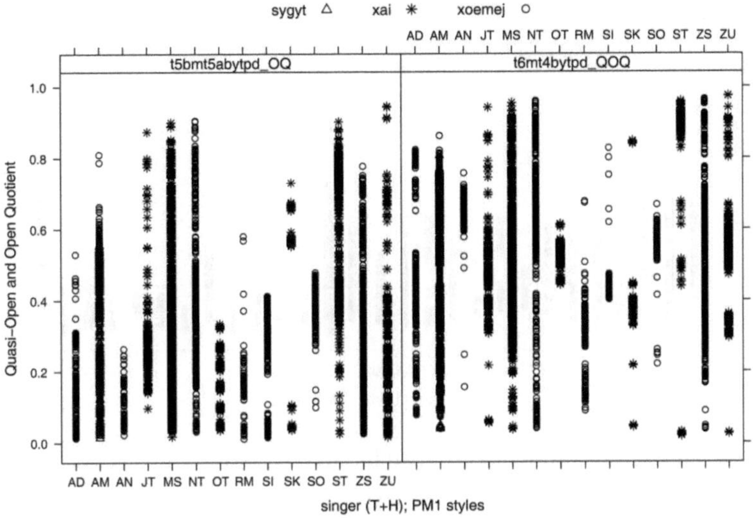

Figure A.3: Lx open quotient and quasi open quotient grouped by singer for PM1; xoemej & sygyt = Tuva, xai = Hakas

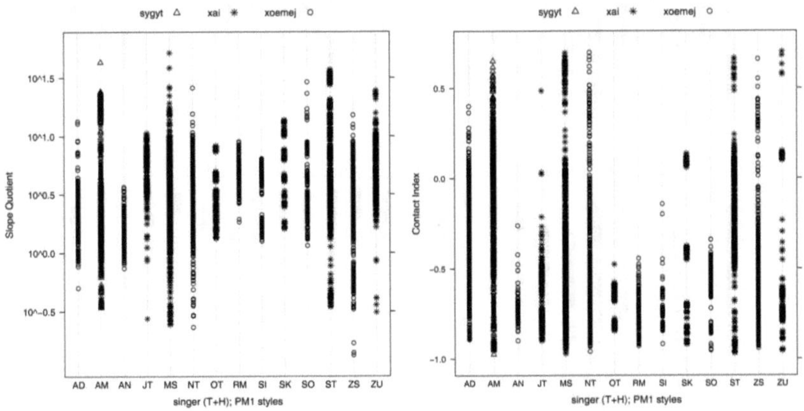

Figure A.4: Lx speed (slope) quotient grouped by singer for PM1;y-axis log 10 (left) and Lx Contact Index grouped by singer for PM1 (right); xoemej & sygyt = Tuva, xai = Hakas

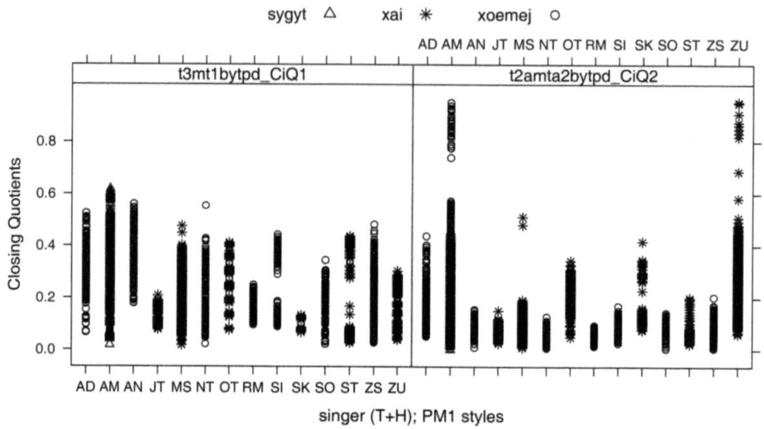

Figure A.5: Lx closing quotient grouped by singers PM1; xoemej & sygyt = Tuva, xai = Hakas

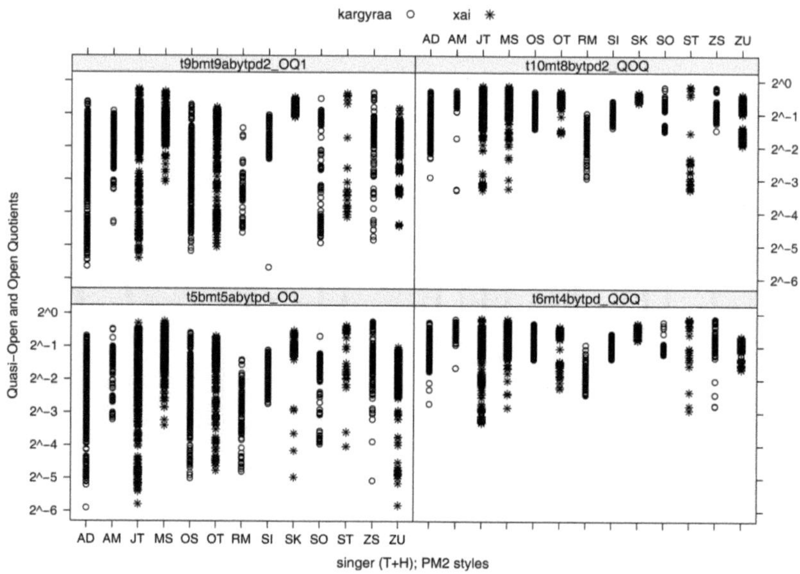

Figure A.6: Lx open quotient and quasi open quotient of first and second cycle in PM2; kargyraa = Tuva, xai = Hakas

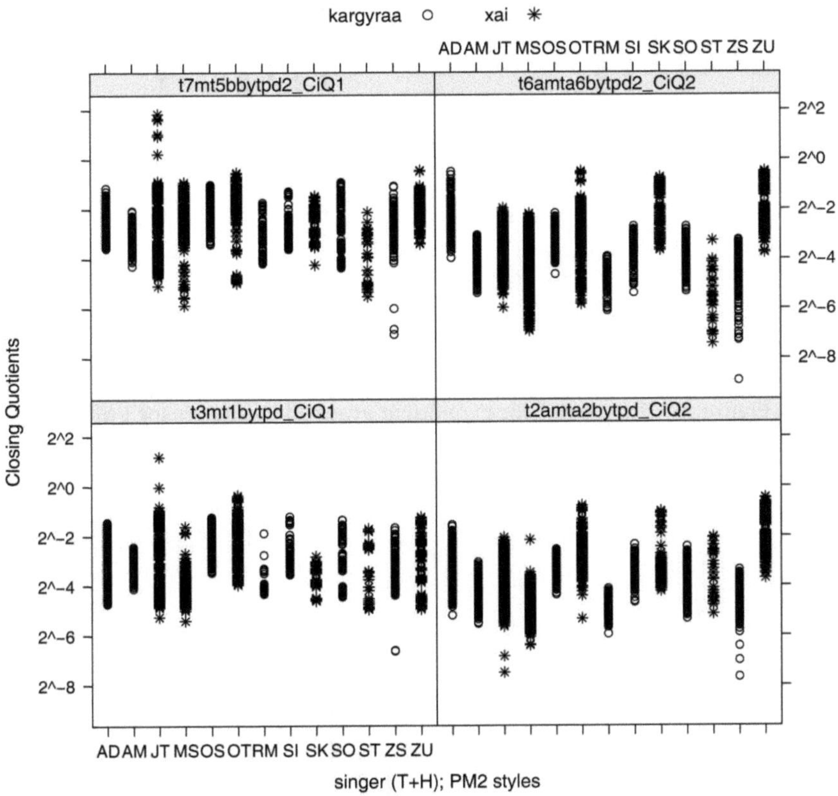

Figure A.7: Lx closing quotients grouped by singers in PM2

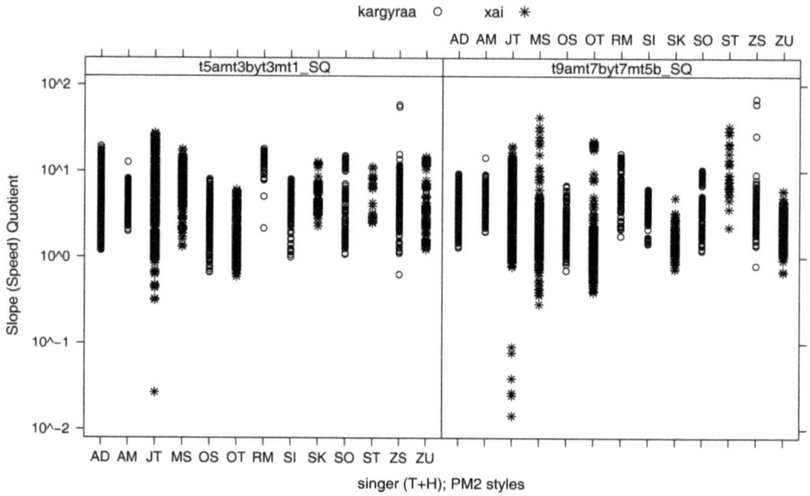

Figure A.8: Lx speed (slope) quotient grouped by singers for PM2

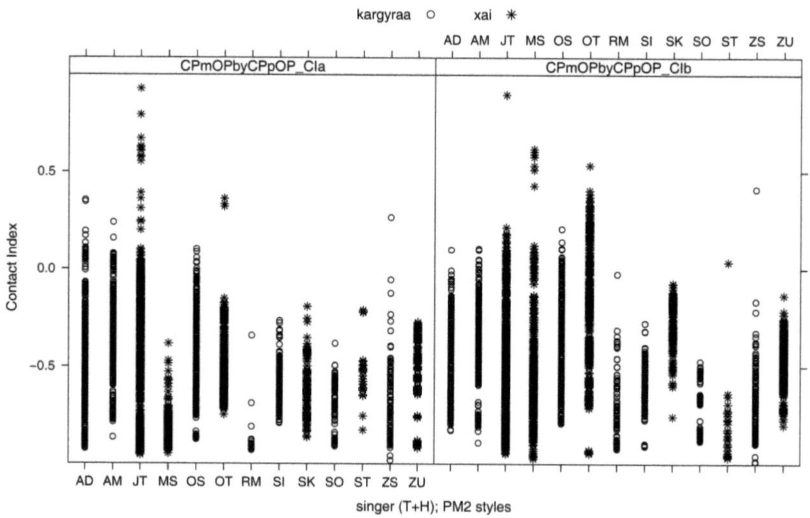

Figure A.9: Lx contact indeces grouped by singer in PM2

A.2.2 Spectra and Spectrograms

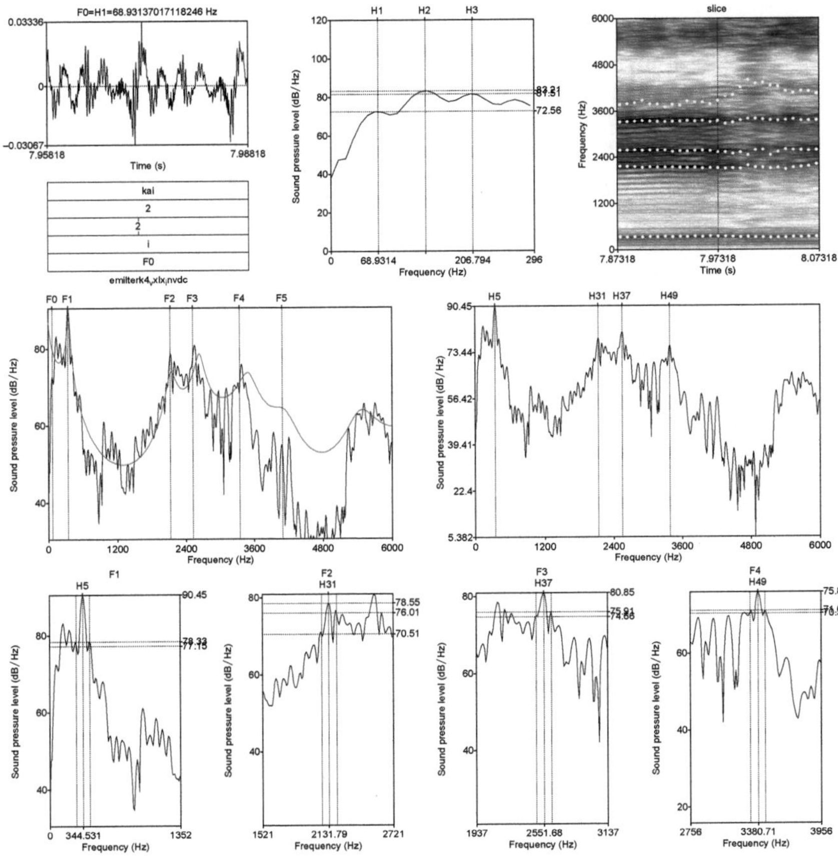

Figure A.10: Formant spectra and spectrograms *emilterk4_vxlx_invdct_2* (ET(A)); Note the extreme low H1 of 68.9Hz; The five tiers at the bottom of the panel in the upper left corner contain information about (1) style name, (2) phonation mode, (3) measure point, (4) vowel quality or harmonic, and (5) comments.

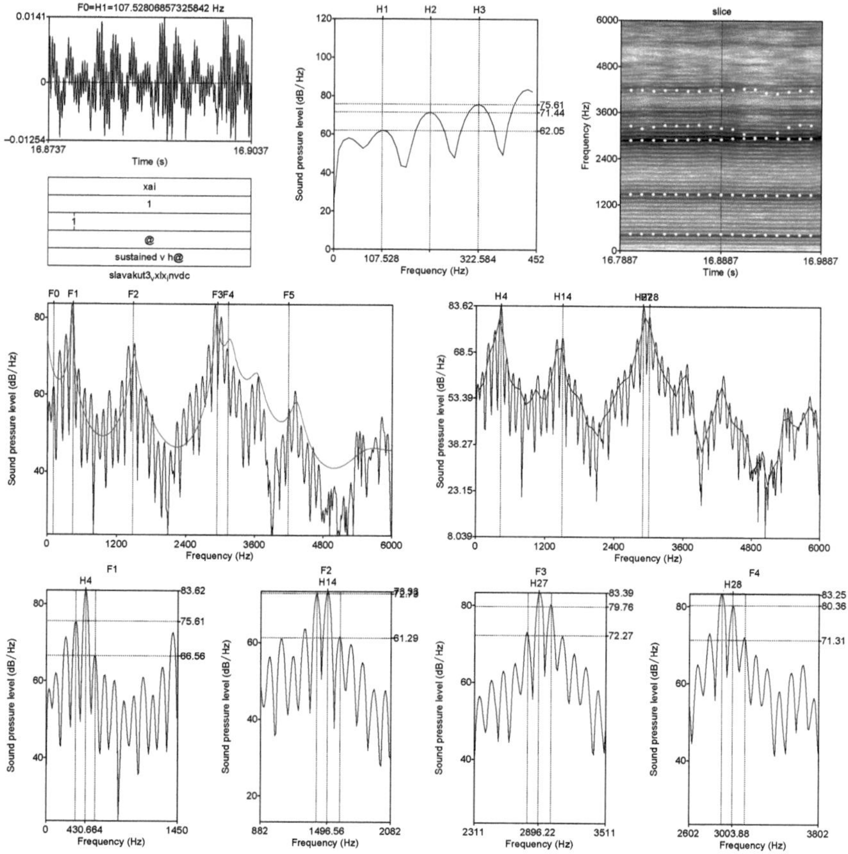

Figure A.11: Formant spectra and spectrograms *slavakut3_vxlx_invdcf_01* (SK(H)); This sample represents a case where F3(/F4) is very wide and prominent and the detection of the upper formants (F5 etc.) has been confused by the tracking algorithm.

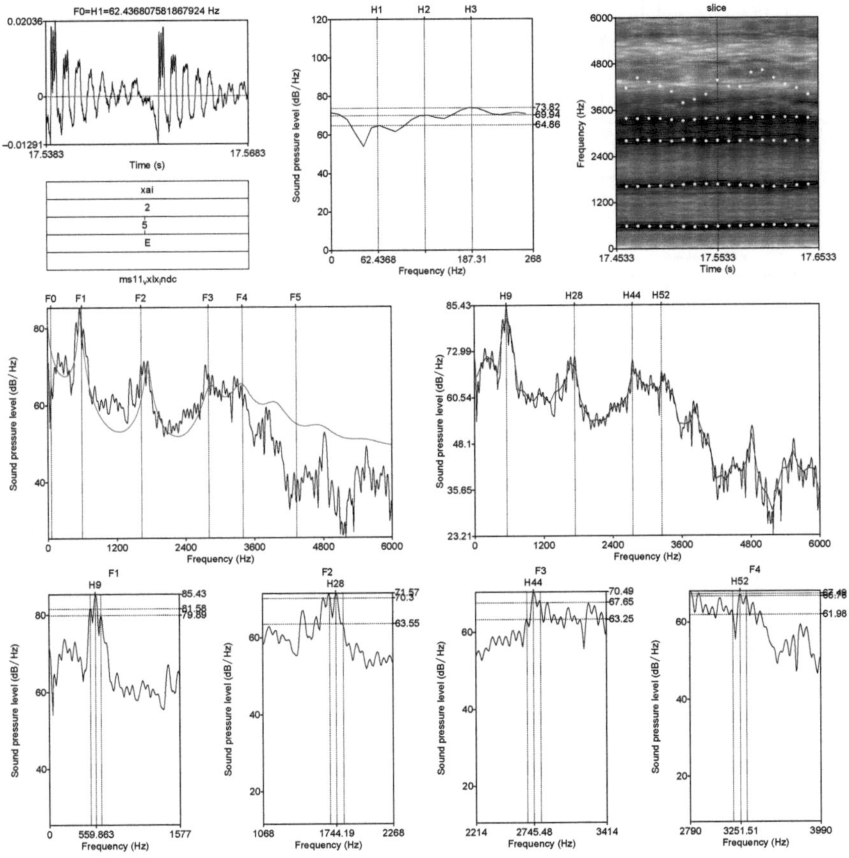

Figure A.12: Formant spectra and spectrograms *ms*11_*vxlx*_*indcf*_05 (MS(H))

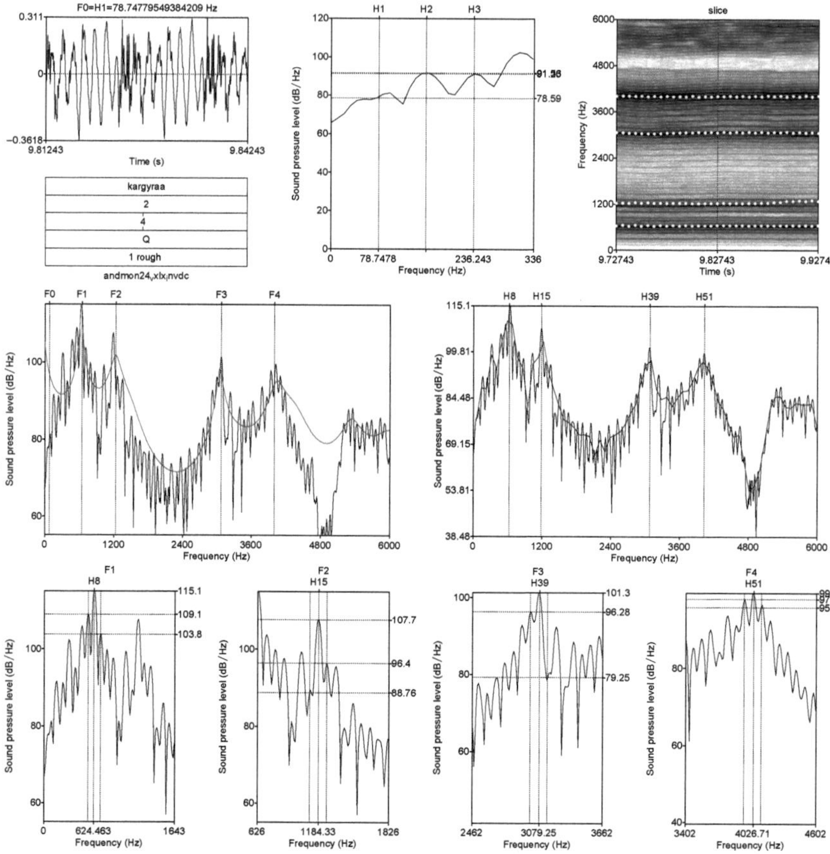

Figure A.13: Formant spectra and spectrograms *andmon24_vxlx_invdct_4* (AM(T))

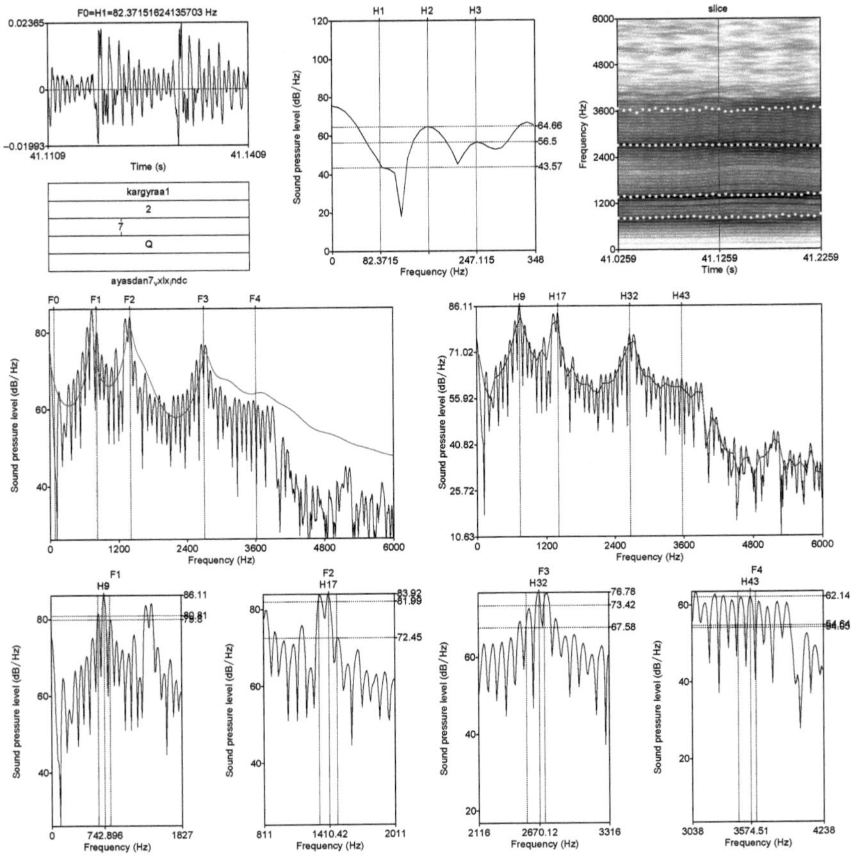

Figure A.14: Formant spectra and spectrograms *ayasdan7_vxlx_indcf_07* (AD(T))

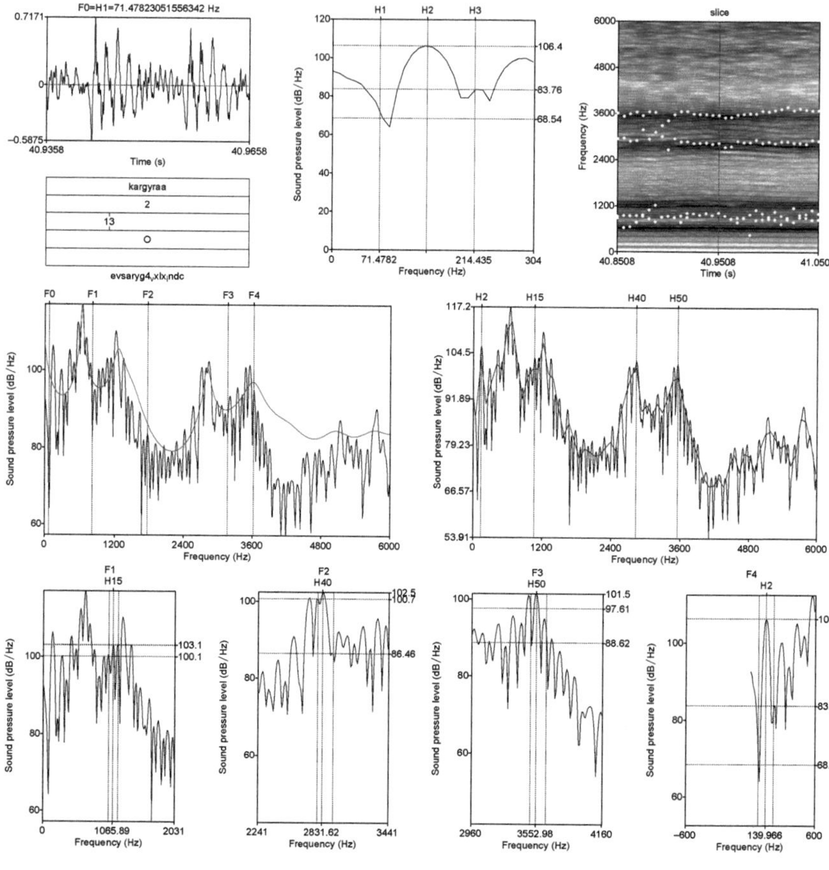

Figure A.15: Formant spectra and spectrograms *evsaryg4_vxlx_indcf*_013 (ES(T))

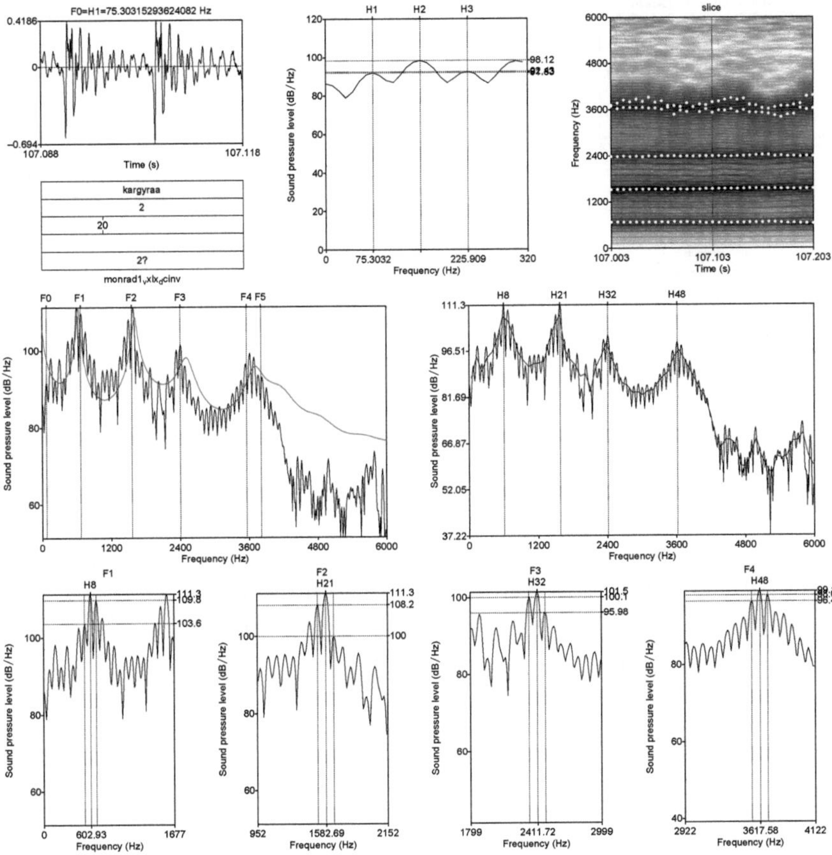

Figure A.16: Formant spectra and spectrograms *monrad1_vxlx_dcinvf_020* (MR(T))

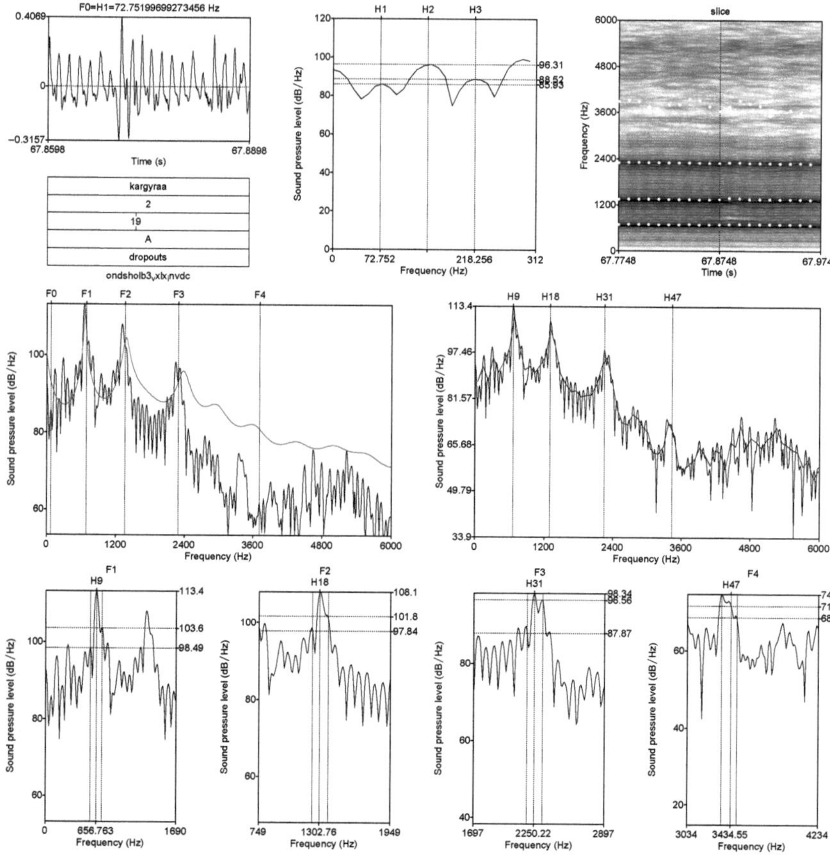

Figure A.17: Formant spectra and spectrograms *ondsholb3_vxlx_invdcf_*019 (OS(T))

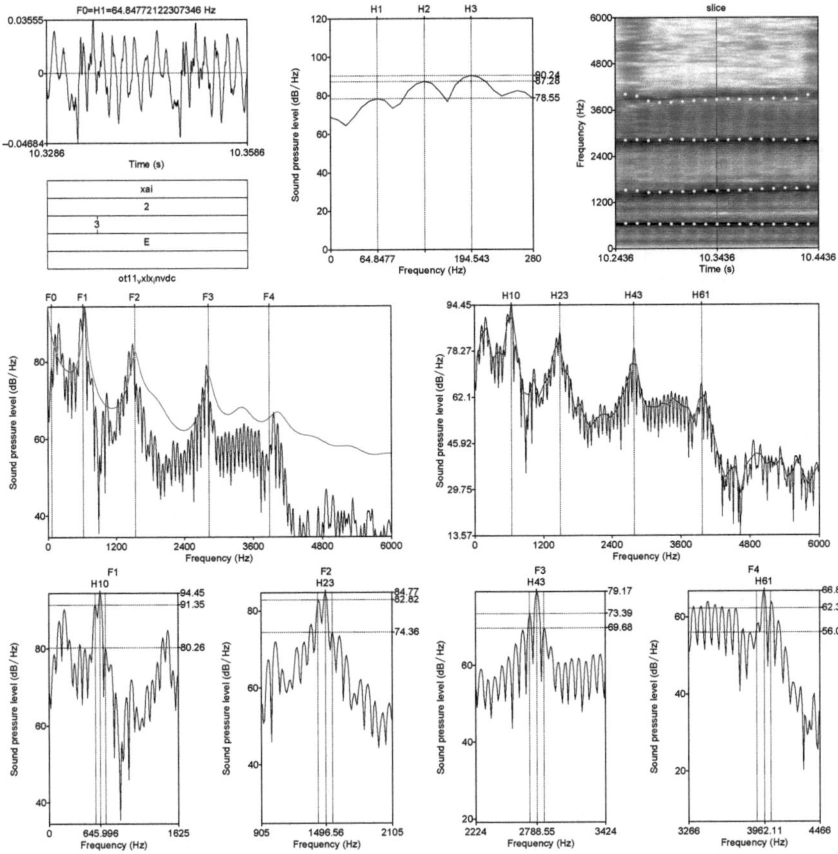

Figure A.18: Formant spectra and spectrograms *ot*11_*vxlx*_*invdcf*_03 (OT(T))

A.2.3 Waveform and Waterfall Plots

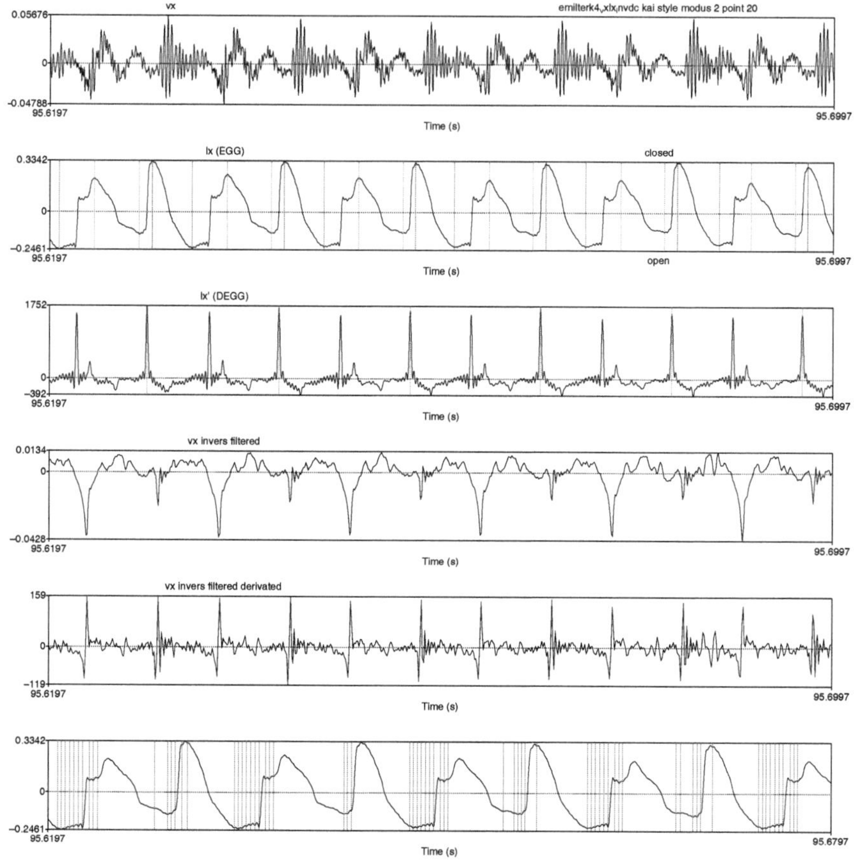

Figure A.19: Vx, Lx, dLx, invfilVx, and derivated-inverse-filtered-vx waveform of sample *emilterk4_vxlx_invdc_20* (ET(A)); the lowest panel shows the detected maxima during contacting phase

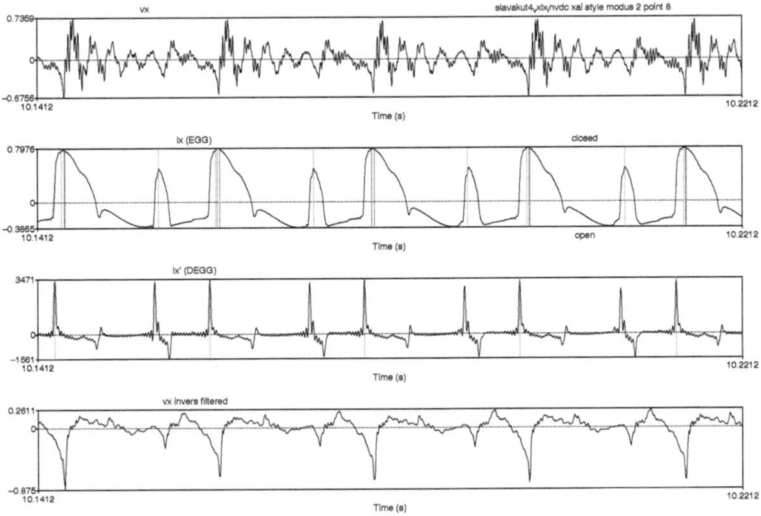

Figure A.20: Vx, Lx, dLx, invfilVx, and derivated-inverse-filtered-vx waveform of sample *slavakut4_vxlx_invdc_8* (SK(H))

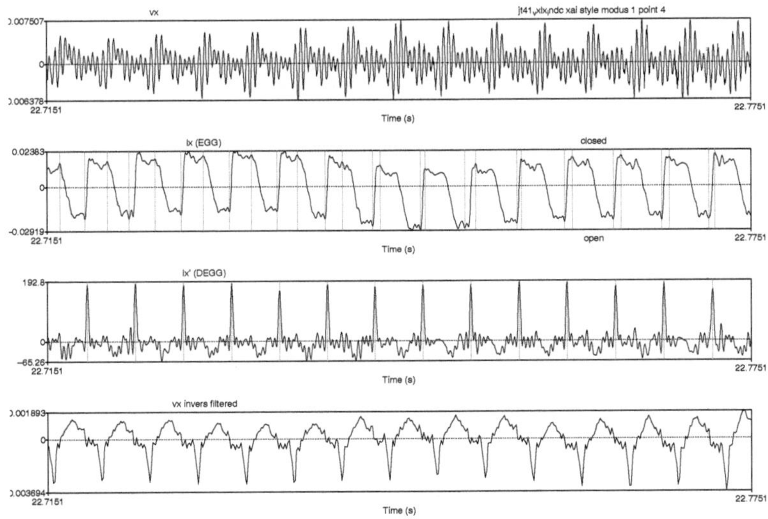

Figure A.21: Vx, Lx, dLx, invfilVx, and derivated-inverse-filtered-vx waveform of sample *jt41_vxlx_indc_4* (JT(H))

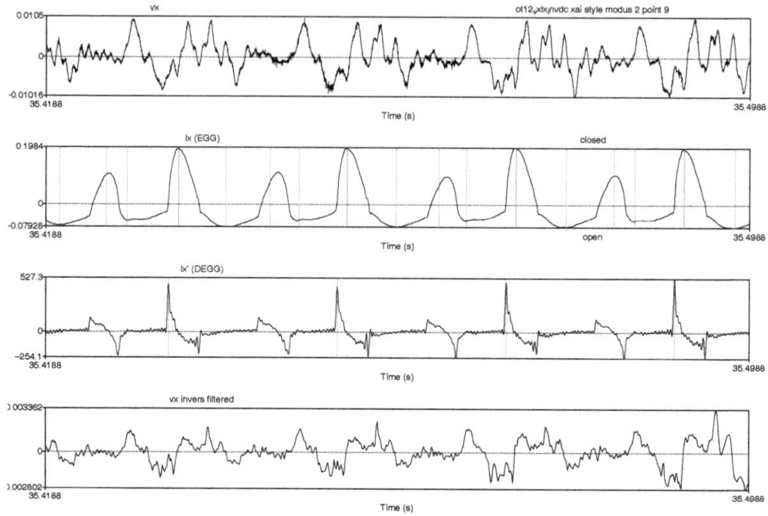

Figure A.22: Vx, Lx, dLx, invfilVx, and derivated-inverse-filtered-vx waveform of sample *ot12_vxlx_invdc_9* (OT(H))

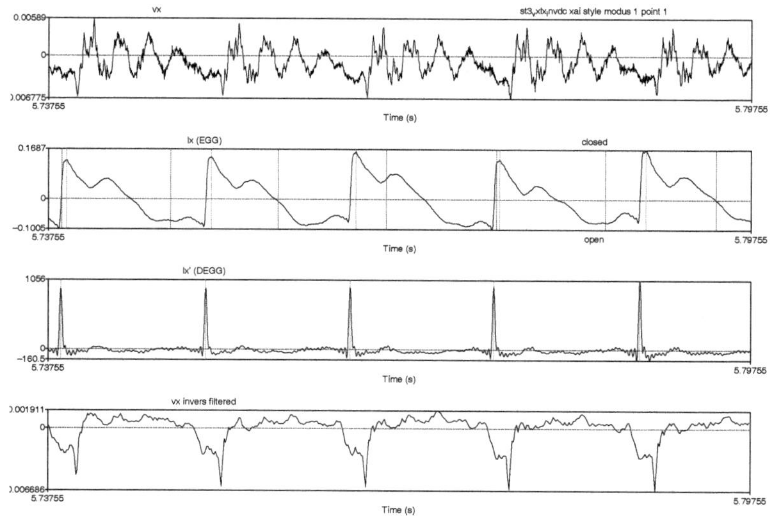

Figure A.23: Vx, Lx, dLx, invfilVx, and derivated-inverse-filtered-vx waveform of sample *st3_vxlx_invdc_1* (ST(H))

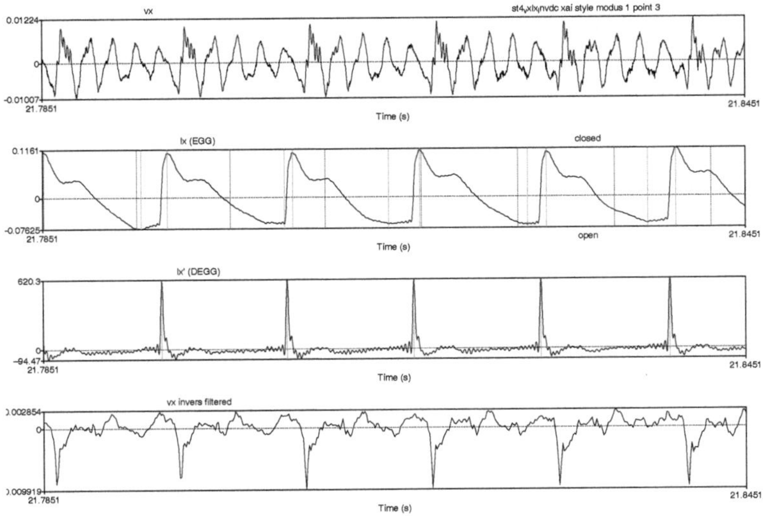

Figure A.24: Vx, Lx, dLx, invfilVx, and derivated-inverse-filtered-vx waveform of sample *st4_vxlx_invdc_3* (ST(H))

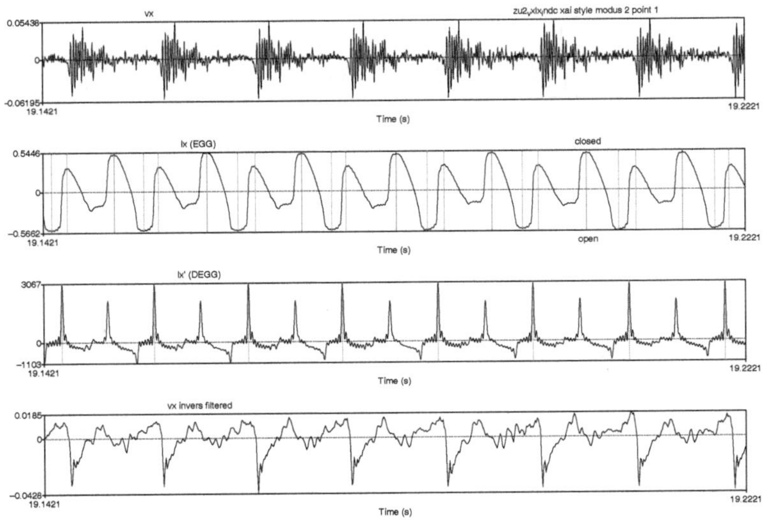

Figure A.25: Vx, Lx, dLx, invfilVx, and derivated-inverse-filtered-vx waveform of sample *zu2_vxlx_indc_1* (ZU(H))

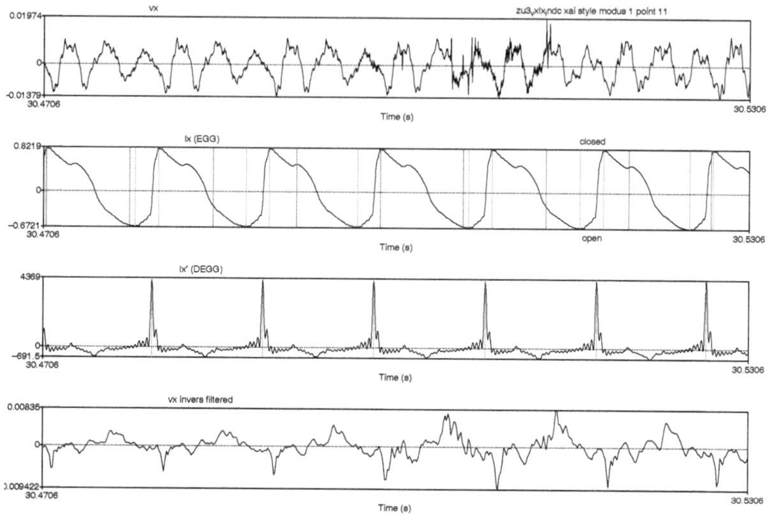

Figure A.26: Vx, Lx, dLx, invfilVx, and derivated-inverse-filtered-vx waveform of sample *zu3_vxlx_indc*_11 (ZU(H))

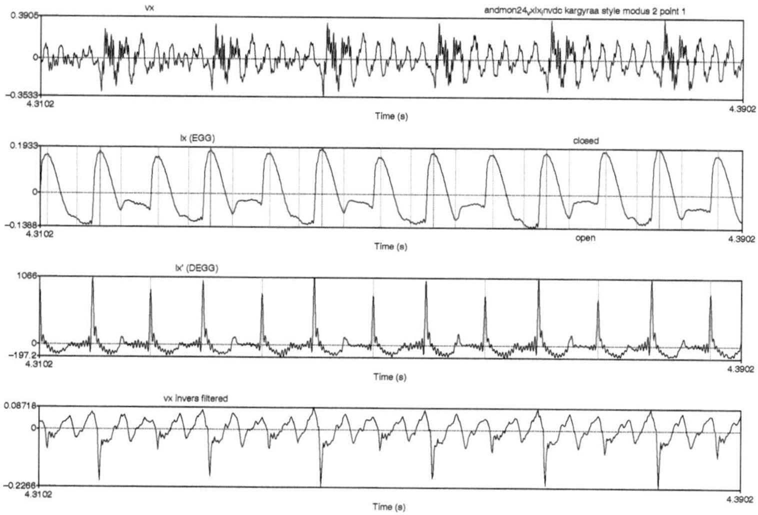

Figure A.27: Vx, Lx, dLx, invfilVx, and derivated-inverse-filtered-vx waveform of sample *andmon24_vxlx_invdc*_1 (AM(T))

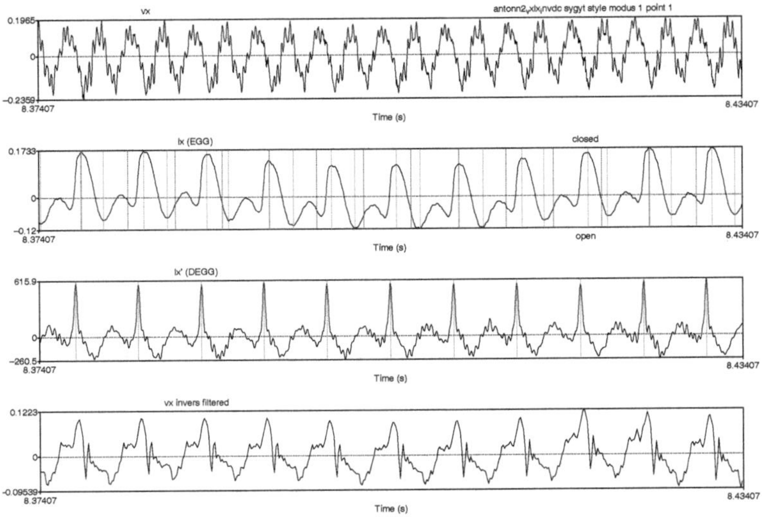

Figure A.28: Vx, Lx, dLx, invfilVx, and derivated-inverse-filtered-vx waveform of sample *antonn2_vxlx_invdc_1* (AN(T))

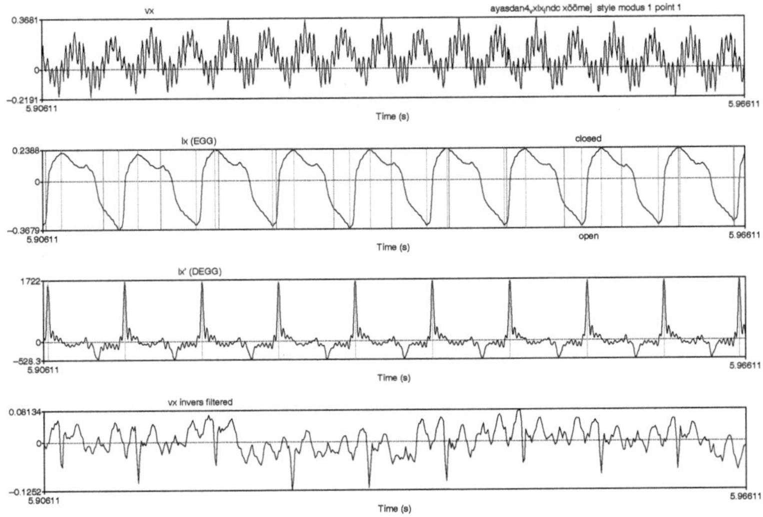

Figure A.29: Vx, Lx, dLx, invfilVx, and derivated-inverse-filtered-vx waveform of sample *ayasdan4_vxlx_indc_1* (AD(T))

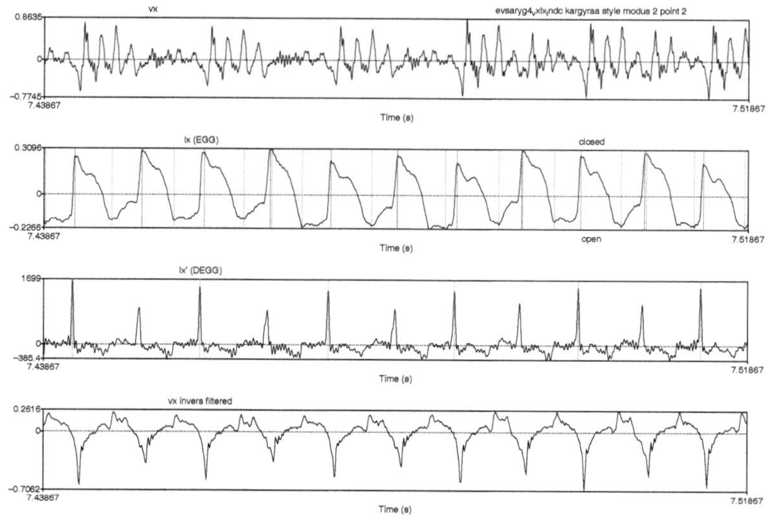

Figure A.30: Vx, Lx, dLx, invfilVx, and derivated-inverse-filtered-vx waveform of sample *evsaryg4_vxlx_indc_2* (ES(T))

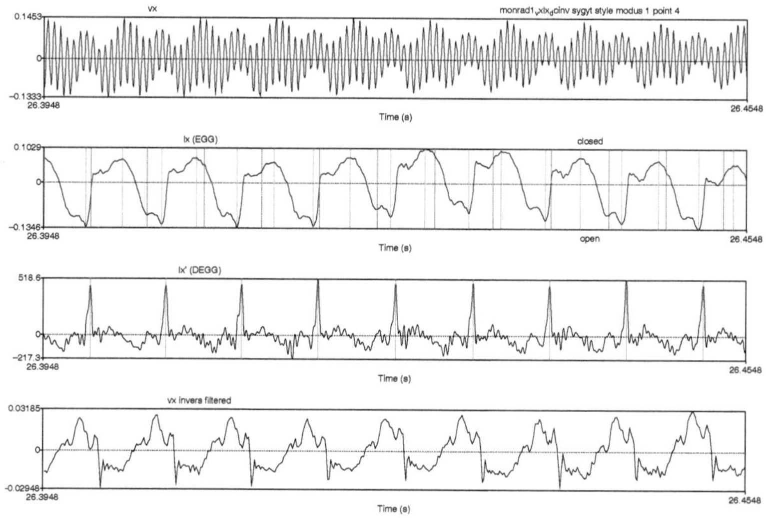

Figure A.31: Vx, Lx, dLx, invfilVx, and derivated-inverse-filtered-vx waveform of sample *monrad1_vxlx_dcinv_4* (MR(T))

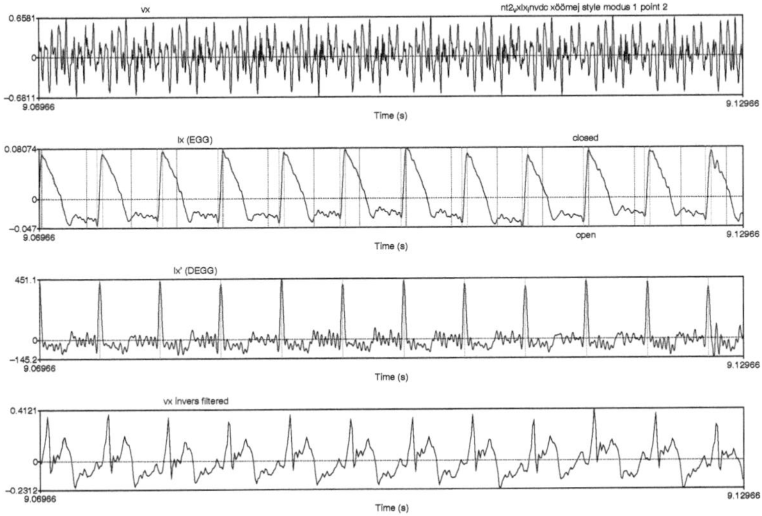

Figure A.32: Vx, Lx, dLx, invfilVx, and derivated-inverse-filtered-vx waveform of sample *nt2_vxlx_invdc_2* (NT(H))

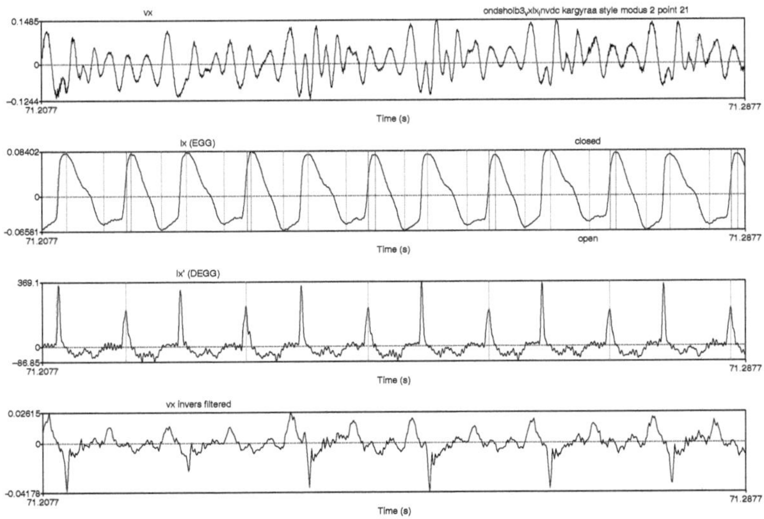

Figure A.33: Vx, Lx, dLx, invfilVx, and derivated-inverse-filtered-vx waveform of sample *ondsholb3_vxlx_invdc_21* (OS(T))

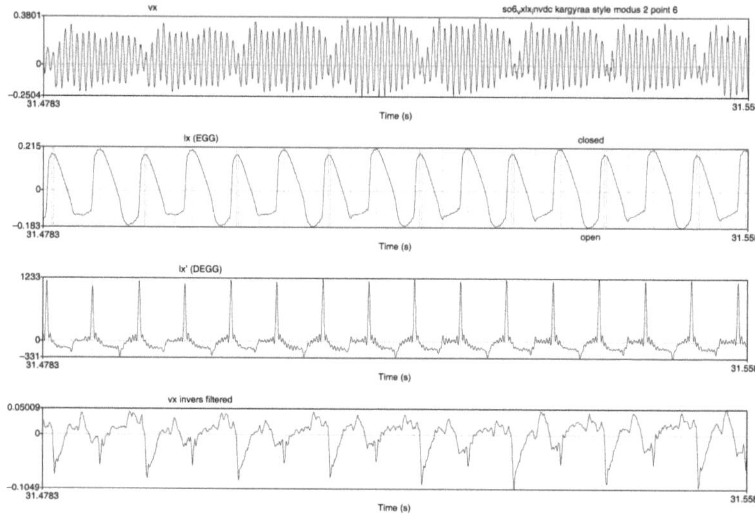

Figure A.34: Vx, Lx, dLx, invfilVx, and derivated-inverse-filtered-vx waveform of sample *so6_vxlx_invdc*_6 (SO(T))

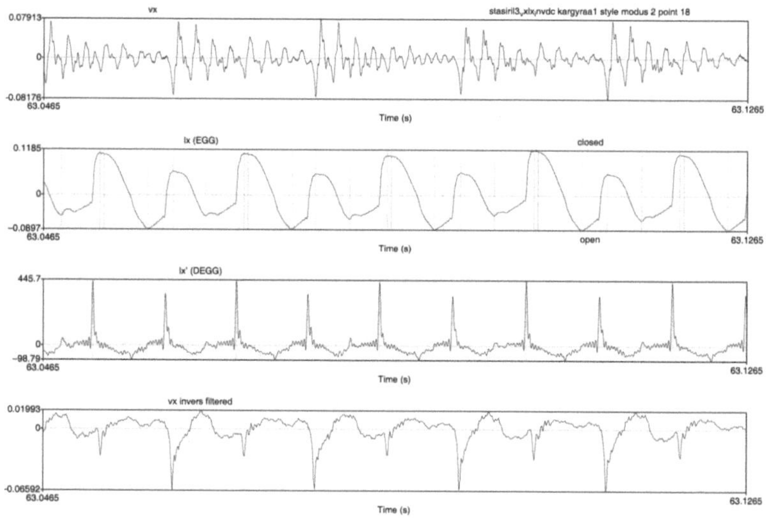

Figure A.35: Vx, Lx, dLx, invfilVx, and derivated-inverse-filtered-vx waveform of sample *stasiril3_vxlx_invdc*_18 (SI(T))

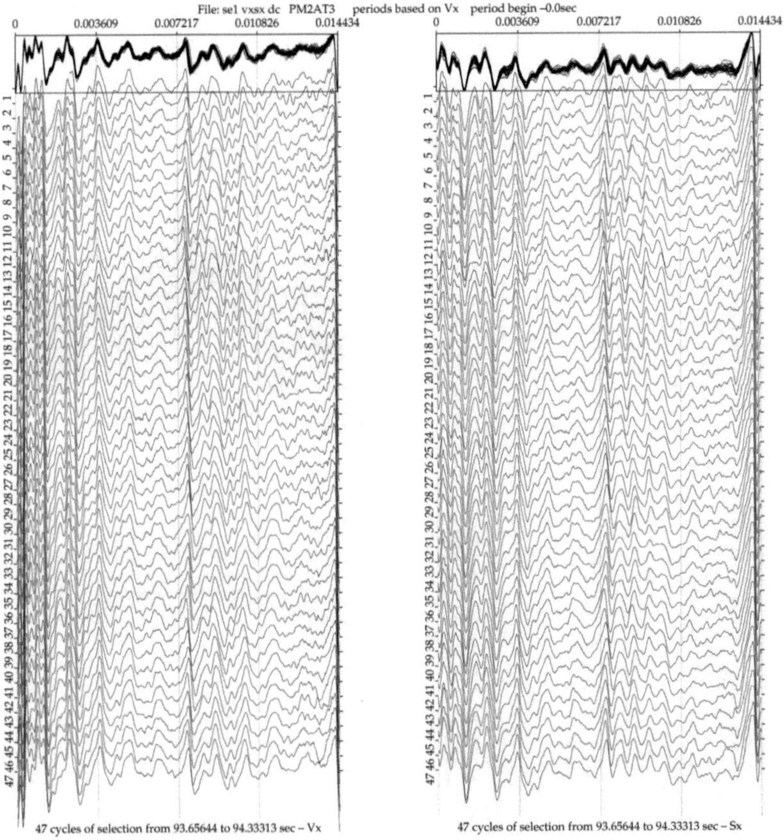

Figure A.36: SxVx waterfall plot phonation mode 2 SE(T)

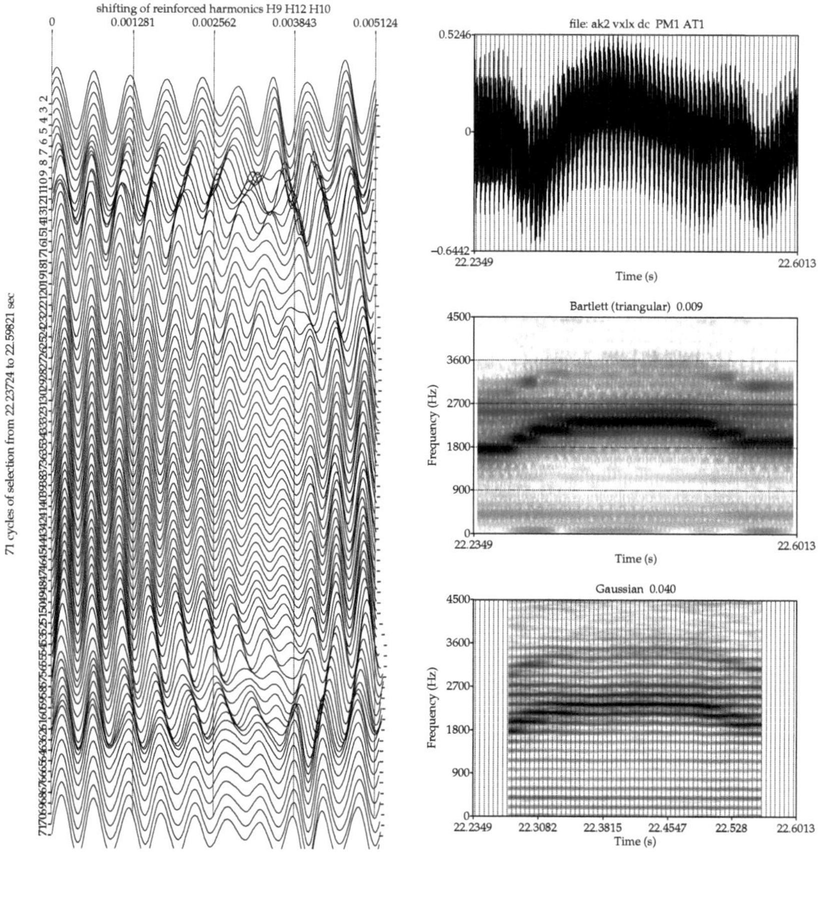

Figure A.37: waterfall plot and spectra of Vx sample singer AK(T)

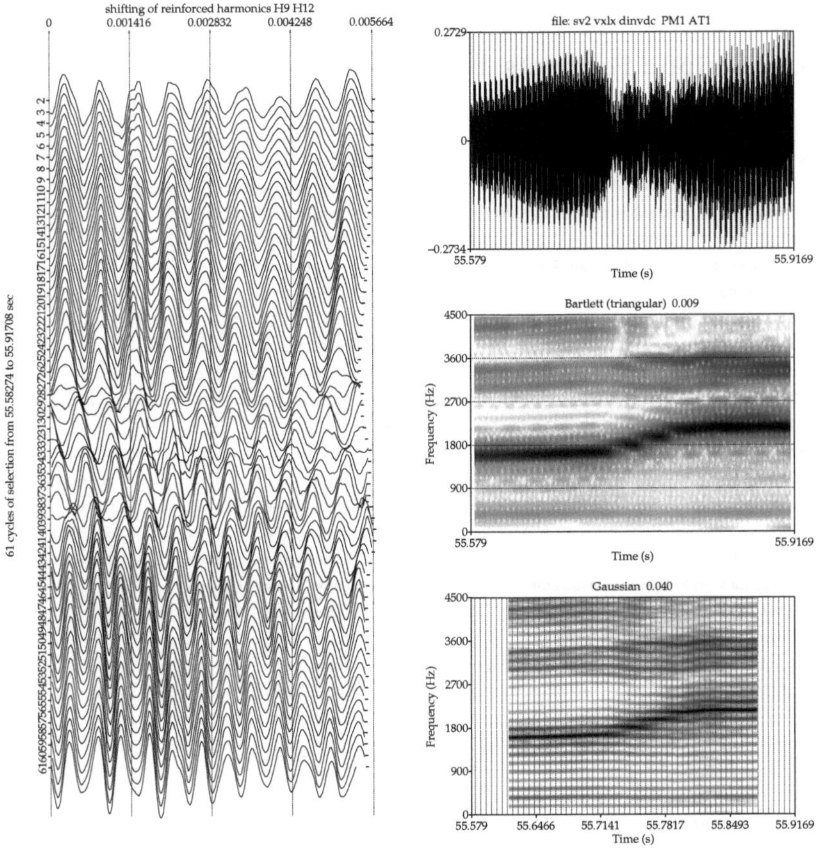

Figure A.38: waterfall plot and spectra of Vx sample singer SV(T)

A.3 Scripts

In order to perform recurrent analysis steps in a semi-automatical way PRAAT allows a number of commands that are available via script. The scripts used for analysis in the present study are given here:

A.3.1 Script 1: Formants, Bandwidths, Harmonics

```
#Spectra (Sona, Spectrum, Ltas) of
#chosen points ##########Formants
#IntervalTier #1phonationtyp/singing style
#IntervalTier #2 modus
#Vowel Token selected by labeled Points in
#PointTier #3
#IntervalTier#4 vowel/musical note or
#prominent overtone
####IntervalTier#5 comment
#SD, Mn & Md of F1 F2 F3 F4 F5 from Point
#the following objects must already exist:
#Sound
#TextGrid
#Formant
#FormantTier
#Pitch ==> F0
#Spectrogramm --> Spectrum slice --> Ltas
name$="st2_vxlx_invdc"
input_directory$="E:\...\'name$'"
output_directory$="E:\...\'name$'\form4spec"
singer$="ST"
Read two Sounds from stereo file...
...'input_directory$'\'name$'.wav
select Sound right
Remove
select Sound left
Rename... 'name$'
select Sound 'name$'
To Formant (burg)... 0 5 5000 0.045 50
Down to FormantTier
select Sound 'name$'
To Pitch (cc)...
...0 45 15 yes 0.03 0.45 0.01 0.35 0.14 300
select Sound 'name$'
To Spectrogram...
...0.035 6000 0.002 20 Hamming
...(raised sine-squared)
##in case of re-initiation#############
name$="emilterk5_vxlx_invdc"
input_directory$="E:\...\'name$'2"
output_directory$="E:\..\'name$'2\form4spec"
singer$="ET"
Erase all
select TextGrid 'name$'
########Insert new tiers
anzahlpoints=Get number of points... 3
####Table
Create Table... 'name$'_h 'anzahlpoints' 87
Set column label (index)... 1 indeces
Set column label (index)... 2 token
Set column label (index)... 3 pointtime
Set column label (index)... 4 timehindex
Set column label (index)... 5 F0
Set column label (index)... 6 F1
Set column label (index)... 7 F2
Set column label (index)... 8 F3
Set column label (index)... 9 F4
Set column label (index)... 10 F5
Set column label (index)... 11 F1mn
Set column label (index)... 12 F2mn
Set column label (index)... 13 F3mn
Set column label (index)... 14 F4mn
Set column label (index)... 15 F5mn
Set column label (index)... 16 F1md
Set column label (index)... 17 F2md
Set column label (index)... 18 F3md
Set column label (index)... 19 F4md
Set column label (index)... 20 F5md
Set column label (index)... 21 F1_H
Set column label (index)... 22 F1_H_F
Set column label (index)... 23 F1_H_A
Set column label (index)... 24 F1_Hm1
```

```
Set column label (index)... 25 F1_Hm1_F
Set column label (index)... 26 F1_Hm1_A
Set column label (index)... 27 F1_Hp1
Set column label (index)... 28 F1_Hp1_F
Set column label (index)... 29 F1_Hp1_A
Set column label (index)... 30 F2_H
Set column label (index)... 31 F2_H_F
Set column label (index)... 32 F2_H_A
Set column label (index)... 33 F2_Hm1
Set column label (index)... 34 F2_Hm1_F
Set column label (index)... 35 F2_Hm1_A
Set column label (index)... 36 F2_Hp1
Set column label (index)... 37 F2_Hp1_F
Set column label (index)... 38 F2_Hp1_A
Set column label (index)... 39 F3_H
Set column label (index)... 40 F3_H_F
Set column label (index)... 41 F3_H_A
Set column label (index)... 42 F3_Hm1
Set column label (index)... 43 F3_Hm1_F
Set column label (index)... 44 F3_Hm1_A
Set column label (index)... 45 F3_Hp1
Set column label (index)... 46 F3_Hp1_F
Set column label (index)... 47 F3_Hp1_A
Set column label (index)... 48 F4_H
Set column label (index)... 49 F4_H_F
Set column label (index)... 50 F4_H_A
Set column label (index)... 51 F4_Hm1
Set column label (index)... 52 F4_Hm1_F
Set column label (index)... 53 F4_Hm1_A
Set column label (index)... 54 F4_Hp1
Set column label (index)... 55 F4_Hp1_F
Set column label (index)... 56 F4_Hp1_A
Set column label (index)... 57 globmax_F
Set column label (index)... 58 globmax_A
Set column label (index)... 59 globmax_N
Set column label (index)... 60 H1_F
Set column label (index)... 61 H2_F
Set column label (index)... 62 H1_A
Set column label (index)... 63 H2_A
Set column label (index)... 64 H1-H2
Set column label (index)... 65 H3_F
Set column label (index)... 66 H3_A
Set column label (index)... 67 H1-H3
Set column label (index)... 68 B1
Set column label (index)... 69 B2
Set column label (index)... 70 B3
Set column label (index)... 71 B4
Set column label (index)... 72 B5
Set column label (index)... 78 vowtone
Set column label (index)... 79 style
Set column label (index)... 80 mode
Set column label (index)... 81 singer
Set column label (index)... 82 file
####################
select TextGrid 'name$'
for i from 1 to 'anzahlpoints'
pointtime=Get time of point... 3 i
intervnr=Get interval at time... 2 'pointtime'
intervt$=Get label of interval... 2 'intervnr'
style$=Get label of interval... 1 'intervnr'
intervnr4=Get interval at time... 4 'pointtime'
vowtone$=Get label of interval... 4 'intervnr4'
#####Token label: Nummer$$Vokal
#####oder nur TokenNummer
#Set point text... 3 i 'i'$$'intervt$'
Set point text... 3 i 'i'
pointlebel$=Get label of point... 3 i
#########get formant values##############
select FormantTier 'name$'
hindex=Get high index from time... 'pointtime'
### hindex means high index =
###following next right point (index)
### in the pointtier
timehindex=Get time from index... 'hindex'
timehindexplus2=Get time from index... hindex+2
timehindexplus4=Get time from index... hindex+4
timehindexplus8=Get time from index... hindex+8
###### F1-5 an 3 points ########
formant11=Get value at time... 1 'timehindex'
...
formant51=Get value at time... 5 'timehindex'

formant11$ = fixed$ (formant11, 2)
if formant11$ = "--undefined--"
formant11$ = "0"
endif
...
formant51$ = fixed$ (formant51, 2)
if formant51$ = "--undefined--"
formant51$ = "0"
endif
select Formant 'name$'
bandw11=Get bandwidth at time... 1
...'timehindex' Hertz Linear
...
bandw51=Get bandwidth at time... 5
```

```
...'timehindex' Hertz Linear
###formating numeric values###
bandw11$ = fixed$ (bandw11, 2)
if bandw11$ = "--undefined--"
bandw11$ = "0"
endif
...
bandw51$ = fixed$ (bandw51, 2)
if bandw51$ = "--undefined--"
bandw51$ = "0"
endif
####
formant1mn=Get mean... 1
...'timehindex' 'timehindexplus8' Hertz
...
formant5mn=Get mean... 5
...'timehindex' 'timehindexplus8' Hertz
####
formant1md=Get quantile... 1
...'timehindex' 'timehindexplus8' Hertz 0.5
...
formant5md=Get quantile... 5
...'timehindex' 'timehindexplus8' Hertz 0.5
###
formant1mn$ = fixed$ (formant1mn, 2)
if formant1mn$ = "--undefined--"
formant1mn$ = "0"
endif
...
formant5mn$ = fixed$ (formant5mn, 2)
if formant5mn$ = "--undefined--"
formant5mn$ = "0"
endif
formant1md$ = fixed$ (formant1md, 2)
if formant1md$ = "--undefined--"
formant1md$ = "0"
endif
...
formant5md$ = fixed$ (formant5md, 2)
if formant5md$ = "--undefined--"
formant5md$ = "0"
endif
########spectra###########
select Spectrogram 'name$'
To Spectrum (slice)... 'timehindex'
LPC smoothing... 9 50
Rename... 'name$'lpc
select Spectrum 'name$'
To Ltas (1-to-1)
select Spectrum 'name$'
To Ltas... 90
Rename... 'name$'1
#######cut beginning end
cutb='timehindex'-0.015
cute='timehindex'+0.015
#########
select Pitch 'name$'
f0=Get value at time...
...'timehindex' Hertz Linear
f0r=round(f0)
#########
Viewport... 0 4 0 2.5
select Sound 'name$'
Draw... 'cutb' 'cute' 0 0 yes curve
Text top... no F0=H1='f0' Hz
########
Viewport... 0 4 1.25 4.25
select  TextGrid 'name$'
Draw... 'cutb' 'cute' no yes no
Text bottom... no 'name$'

lowerbh1 = 'f0r' - 10
upperbh1 = 'f0r' + 10
lowerbh2 = ('f0r' * 2) - 10
upperbh2 = ('f0r' * 2) + 10
select Spectrogram 'name$'
Viewport... 8 12 0 4
sonab='timehindex'-0.1
sonae='timehindex'+0.1
Paint... 'sonab' 'sonae'
...0 0 100 yes 70 6 0 yes
One mark bottom...
...'timehindex' yes yes yes
Marks left... 6 yes yes no
Text top... no slice
select Formant 'name$'
Red
Speckle... 'sonab' 'sonae' 6000 30 no
Black
Viewport... 0 6 4 8
select Spectrum 'name$'
Draw... 0 0 0 0 yes
Marks bottom... 6 yes yes no
select Spectrum 'name$'lpc
Red
Draw... 0 0 0 0 no
```



```
Black
select Spectrum 'name$'
One mark top... 'f0r' no yes yes F0
if 'formant1mn$'>0
One mark top... 'formant1mn$' no yes yes F1
endif
...
if 'formant5mn$'>0
One mark top... 'formant5mn$' no yes yes F5
endif
Viewport... 6 12 4 8
select Ltas 'name$'
glmaxfq=Get frequency of maximum... 0 0 None
glminfq=Get frequency of minimum... 0 0 None
globmax=Get maximum... 0 0 None
globmin=Get minimum... 0 0 None
gn='glmaxfq'/'f0'
gn=round (gn)
f2_h_b1='formant21$'-100
#-0.5*'bandw21$'
f2_h_b2='formant21$'+100
#+0.5*'bandw21$'
f2_h_f=Get frequency of maximum...
...'f2_h_b1' 'f2_h_b2' None
f2_h_a=Get maximum... 'f2_h_b1' 'f2_h_b2' None
f2_h='f2_h_f'/'f0'
f2_h=round(f2_h)
f2_hm1='f2_h'-1
f2_hm1_f='f0'*'f2_hm1'
f2_hm1_a=Get value at frequency...
...'f2_hm1_f' Nearest
f2_hp1='f2_h'+1
f2_hp1_f='f0'*'f2_hp1'
f2_hp1_a=Get value at frequency...
...'f2_hp1_f' Nearest
Draw... 0 0 'globmin' 'globmax' yes curve
Marks left... 6 yes yes no
Marks bottom... 6 yes yes no
One mark top... 'f2_h_f' no yes yes H'f2_h'
##lower border gl maxim fq######
hbandw2='bandw21$'/2
lwbglmaxfq='formant11$'+'bandw11$'
f1_h_b1='formant11$'-100
if 'formant11$'<100
f1_h_b1=0
endif
#-0.5*'bandw11$'
f1_h_b2='formant11$'+100
#+0.5*'bandw11$'
f1_h_f=Get frequency of maximum...
...'f1_h_b1' 'f1_h_b2' None
f1_h_a=Get maximum...
...'f1_h_b1' 'f1_h_b2' None
f1_h='f1_h_f'/'f0'
f1_h=round(f1_h)
f1_hm1='f1_h'-1
f1_hm1_f='f0'*'f1_hm1'
f1_hm1_a=Get value at frequency...
...'f1_hm1_f' Nearest
f1_hp1='f1_h'+1
f1_hp1_f='f0'*'f1_hp1'
f1_hp1_a=Get value at frequency...
...'f1_hp1_f' Nearest
#H1, H2, H1-H2
h1_db = Get value at frequency...
...'f0' Nearest
h1_f = 'f0'
h2_f = 2*'f0'
h2_db = Get value at frequency...
...'h2_f' Nearest
h1_h2 = 'h1_db'-'h2_db'
h3_f = 3*'f0'
h3_db = Get value at frequency...
...'h3_f' Nearest
h1_h3 = 'h1_db'-'h3_db'
##higher border #####
hgbglmaxfq='formant31$'-2*'bandw31$'
hgbglmaxfq2='formant31$'+2*'bandw31$'
highrmaxfq=Get frequency of maximum...
...'hgbglmaxfq' 'hgbglmaxfq2' None
highrmaxdb=Get maximum...
...'hgbglmaxfq' 'hgbglmaxfq2' None
f3_h_b1='formant31$'-200
#-0.5*'bandw31$'
f3_h_b2='formant31$'+100
#+0.5*'bandw31$'
f3_h_f=Get frequency of maximum...
...'f3_h_b1' 'f3_h_b2' None
f3_h_a=Get maximum...
...'f3_h_b1' 'f3_h_b2' None
f3_h='f3_h_f'/'f0'
f3_h=round(f3_h)
f3_hm1='f3_h'-1
f3_hm1_f='f0'*'f3_hm1'
f3_hm1_a=Get value at frequency...
...'f3_hm1_f' Nearest
```

```
f3_hp1='f3_h'+1
f3_hp1_f='f0'*'f3_hp1'
f3_hp1_a=Get value at frequency...
...'f3_hp1_f' Nearest
f4_h_b1='formant41$'-200
#-0.5*'bandw41$'
f4_h_b2='formant41$'+200
#+0.5*'bandw41$'
f4_h_f=Get frequency of maximum...
...'f4_h_b1' 'f4_h_b2' None
f4_h_a=Get maximum...
...'f4_h_b1' 'f4_h_b2' None
f4_h='f4_h_f'/'f0'
f4_h=round(f4_h)
f4_hm1='f4_h'-1
f4_hm1_f='f0'*'f4_hm1'
f4_hm1_a=Get value at frequency...
...'f4_hm1_f' Nearest
f4_hp1='f4_h'+1
f4_hp1_f='f0'*'f4_hp1'
f4_hp1_a=Get value at frequency...
...'f4_hp1_f' Nearest
One mark top... 'f1_h_f' no yes yes H'f1_h'
if 'formant31$'>0
One mark top... 'f3_h_f' no yes yes H'f3_h'
endif
if 'formant41$'>0
One mark top... 'f4_h_f' no yes yes H'f4_h'
endif
select Ltas 'name$'1
#Select outer viewport... 6 12 4 8
Blue
Draw... 0 0 'globmin' 'globmax' no curve
Black
#####the lower three spectra#########
#lb low border # hb high border
lb1='formant11$'-1000
lb1=round(lb1)
hb1='formant11$'+1000
hb1=round(hb1)
lb2='formant21$'-600
lb2=round(lb2)
hb2='formant21$'+600
hb2=round(hb2)
lb3='formant31$'-600
lb3=round(lb3)
hb3='formant31$'+600
hb3=round(hb3)
lb4='formant41$'-600
lb4=round(lb4)
hb4='formant41$'+600
hb4=round(hb4)
select Spectrum 'name$'
Viewport... 4 8 0 4
Draw... 0 2*'upperbh2' 0 120 yes curve
One mark bottom... 'h1_f' yes yes yes
One mark bottom... 'h2_f' no yes yes
One mark bottom... 3*'f0' yes yes yes
One mark top... 'h1_f' no yes no H1
One mark top... 'h2_f' no yes no H2
One mark top... 'h3_f' no yes no H3
One mark right... 'h1_db' yes yes yes
One mark right... 'h2_db' yes yes yes
One mark right... 'h3_db' yes yes yes
Viewport... 0 3 8 12
Draw... 0 'hb1' 0 0 yes curve
One mark bottom... 'f1_h_f' yes yes yes
One mark bottom... 'f1_hm1_f' no no yes
One mark bottom... 'f1_hp1_f' no no yes
One mark top... 'f1_h_f' no yes no H'f1_h'
One mark right... 'f1_h_a' yes yes yes
One mark right... 'f1_hm1_a' yes yes yes
One mark right... 'f1_hp1_a' yes yes yes
Text top... yes F1
Viewport... 3 6 8 12
Draw... 'lb2' 'hb2' 0 0 yes curve
One mark bottom... 'f2_h_f' yes yes yes
One mark bottom... 'f2_hm1_f' no no yes
One mark bottom... 'f2_hp1_f' no no yes
One mark top... 'f2_h_f' no yes no H'f2_h'
One mark right... 'f2_h_a' yes yes yes
One mark right... 'f2_hm1_a' yes yes yes
One mark right... 'f2_hp1_a' yes yes yes
Text top... yes F2
Viewport... 6 9 8 12
Draw... 'lb3' 'hb3' 0 0 yes
One mark bottom... 'f3_h_f' yes yes yes
One mark bottom... 'f3_hm1_f' no no yes
One mark bottom... 'f3_hp1_f' no no yes
One mark top... 'f3_h_f' no yes no H'f3_h'
One mark right... 'f3_h_a' yes yes yes
One mark right... 'f3_hm1_a' yes yes yes
One mark right... 'f3_hp1_a' yes yes yes
Text top... yes F3
if 'formant41$'>0
Viewport... 9 12 8 12
```



```
Draw... 'lb4' 'hb4' 0 0 yes curve
One mark bottom... 'f4_h_f' yes yes yes
One mark bottom... 'f4_hm1_f' no no yes
One mark bottom... 'f4_hp1_f' no no yes
One mark top... 'f4_h_f' no yes no H'f4_h'
One mark right... 'f4_h_a' yes yes yes
One mark right... 'f4_hm1_a' yes yes yes
One mark right... 'f4_hp1_a' yes yes yes
Text top... yes F4
endif
pause ok?
########fill table########################
select Table 'name$'_h
Set numeric value... i indeces 'i'
...
Set string value... i file 'name$'
########Save & Remove #############
Viewport... 0 12 0 12
if 'i'<=9
Write to praat picture file...
...'output_directory$'\'name$'f_0'i'.prapic
Write to EPS file...
...'output_directory$'\'name$'f_0'i'.eps
Write to Windows metafile...
...'output_directory$'\'name$'f_0'i'.emf
else
Write to praat picture file...
...'output_directory$'\'name$'f_'i'.prapic
Write to EPS file...
...'output_directory$'\'name$'f_'i'.eps
Write to Windows metafile...
...'output_directory$'\'name$'f_'i'.emf
endif
Erase all
select Ltas 'name$'
Remove
select Ltas 'name$'1
Remove
select Spectrum 'name$'lpc
Remove
select Spectrum 'name$'
Remove
select TextGrid 'name$'
endfor
select Table 'name$'_h
Write to table file...
...'output_directory$'\'name$'_h.txt
```

A.3.2 Script 2: Obtaining Jitter, Shimmer, HNR, NHR, etc.

```
name$="ms13_vxlx_indc"
input_directory$="E:\...\'name$'"
output_directory$="E:\...\'name$'\"
singer$="MS"
#Read two Sounds from stereo file...
...'input_directory$'\'name$'.wav
#select Sound right
#Remove
#select Sound left
#Rename... 'name$'
select Sound 'name$'
To Pitch (cc)... 0 45 15 yes
...0.03 0.45 0.01 0.35 0.14 300
To PointProcess
###
Erase all
select TextGrid 'name$'
nrinterv=Get number of points... 3
Create Table... 'name$'_vJ 'nrinterv' 30
Set column label (index)... 1 intervindex
Set column label (index)... 2 intervbeg
Set column label (index)... 3 intervend
Set column label (index)... 4 nr_pd_interv
Set column label (index)... 5 nr_pt_interv
Set column label (index)... 6 modus
Set column label (index)... 7 periodmn
Set column label (index)... 8 periodsd
Set column label (index)... 9 pitchmn
Set column label (index)... 10 pitchmd
Set column label (index)... 11 jitterLoc
Set column label (index)... 12 jitterRAP
Set column label (index)... 13 jitterppq5
Set column label (index)... 14 shimmerLoc
Set column label (index)... 15 shimmerapq3
Set column label (index)... 16 shimmerapq5
Set column label (index)... 17 shimmerapq11
Set column label (index)... 18 HNRmn
Set column label (index)... 19 NHRmn
```

```
Set column label (index)... 20 autocorr
Set column label (index)... 21 ltasmn02
Set column label (index)... 22 ltasmn25
Set column label (index)... 23 ltasmn58
Set column label (index)... 24 ltasslope1
Set column label (index)... 25 ltasslope2
Set column label (index)... 26 ltasslope3
Set column label (index)... 27 vowtone
Set column label (index)... 28 style
Set column label (index)... 29 singer
Set column label (index)... 30 file
################################
for i from 1 to 'nrinterv'
select TextGrid 'name$'
intervbeg=Get time of point... 3 'i'
#Set the time of interval behind
#the plus (1=1second)
##number of intervals should be between
##40 and 100 otherwise jitter values
##become instable
intervend='intervbeg'+0.45
### read labels
interv_number=Get interval at time...
...2 'intervbeg'
interv_lab2=Get label of interval...
...2 'interv_number'
interv_number_tier4=Get interval at time...
...4 'intervbeg'
vowtone$=Get label of interval...
...4 'interv_number_tier4'
interv_number_tier1=Get interval at time...
...1 'intervbeg'
style_lab$=Get label of interval...
...1 'interv_number_tier1'
############
select Sound 'name$'
plus Pitch 'name$'
plus PointProcess 'name$'
report$ = Voice report...
...'intervbeg' 'intervend'
...45 300 1.3 1.6 0.03 0.45
autocorr = extractNumber (report$,
... "Mean autocorrelation: ")
hnrmn = extractNumber (report$,
..."Mean harmonics-to-noise ratio: ")
nhrmn = extractNumber (report$,
..."Mean noise-to-harmonics ratio: ")
select PointProcess 'name$'
periodmn=Get mean period...
...'intervbeg' 'intervend' 0.0001 0.02 1.8
periodmn$ = fixed$ (periodmn, 6)
if periodmn$ = "--undefined--"
periodmn$ = "0"
endif
periodsd=Get stdev period...
...'intervbeg' 'intervend' 0.0003 0.03 1.8
periodsd$ = fixed$ (periodsd, 6)
if periodsd$ = "--undefined--"
periodsd$ = "0"
endif
jitterLoc = Get jitter (local)...
...'intervbeg' 'intervend' 0.0003 0.03 1.8
jitterLoc$ = fixed$ (jitterLoc, 6)
if jitterLoc$ = "--undefined--"
jitterLoc$ = "0"
endif
jitterRAP = Get jitter (rap)...
...'intervbeg' 'intervend' 0.0003 0.03 1.8
jitterRAP$ = fixed$ (jitterRAP, 6)
if jitterRAP$ = "--undefined--"
jitterRAP$ = "0"
endif
jitterppq5 = Get jitter (ppq5)...
...'intervbeg' 'intervend' 0.0003 0.03 1.8
jitterppq5$ = fixed$ (jitterppq5, 6)
if jitterppq5$ = "--undefined--"
jitterppq5$ = "0"
endif
select Sound 'name$'
plus PointProcess 'name$'
shimmerLoc=Get shimmer (local)...
...'intervbeg' 'intervend' 0.0003 0.03 1.8 2
shimmerLoc$ = fixed$ (shimmerLoc, 6)
if shimmerLoc$ = "--undefined--"
shimmerLoc$ = "0"
endif
shimapq3=Get shimmer (apq3)...
...'intervbeg' 'intervend' 0.0003 0.03 1.8 2
shimapq3$ = fixed$ (shimapq3, 6)
if shimapq3$ = "--undefined--"
shimapq3$ = "0"
endif
shimapq5=Get shimmer (apq5)...
...'intervbeg' 'intervend' 0.0003 0.03 1.8 2
shimapq5$ = fixed$ (shimapq5, 6)
if shimapq5$ = "--undefined--"
```

```
shimapq5$ = "0"
endif
shimapq11=Get shimmer (apq11)...
...'intervbeg' 'intervend' 0.0003 0.03 1.8 2.4
shimapq11$ = fixed$ (shimapq11, 6)
if shimapq11$ = "--undefined--"
shimapq11$ = "0"
endif
autocorr$ = fixed$ (autocorr, 6)
if autocorr$ = "--undefined--"
autocorr$ = "0"
endif
hnrmn$ = fixed$ (hnrmn, 6)
if hnrmn$ = "--undefined--"
hnrmn$ = "0"
endif
nhrmn$ = fixed$ (nhrmn, 6)
if nhrmn$ = "--undefined--"
nhrmn$ = "0"
endif
####################
select Sound 'name$'
Edit
editor Sound 'name$'
Select... 'intervbeg' 'intervend'
Extract windowed selection...
...slice Hamming 1 yes
#endeditor
Close
select Sound slice
To Spectrum... yes
select Spectrum slice
To Ltas (1-to-1)
select Ltas slice
Rename... slice1
###########
select PointProcess 'name$'
plus Sound slice
To Ltas (only harmonics)...
...35 0.0001 0.02 1.4
Rename... slice2
############################
select Sound slice
To Ltas... 90
Select outer viewport... 0 6 8 12
select Sound slice
To Spectrogram... 0.025 8000 0.002 20
...Hamming (raised sine-squared)
Paint... 0 0 0 0 100 yes 50 6 0 yes
Marks left... 6 yes yes yes
Text top... no
.Hamming windowed selection
... - Vowel/Tone 'vowtone$'
############################
Select outer viewport... 0 6 0 4
select Spectrum slice
Draw... 0 8000 0 0 yes
Text top...
...no Spectrum at 'intervbeg' point 'i'
Select outer viewport... 6 12 0 4
select Ltas slice1
Draw... 0 4000 -20 80 yes curve
Marks bottom... 6 yes yes yes
Text top... no Ltas 1-to-1 - file
...name 'name$' -
...singer 'singer$' - 'style_lab$'
Select outer viewport... 6 12 4 8
select Ltas slice
Draw... 0 8000 -50 80 yes curve
One mark bottom... 2000 yes yes yes
One mark bottom... 5000 yes yes yes
Text top... no Ltas Band 90
################
select Ltas slice2
Select outer viewport... 6 12 8 12
ltasmin=Get minimum... 0 0 None
ltasmax=Get maximum... 0 0 None
ltashmin=Get frequency of minimum... 0 0 None
ltashmax=Get frequency of maximum... 0 0 None
Draw... 0 0 'ltasmin'-20 'ltasmax'+20 yes curve
Text top... no Ltas (only harmonics)
#One mark bottom... 'ltashmin' yes yes yes
One mark bottom... 'ltashmax' yes yes yes
#
Select outer viewport... 0 6 4 8
select Spectrum slice
Draw (log freq)... 10 10000 0 0 yes
Text top... no Log. Spectrum
#
select Ltas slice
ltasmn02 = Get mean... 0 2000 energy
ltasmn25 = Get mean... 2000 5000 energy
ltasmn58 = Get mean... 5000 8000 energy
ltasmn02db = Get mean... 0 2000 dB
ltasmn25db = Get mean... 2000 5000 dB
ltasmn58db = Get mean... 5000 8000 dB
```

```
# quasi SPI
ltasslope1 = Get slope...
...0 2000 2000 5000 energy
ltasslope2 = Get slope...
...0 2000 5000 8000 energy
ltasslope3 = Get slope...
...2000 5000 5000 8000 energy
#
Viewport... 6 12 4 8
One mark left... 'ltasmn02db' yes yes yes
One mark right... 'ltasmn02db' no yes no mn02
select Ltas slice
if 'i'<=9
Write to binary file... 'output_directory$'
...\Ltas\'name$'slice0'i'.Ltas
else
Write to binary file... 'output_directory$'
...\Ltas\'name$'slice'i'.Ltas
endif
#pause ok?
Viewport... 0 12 0 12
if 'i'<=9
Write to praat picture file...
...'output_directory$'
...\'name$'ltas_0'i'.prapic
Write to EPS file...
...'output_directory$'\'name$'ltas_0'i'.eps
Write to Windows metafile...
...'output_directory$'\'name$'ltas_0'i'.emf
else
Write to praat picture file...
...'output_directory$'
...\'name$'ltas_'i'.prapic
Write to EPS file...
...'output_directory$'\'name$'ltas_'i'.eps
Write to Windows metafile...
...'output_directory$'\'name$'ltas_'i'.emf
endif
Erase all
##############
select Sound slice
plus Spectrum slice
plus Spectrogram slice
plus Ltas slice
plus Ltas slice1
plus Ltas slice2
Remove
##############
select Table 'name$'_vJ
Set numeric value... i intervindex 'i'
...
Set string value... i file 'output_directory$'
endfor
###############
select Table 'name$'_vJ
Write to table file...
...'output_directory$'\'name$'_vJ.txt
```

A.3.3 Script 3: Vx, Lx, Inverse Filtering of Vx, EGG-Quotients

```
##Script for measuring in egg signal
##with double source mode
##at a ajustible time interval from a
##determinded pt
##(textgrid token pt in pttier)
##source is a stereo file with
##left vx channel and right lx channel
##Text grid must already exist as object
##(it1: style it2: mode pt3: token)
name$="ayasdan6_vxlx_indc"
input_directory$="D:\...\'name$'"
output_directory$="D:\...\'name$'"
singer$="AD"
##only activate the following line if
##stereo sound does not load the first time
Read two Sounds from stereo file...
...'input_directory$'\'name$'.wav
select Sound left
Rename... 'name$'_vx
select Sound right
Rename... 'name$'_lx
Read two Sounds from stereo file...
...'input_directory$'\'name$'.wav
select Sound right
Rename... 'name$'_dlx
select Sound left
Rename... 'name$'_vx_inv
Resample... 8000 50
```

```
To LPC (burg)... 20 0.035 0.005 100
select LPC 'name$'_vx_inv_8000

select Sound 'name$'_vx_inv_8000
plus LPC 'name$'_vx_inv_8000
Filter (inverse)
Rename... 'name$'_vx_invf_8000
Filter (pass Hann band)... 20 3100 10
Formula... (self[col+1]-self[col])/dx
Rename... 'name$'_vx_invf_8000_band_der
select Sound 'name$'_vx_invf_8000
Filter (pass Hann band)... 25 3100 10

select Sound 'name$'_lx
Filter (pass Hann band)... 20 3100 10
select Sound 'name$'_lx_band
##PProc  based on Minimum peaks for
##CQ ect. estimation
To PointProcess (periodic, peaks)...
...85 260 no yes
select Sound 'name$'_lx_band
##PProc based on Maximum peaks for
##jitter shimmer measures
To PointProcess (periodic, peaks)...
...75 260 yes no
Rename... 'name$'_lx_banda
##if the two above would contain no points
select Sound 'name$'_lx_band
To PointProcess (periodic, cc)... 45 200
Rename... 'name$'_lx_bandb

##adjustment for second long ##########
##not necessary for samples with only mode 1
select Sound 'name$'_lx_band
To PointProcess (periodic, peaks)...
...40 96 yes no
Rename... 'name$'_lx_band_2
select Sound 'name$'_dlx
Filter (pass Hann band)... 10 3100 10
select Sound 'name$'_dlx_band
Formula... (self[col+1]-self[col])/dx
To PointProcess (periodic, peaks)...
...40 250 yes no
select Sound 'name$'_dlx
To PointProcess (extrema)... no yes Sinc70
Rename... 'name$'_dlx_band_pi
###
select Sound 'name$'_lx_band
To PointProcess (extrema)... no yes Sinc70
Rename... 'name$'_lx_band_pi
select Sound 'name$'_lx_band
To PointProcess (extrema)... yes no Sinc70
Rename... 'name$'_lx_band_pa
select Sound 'name$'_lx_band
To PointProcess (zeroes)... yes no
Rename... 'name$'_lx_band_pzr
select Sound 'name$'_lx_band
To PointProcess (zeroes)... no yes
Rename... 'name$'_lx_band_pzf
pause ok?
## in case ##
name$="ayasdan6_vxlx_indc"
input_directory$="D:\...\'name$'"
output_directory$="D:\...\'name$'"
singer$="AD"
select PointProcess 'name$'_dlx_band
nrpoints=Get number of points
select TextGrid 'name$'
nrinterv=Get number of points... 3
Create Table... 'name$' 'nrpoints' 58
Set column label (index)... 1 pt
Set column label (index)... 2 loopnr
#points
Set column label (index)... 3 t1
Set column label (index)... 4 ta2
Set column label (index)... 5 t2
Set column label (index)... 6 t2a
Set column label (index)... 7 t3
Set column label (index)... 8 t4
Set column label (index)... 9 t5a
Set column label (index)... 10 t5b
Set column label (index)... 11 ta6
Set column label (index)... 12 t6
Set column label (index)... 13 t6a
Set column label (index)... 14 t7
Set column label (index)... 15 t8
Set column label (index)... 16 t9a
Set column label (index)... 17 t9b
Set column label (index)... 18 t10
#zero crossings
Set column label (index)... 19 t22
Set column label (index)... 20 t44
Set column label (index)... 21 t66
Set column label (index)... 22 t88
Set column label (index)... 23 t00
#first period
```

```
Set column label (index)... 24 t_pd
#second period
Set column label (index)... 25 t_pd2
#whole double period
Set column label (index)... 26 t_pd3
#OP1 A
Set column label (index)... 27 t4_t5b
#OP2 A
Set column label (index)... 28 t5a_t5b
#OP3 A
Set column label (index)... 29 t4_t6
#open phase1 B
Set column label (index)... 30 t8_t9b
#open phase2 B
Set column label (index)... 31 t9a_t9b
#open phase 3 B
Set column label (index)... 32 t8_t10
#CiP1 A
Set column label (index)... 33 t1_t3
#CiP2 A
Set column label (index)... 34 ta2_t2a
#CiP1 B cycle
Set column label (index)... 35 t5b_t7
#CiP2 B cycle
Set column label (index)... 36 ta6_t6a
#CdP1 A
Set column label (index)... 37 t2_t4
#CdP2 A
Set column label (index)... 38 t1_t4
#CdP3 A
Set column label (index)... 39 t3_t4
#CdP1 B
Set column label (index)... 40 t6_t8
#CdP2 B
Set column label (index)... 41 t5b_t8
#CdP3 B
Set column label (index)... 42 t7_t8
######## A Cycle####################
Set column label (index)... 43
... t3mt1/tpd_CiQ1
Set column label (index)... 44
... t2amta2/tpd_CiQ2
#open q
Set column label (index)... 45
... t5bmt5a/tpd_OQ
#pseudo SQ closed / open p or
#QOQ Quasi OpenQuotient
Set column label (index)... 46
... t6mt4/tpd_QOQ
#(SQ2) quasi opening / closing
Set column label (index)... 47
... t5amt3/t3mt1_SQ
Set column label (index)... 48
... CPmOP/CPpOP_CIa
########## B Cycle ###############
Set column label (index)... 49
... t7mt5b/tpd2_CiQ1
Set column label (index)... 50
... t6amta6/tpd2_CiQ2
Set column label (index)... 51
... t9bmt9a/tpd2_OQ1
Set column label (index)... 52
... t10mt8/tpd2_QOQ
Set column label (index)... 53
... t9amt7/t7mt5b_SQ
Set column label (index)... 54
... CPmOP/CPpOP_CIb
########################
Set column label (index)... 55 style
Set column label (index)... 56 modus
Set column label (index)... 57 singer
Set column label (index)... 58 intervindex
#########################
Create Table... 'name$'_J 'nrinterv' 34
Set column label (index)... 1 intervindex
Set column label (index)... 2 intervbeg
Set column label (index)... 3 intervend
Set column label (index)... 4 nr_pd_interv
Set column label (index)... 5 nr_pt_interv
Set column label (index)... 6 modus
Set column label (index)... 7 periodmn1
Set column label (index)... 8 periodsd1
Set column label (index)... 9 periodmn2
Set column label (index)... 10 periodsd2
#### by means of PProc with all Points
Set column label (index)... 11 jitterLoc
Set column label (index)... 12 jitterLocA
Set column label (index)... 13 jitterRAP
Set column label (index)... 14 jitterppq5
Set column label (index)... 15 jitterddp
Set column label (index)... 16 shimmerLoc
Set column label (index)... 17 shimmerLocdB
Set column label (index)... 18 shimmerapq3
Set column label (index)... 19 shimmerapq5
Set column label (index)... 20 shimmerapq11
Set column label (index)... 21 shimmerdda
```



```
#by means of PProc with only the long period
Set column label (index)... 22 jitterLoc2
Set column label (index)... 23 jitterLocA2
Set column label (index)... 24 jitterRAP2
Set column label (index)... 25 jitterppq52
Set column label (index)... 26 jitterddp2
Set column label (index)... 27 shimmerLoc2
Set column label (index)... 28 shimmerLocdB2
Set column label (index)... 29 shimmerapq32
Set column label (index)... 30 shimmerapq52
Set column label (index)... 31 shimmerapq112
Set column label (index)... 32 shimmerdda2
Set column label (index)... 33 style
Set column label (index)... 34 singer

for z from 1 to 'nrpoints'
select Table 'name$'
Set numeric value... 'z' pt 'z'
endfor

for i from 1 to 'nrinterv'
select TextGrid 'name$'
intervbeg=Get time of point... 3 'i'
#Set the time of interval behind the plus
#(1=1second)
#number of intervals should be
#between 40 and 100 otherwise
#jitter values  become instable
intervend='intervbeg'+0.45
interv_number=Get interval at time...
...2 'intervbeg'
interv_lab=Get label of interval...
...2 'interv_number'
interv_number_tier1=Get interval at time...
...1 'intervbeg'
style_lab$=Get label of interval...
...1 'interv_number_tier1'

####Double cycle######## outer loop ####

if 'interv_lab'=2
#peak max
select PointProcess 'name$'_lx_banda
#cc
#select PointProcess 'name$'_lx_bandb

pnexttobeg=Get high index... 'intervbeg'
```

```
pnexttoend=Get low index... 'intervend'
ptnr1='pnexttoend'-'pnexttobeg'+1
pdnr1='pnexttoend'-'pnexttobeg'
pdmn1=Get mean period...
...'intervbeg' 'intervend' 0.0001 0.02 1.8
pdmn1$ = fixed$ (pdmn1, 6)
if pdmn1$ = "--undefined--"
pdmn1$ = "0"
endif
...
select Sound 'name$'_lx_band
plus PointProcess 'name$'_lx_banda
#plus PointProcess 'name$'_lx_bandb
##amplitude factor from 1.3 to 2

shimLoc=Get shimmer (local)...
...'intervbeg' 'intervend' 0.0003 0.03 1.8 2
shimLoc$ = fixed$ (shimLoc, 6)
if shimLoc$ = "--undefined--"
shimLoc$ = "0"
endif
...

select PointProcess 'name$'_lx_band_2
#cc if the PP isn't succesfull
#select PointProcess 'name$'_lx_bandb
pnexttobeg2=Get high index... 'intervbeg'
pnexttoend2=Get low index... 'intervend'
tpnexttobeg2=Get time from index...
...'pnexttobeg2'
ptnr2='pnexttoend2'-'pnexttobeg2'+1
pdnr2='pnexttoend2'-'pnexttobeg2'
pdmn2=Get mean period...
...'intervbeg' 'intervend' 0.0003 0.03 1.6
pdmn2$ = fixed$ (pdmn2, 6)
if pdmn2$ = "--undefined--"
pdmn2$ = "0"
endif
pdsd2=Get stdev period...
...'intervbeg' 'intervend' 0.0003 0.03 1.6
pdsd2$ = fixed$ (pdsd2, 6)
if pdsd2$ = "--undefined--"
pdsd2$ = "0"
endif
jitLoc2=Get jitter (local)...
...'intervbeg' 'intervend' 0.0003 0.03 1.6
jitLoc2$ = fixed$ (jitLoc2, 6)
if jitLoc2$ = "--undefined--"
```

```
jitLoc2$ = "0"
endif
jitLocA2=Get jitter (local, absolute)...
...'intervbeg' 'intervend' 0.0003 0.03 1.6
jitLocA2$ = fixed$ (jitLocA2, 6)
if jitLocA2$ = "--undefined--"
jitLocA2$ = "0"
endif
jitRAP2=Get jitter (rap)...
...'intervbeg' 'intervend' 0.0003 0.03 1.6
jitRAP2$ = fixed$ (jitRAP2, 6)
if jitRAP2$ = "--undefined--"
jitRAP2$ = "0"
endif
jitppq52=Get jitter (ppq5)...
...'intervbeg' 'intervend' 0.0003 0.03 1.6
jitppq52$ = fixed$ (jitppq52, 6)
if jitppq52$ = "--undefined--"
jitppq52$ = "0"
endif
jitddp2=Get jitter (ddp)...
...'intervbeg' 'intervend' 0.0003 0.03 1.6
jitddp2$ = fixed$ (jitddp2, 6)
if jitddp2$ = "--undefined--"
jitddp2$ = "0"
endif
select Sound 'name$'_lx_band
plus PointProcess 'name$'_lx_band_2
shimLoc2=Get shimmer (local)... 'intervbeg'
... 'intervend' 0.0003 0.03 1.4 1.8
shimLoc2$ = fixed$ (shimLoc2, 6)
if shimLoc2$ = "--undefined--"
shimLoc2$ = "0"
endif
shimLocdB2=Get shimmer (local_dB)...
...'intervbeg' 'intervend'
...0.0003 0.03 1.4 1.8
shimLocdB2$ = fixed$ (shimLocdB2, 6)
if shimLocdB2$ = "--undefined--"
shimLocdB2$ = "0"
endif
shimapq32=Get shimmer (apq3)... 'intervbeg'
... 'intervend' 0.0003 0.03 1.4 1.8
shimapq32$ = fixed$ (shimapq32, 6)
if shimapq32$ = "--undefined--"
shimapq32$ = "0"
endif
shimapq52=Get shimmer (apq5)...
...'intervbeg' 'intervend' 0.0003 0.03 1.4 2
shimapq52$ = fixed$ (shimapq52, 6)
if shimapq52$ = "--undefined--"
shimapq52$ = "0"
endif
shimapq112=Get shimmer (apq11)... 'intervbeg'
... 'intervend' 0.0003 0.03 1.4 2.2
shimapq112$ = fixed$ (shimapq112, 6)
if shimapq112$ = "--undefined--"
shimapq112$ = "0"
endif
shimdda2=Get shimmer (dda)... 'intervbeg'
... 'intervend' 0.0003 0.03 1.4 1.9
shimdda2$ = fixed$ (shimdda2, 6)
if shimdda2$ = "--undefined--"
shimdda2$ = "0"
endif

select Table 'name$'_J
Set numeric value... i intervindex 'i'
Set numeric value... i intervbeg 'intervbeg'
Set numeric value... i intervend 'intervend'
...
Set numeric value... i shimmerdda 'shimdda$'
############
Set numeric value... i jitterLoc2 'jitLoc2$'
...
Set numeric value... i shimmerdda2 'shimdda2$'
Set string value... i style 'style_lab$'
Set string value... i singer 'singer$'
Set numeric value... i modus 'interv_lab'
printline 'i'

###### Drawing ##### double modus ######
Erase all
Select outer viewport... 0 12 0 2
select Sound 'name$'_vx
Draw... 'intervbeg'
...'intervbeg'+0.08 0 0 yes curve
Select outer viewport... 6 12 0 2
Text top... no 'name$' 'style_lab$'
... style modus 'interv_lab' point 'i'

Select outer viewport... 0 12 2 4
select Sound 'name$'_lx_band
Draw... 'intervbeg'
...'intervbeg'+0.08 0 0 yes curve
Red
```

```
select PointProcess 'name$'_lx_band
Draw... 'intervbeg' 'intervbeg'+0.08 0 0 no
Green
...

#### Double cycle #### inner loop #######

select PointProcess 'name$'_dlx_band
# assumed that only double cycles
#(long periods) are marked in PP cc dlx
pnexttobeg3=Get high index... 'intervbeg'
pnexttoend3=Get low index... 'intervend'

for n from 'pnexttobeg3' to 'pnexttoend3'-1
#intvnr is here the number of intervals
#defined by points in tier 3 inner
#the given interval in tier 2
intvnr='pdnr1'
x='n'-'pnexttobeg3'+1
######
select PointProcess 'name$'_dlx_band
t2=Get time from index... 'n'
t10=Get time from index... 'n'+1
po=('t10' - 't2')/10
######
select Sound 'name$'_dlx_band
t6=Get time of maximum... 't2'+'po'
...'t10'-'po' Sinc70
po1=('t6' - 't2')/10
t4=Get time of minimum... 't2'+'po1'
...'t6'-'po1' Sinc70
po2=('t10' - 't6')/10
t8=Get time of minimum... 't6'+'po2'
...'t10'-'po2' Sinc70
####
select PointProcess 'name$'_dlx_band_pi
#ta2= minimum before max peak (t2) in dlx
#t2a= minimum after max peak (t2) in dlx
p_ta2=Get low index... 't2'
ta2=Get time from index... 'p_ta2'
p_t2a=Get high index... 't2'
t2a=Get time from index... 'p_t2a'
p_ta6=Get low index... 't6'
ta6=Get time from index... 'p_ta6'
p_t6a=Get high index... 't6'
t6a=Get time from index... 'p_t6a'
###
select PointProcess 'name$'_lx_band_pi
p_t1=Get low index... 't2'
t1=Get time from index... 'p_t1'
p_t5b=Get low index... 't6'
t5b=Get time from index... 'p_t5b'
p_t5a=Get high index... 't4'
t5a=Get time from index... 'p_t5a'
p_t9b=Get low index... 't10'
t9b=Get time from index... 'p_t9b'
p_t9a=Get high index... 't8'
t9a=Get time from index... 'p_t9a'
###
select PointProcess 'name$'_lx_band_pa
p_t3=Get high index... 't2'
t3=Get time from index... 'p_t3'
p_t7=Get high index... 't6'
t7=Get time from index... 'p_t7'
###
select PointProcess 'name$'_lx_band_pzr
#raising 22, 66, 00
#falling 44, 88
p_t22=Get nearest index... 't2'
p_t00=Get nearest index... 't10'
p_t66='p_t22'+1
t22=Get time from index... 'p_t22'
t00=Get time from index... 'p_t00'
t66=Get time from index... 'p_t66'
###
select PointProcess 'name$'_lx_band_pzf
p_t44=Get high index... 't22'
p_t88=Get low index... 't00'
t44=Get time from index... 'p_t44'
t88=Get time from index... 'p_t88'
#OP
t4_t5b='t5b'-'t4'
t8_t9b='t9b'-'t8'
t5a_t5b='t5b'-'t5a'
t9a_t9b='t9b'-'t9a'
t4_t6='t6'-'t4'
t8_t10='t10'-'t8'
#CiP
t1_t3='t3'-'t1'
t5b_t7='t7'-'t5b'
ta2_t2a='t2a'-'ta2'
ta6_t6a='t6a'-'ta6'
#CdP
t2_t4='t4'-'t2'
t1_t4='t4'-'t1'
t3_t4='t4'-'t3'
```

```
t6_t8='t8'-'t6'
t5b_t8='t8'-'t5b'
t7_t8='t8'-'t7'
#first period
t_pd='t6'-'t2'
#second period
t_pd2='t10'-'t6'
#the whole period
t_pd3='t10'-'t2'

########## A Cycle#####################
# (CiQ1)
t3mt1_tpd=('t3'-'t1')/'t_pd'
# (CiQ2)
t2amta2_tpd=('t2a'-'ta2')/'t_pd'
# (OQ)
t5bmt5a_tpd=('t5b'-'t5a')/'t_pd'
# QOQ Quasi OpenQuotient
t6mt4_tpd=('t6'-'t4')/'t_pd'
#(SQ2) quasi opening / closing q.
t5amt3_t3mt1=('t5a'-'t3')/('t3'-'t1')
#CI
cia=(('t3'-'t2')-('t4'-'t3'))/('t4'-'t2')
############## B Cycle ###############
#CiQ1
t7mt5b_tpd2=('t7'-'t5b')/'t_pd2'
#CiQ2
t6amta6_tpd2=('t6a'-'ta6')/'t_pd2'
#OiQ
t9bmt9a_tpd2=('t9b'-'t9a')/'t_pd2'
#QOQ
t10mt8_tpd2=('t10'-'t8')/'t_pd2'
#SQ
t9amt7_t7mt5b=('t9a'-'t7')/('t7'-'t5b')
#CI
cib=(('t7'-'t6')-('t8'-'t7'))/('t8'-'t6')

############double cycle###########
select Table 'name$'
Set numeric value... n pt 'n'
...
Set numeric value... n modus 'interv_lab'
print 'n'
endfor

####single cycle #### outer loop ########
elsif 'interv_lab'=1
select Sound 'name$'_lx_band
interv_min=Get minimum...
...'intervbeg' 'intervend' Sinc70
interv_max=Get maximum...
...'intervbeg' 'intervend' Sinc70
#####
select PointProcess 'name$'_lx_banda
#cc
#select PointProcess 'name$'_lx_bandb
pnexttobeg=Get high index... 'intervbeg'
pnexttoend=Get low index... 'intervend'
ptnr1='pnexttoend'-'pnexttobeg'+1
pdnr1='pnexttoend'-'pnexttobeg'
pdmn1=Get mean period...
...'intervbeg' 'intervend' 0.0001 0.02 1.6
pdmn1$ = fixed$ (pdmn1, 6)
if pdmn1$ = "--undefined--"
pdmn1$ = "0"
endif
pdsd1=Get stdev period...
...'intervbeg' 'intervend' 0.0001 0.02 1.6
pdsd1$ = fixed$ (pdsd1, 6)
if pdsd1$ = "--undefined--"
pdsd1$ = "0"
endif
jitLoc=Get jitter (local)...
...'intervbeg' 'intervend' 0.0003 0.03 1.8
jitLoc$ = fixed$ (jitLoc, 6)
if jitLoc$ = "--undefined--"
jitLoc$ = "0"
endif
jitLocA=Get jitter (local, absolute)...
...'intervbeg' 'intervend' 0.0003 0.03 1.8
jitLocA$ = fixed$ (jitLocA, 6)
if jitLocA$ = "--undefined--"
jitLocA$ = "0"
endif
jitRAP=Get jitter (rap)...
...'intervbeg' 'intervend' 0.0003 0.03 1.8
jitRAP$ = fixed$ (jitRAP, 6)
if jitRAP$ = "--undefined--"
jitRAP$ = "0"
endif
jitppq5=Get jitter (ppq5)...
...'intervbeg' 'intervend' 0.0003 0.03 1.8
jitppq5$ = fixed$ (jitppq5, 6)
if jitppq5$ = "--undefined--"
jitppq5$ = "0"
endif
```



```
jitddp=Get jitter (ddp)...
...'intervbeg' 'intervend' 0.0003 0.03 1.8
jitddp$ = fixed$ (jitddp, 6)
if jitddp$ = "--undefined--"
jitddp$ = "0"
endif
select Sound 'name$'_lx_band
plus PointProcess 'name$'_lx_banda
#cc
#plus PointProcess 'name$'_lx_bandb
shimLoc=Get shimmer (local)... 'intervbeg'
... 'intervend' 0.0003 0.03 1.4 1.8
shimLoc$ = fixed$ (shimLoc, 6)
if shimLoc$ = "--undefined--"
shimLoc$ = "0"
endif
shimLocdB=Get shimmer (local_dB)...
...'intervbeg' 'intervend'
...0.0003 0.04 1.3 1.8
shimLocdB$ = fixed$ (shimLocdB, 6)
if shimLocdB$ = "--undefined--"
shimLocdB$ = "0"
endif
shimapq3=Get shimmer (apq3)... 'intervbeg'
... 'intervend' 0.0003 0.03 1.4 1.8
shimapq3$ = fixed$ (shimapq3, 6)
if shimapq3$ = "--undefined--"
shimapq3$ = "0"
endif
shimapq5=Get shimmer (apq5)...
...'intervbeg' 'intervend'
...0.0003 0.03 1.4 1.8
shimapq5$ = fixed$ (shimapq5, 6)
if shimapq5$ = "--undefined--"
shimapq5$ = "0"
endif

shimapq11=Get shimmer (apq11)...
...'intervbeg' 'intervend'
...0.0001 0.02 1.3 2
shimapq11$ = fixed$ (shimapq11, 6)
if shimapq11$ = "--undefined--"
shimapq11$ = "0"
endif
shimdda=Get shimmer (dda)...
...'intervbeg' 'intervend'
...0.0003 0.03 1.4 1.9
shimdda$ = fixed$ (shimdda, 6)
if shimdda$ = "--undefined--"
shimdda$ = "0"
endif

select Table 'name$'_J
Set numeric value... i intervindex 'i'
...
Set numeric value... i modus 'interv_lab'
#####Drawing##### single modus#######
Erase all
Select outer viewport... 0 12 0 2
select Sound 'name$'_vx
Draw... 'intervbeg'
...'intervbeg'+0.06 0 0 yes curve
Select outer viewport... 6 12 0 2
Text top... no 'name$' 'style_lab$'
...style modus 'interv_lab' point 'i'
Select outer viewport... 0 12 2 4
select Sound 'name$'_lx_band
Draw... 'intervbeg'
...'intervbeg'+0.06 0 0 yes curve
Red
select PointProcess 'name$'_lx_band
Draw... 'intervbeg' 'intervbeg'+0.06 0 0 no
Green
select PointProcess 'name$'_lx_banda
Draw... 'intervbeg' 'intervbeg'+0.06 0 0 no
Maroon
select PointProcess 'name$'_lx_bandb
Draw... 'intervbeg' 'intervbeg'+0.08 0 0 no
Black
Select outer viewport... 0 12 4 6
select Sound 'name$'_dlx_band
Draw... 'intervbeg'
...'intervbeg'+0.06 0 0 yes curve
select PointProcess 'name$'_dlx_band
Red
Draw... 'intervbeg' 'intervbeg'+0.06 0 0 no
Black
Select outer viewport... 0 12 6 8
select Sound 'name$'_vx_invf_8000_band
Draw... 'intervbeg'
...'intervbeg'+0.06 0 0 yes curve
Select outer viewport... 0 12 8 10
select Sound 'name$'_vx_invf_8000_band_der
Draw... 'intervbeg'
...'intervbeg'+0.06 0 0 yes curve
Select outer viewport... 0 12 10 12
```

```
select Sound 'name$'_lx_band
Draw... 'intervbeg'
...'intervbeg'+0.06 0 0 yes curve
Blue
select PointProcess 'name$'_lx_band_pi
Draw... 'intervbeg' 'intervbeg'+0.06 0 0 no
Black
Select outer viewport... 6 12 2 4
Text top... no closed
Text bottom... no open
Select outer viewport... 0 6 2 4
Text top... no lx (EGG)
Select outer viewport... 0 6 4 6
Text top... no lx' (DEGG)
Select outer viewport... 0 4.5 0 2
Text top... no vx
Select outer viewport... 0 6 6 8
Text top... no vx invers filtered
Select outer viewport... 0 6 8 10
Text top... no vx invers filtered derivated
Select outer viewport... 0 12 0 12
printline 'i'
pause ok?
Write to praat picture file...
...'output_directory$'\'name$'_'i'.prapic
Write to EPS file...
...'output_directory$'\'name$'_'i'.eps
Write to Windows metafile...
...'output_directory$'\'name$'_'i'.emf
############# inner loop ###
#### single cycle #####################
select PointProcess 'name$'_dlx_band
pnexttobeg3=Get high index... 'intervbeg'
pnexttoend3=Get low index... 'intervend'
for n from 'pnexttobeg3' to 'pnexttoend3'-1
#loopnr
y='n'-'pnexttobeg3'+1
select PointProcess 'name$'_dlx_band
t2=Get time from index... 'n'
t6=Get time from index... 'n'+1
select Sound 'name$'_dlx_band
t4=Get time of minimum... 't2' 't6' Sinc70
select PointProcess 'name$'_dlx_band_pi
#ta2= minimum before max peak (t2) in dlx
#t2a= minimum after max peak (t2) in dlx
p_ta2=Get low index... 't2'
ta2=Get time from index... 'p_ta2'
p_t2a=Get high index... 't2'
```

```
t2a=Get time from index... 'p_t2a'
##
select PointProcess 'name$'_lx_band_pi
p_t1=Get low index... 't2'
t1=Get time from index... 'p_t1'
p_t5b=Get low index... 't6'
t5b=Get time from index... 'p_t5b'
p_t5a=Get high index... 't4'
t5a=Get time from index... 'p_t5a'
select PointProcess 'name$'_lx_band_pa
p_t3=Get high index... 't2'
t3=Get time from index... 'p_t3'
select PointProcess 'name$'_lx_band_pzr
#raising 22, 66
#falling 44
p_t22=Get nearest index... 't2'
p_t66=Get nearest index... 't6'
t22=Get time from index... 'p_t22'
t66=Get time from index... 'p_t66'
select PointProcess 'name$'_lx_band_pzf
p_t44=Get high index... 't22'
t44=Get time from index... 'p_t44'
#period
t_pd='t6'-'t2'
#OP
t4_t5b='t5b'-'t4'
t5a_t5b='t5b'-'t5a'
t4_t6='t6'-'t4'
#CiP
t1_t3='t3'-'t1'
ta2_t2a='t2a'-'ta2'
#CdP
t2_t4='t4'-'t2'
t1_t4='t4'-'t1'
t3_t4='t4'-'t3'
####################
# (CiQ1)
t3mt1_tpd=('t3'-'t1')/'t_pd'
# (CiQ2)
t2amta2_tpd=('t2a'-'ta2')/'t_pd'
# (OQ)
t5bmt5a_tpd=('t5b'-'t5a')/'t_pd'
#QOQ Quasi OpenQuotient
t6mt4_tpd=('t6'-'t4')/'t_pd'
#(SQ2) quasi opening / closing
t5amt3_t3mt1=('t5a'-'t3')/('t3'-'t1')
#CI
cia=(('t3'-'t2')-('t4'-'t3'))/('t4'-'t2')
```



```
################################
select Table 'name$'
Set numeric value... n pt 'n'
...
Set numeric value... n modus 'interv_lab'
print 'n'
endfor

####inner loop end#####
endif
printline endloop
endfor

select Table 'name$'
Write to table file...
...'output_directory$'\'name$'.txt
select Table 'name$'_J
Write to table file...
...'output_directory$'\'name$'_J.txt
printline Done!
```

A.3.4 Script 4: Cascading Waveforms

```
#in preparation
#Extract sound selection (preserve times)
#Extract visible pulses
#for one column the number of
#periods should not be over 55
#otherwise step has to be adjusted
#in this script the first period defines
# the horizontal edges, all other orient
#at it but dur will alternate
fenster=1.9
step=0.17
Erase all
select PointProcess untitled
anzahlpunkte=Get number of points
anzahlperioden=anzahlpunkte-1
##########zahl vor / gibt an, bis wohin
fraktion=12/anzahlperioden
pt1=Get time from index... 2
pt1$=fixed$ (pt1, 5)
pt12=Get time from index... 3
pt12$=fixed$ (pt12, 5)
pt2=Get time from index... 'anzahlpunkte'
pt2$=fixed$ (pt2, 5)
d1='pt12'-'pt1'
for i from 2 to anzahlpunkte-1
select PointProcess untitled
periodenanfang=Get time from index... i
periodenende=Get time from index... i+1
d2='periodenende'-'periodenanfang'
gf='d2' / 'd1'
x=6*'gf'
#echo 'x'
#pause ok?
x$=fixed$ (x, 2)
select Sound untitled
if i >1
oben=i*'step'-'step'
unten='oben'+'fenster'
else
oben=i*'fenster'-'fenster'
#oben=0
unten='fenster'
endif
#if i >1
Viewport... 0 'x$' 'oben' 'unten'
#else
#Viewport... 0 6 'oben' 'unten'
#endif
Draw... 'periodenanfang' 'periodenende'
...0.5 -0.6 no curve
Text left... no 'i'
One mark right... 0 no yes no
One mark left... 0 no yes no
if i=2
Viewport... 0 6 0 12
p1=periodenanfang
p2=periodenanfang+
...(periodenende-periodenanfang)/4
p3=periodenanfang+
...(periodenende-periodenanfang)/2
p4=periodenanfang+
...(periodenende-periodenanfang)*0.75
p5=periodenende
t2=(periodenende-periodenanfang)/4
```

```
t2$=fixed$ (t2, 6)
t3=(periodenende-periodenanfang)/2
t3$=fixed$ (t3, 6)
t4=(periodenende-periodenanfang)*0.75
t4$=fixed$ (t4, 6)
t5=p5-periodenanfang
t5$=fixed$ (t5, 6)
#
One mark top... 'p1' no yes yes
One mark top... 'p2' no yes yes
One mark top... 'p3' no yes yes
One mark top... 'p4' no yes yes
One mark top... 'p5' no yes yes
One mark top... 'p1' no no no 0
One mark top... 'p2' no no no 't2$'
One mark top... 'p3' no no no 't3$'
One mark top... 'p4' no no no 't4$'
One mark top... 'p5' no no no 't5$'
endif
endfor
```

Appendix B

REFERENCES

B.1 Glossary

air flow rate: mean glottal flow

double source /cycle phonation: vs. single source/cycle mechanism

jugular fossa (*fossa jugularis*): sometimes also found as jugular notch or suprasternal notch, not to confuse with fossa bulbus superior venae jugularis or short fossa jugularis at os temporale (cf. Waldeyer and Mayet, 1986: 15, 155)

kai: Altaian and Shorian term for ThS, epic singing respectively, both differ in pitch and timbre

kargyraa: low register voice and style in Tuvan ThS, corresponds to xarxiraa in Mongolian ThS and kai in Altaian ThS

mechanism: interaction articulating structures in biomechanical perspective

partial: harmonic; overtone

penetrance power: (Germ. 'Durchdringungsfähigkeit') measure of voice perceivability through a static background noise

perturbation: a disturbance, or small change, in a cyclic variable (period, amplitude, open quotient, etc.) that is constant in regular periodic oscillation (Titze, 1994b).

phase closure: determines in video stroboscopy usually the relation between open phase and closed phase (after Hirano and Bless, 1993)

phonation mode: preferably for perceptual perspective only

phonation: immediate process of voice production inner the vocal tract

register: usually determining areas or ranges of similar sound quality, which are suppose to be connected/correlated to voice source behaviour (vibratory patterns, mass involvement)

respiratory tract: including subglottal airways spectral power density: also power spectral density [Schallleistungsdichte]

sygyt: whistling Tuvan ThS style

technique: vocal technique vs. singing technique

Tyva (Tyvan): refers to the Republic of Tyva located in the Russian Federation; the Russian form of the ethnonym is Tuva, Tuvinian

ventricular folds (*plica ventricularis*): sometimes vestibular folds or false folds

vocal tract: usually only supraglottal space (w.s.) meaning the room between glottis and mouth (incl. nasal cavity)

xai: 1. general and common term for ThS in Hakassia, 2. synonymous to epic-singing

xakas, hakas (hakassian): refers to the Republic of Hakassia [xakas]

xöömej: 1. general and common term for ThS in Tuva, 2. separate throat singing style in Tyva

B.2 Analysed Recordings

B.2.1 Audio-CDs

[A] The list contains all acknowledged and pre-analysed audio data, which comprises in addition to the observations made in the field. The names appear as stated by the singers or as identified in the meta-data of recordings.

Tyva:

1. Melodia C30-14937-42 (3 LPs): Tuvinskij Folklor (1981)
2. Melodia D 030773-74 : Tyva Ajalgalar – Melodii Tuvy (1968)
3. PAN 2005 CD : TUVA – Voices from the Land of the Eagels (1991)
4. PAN 2013 CD: TUVA – VOICES FROM THE SPIRIT WORLD (1992)
5. PAN 2019 CD : UZLYAU – Guttural Singing of the peoples of the Sayan, Altai and Ural Mountains (1993)
6. SHANACHIE 64050 : HUUN-HUUR-TU – 60 Horses in my Herd (1993)
7. SHANACHIE 64058 : HUUN-HUUR-TU – The Orphant's Lament (1994)
8. SHANACHIE 64080 : HUUN-HUUR-TU – If I'd been born an eagle (1997)
9. SHANACHIE 64070 : CHIRGILCHIN: The Wolf & The Kid (1996)
10. SF CD 40017: TUVA- Voices from the Center of Asia (1987) Smithsonian/ Folkways Records Center for Folklife Programs and Cultural Studies
11. wdr-World Network Nr. 21: Tuvinian Singers & Musicians (Xöömej: Throatsinging from the Center of Asia) (1993)
12. Silex Mosaique Y 225222: Musiques Traditionelles d' Asie Central : Chants Harmoniques Touvas (1991, 92, 93)
13. Ellipsis Arts 4080: Deep in the Heart of Tuva: Cowboy Music from the Wild East (1996)
14. Carol 2339-2 Realworld Tuva : SHU-DE – Voices from the distant steppe (1994)
15. GMCD 9504: YAT-KHA : Yenisei-Punk (1995)
16. GR 90-202: YAT-KHA: Yat-Kha (1993)
17. FMP 42: SAINKHO NAMTCHYLAK: Lost Rivers (1992)

18. JARO 4195-2 : The Spirit In Past & Present – Music from one Earth (Sampler: Huun-Huur-Tu, Angelite, Sarband, Gonashvili, M. Alperin, Trinovox, Earborn) (1996)
19. CDLA 96020: Vershki da Koreshki (Sylla, Xovalyg, Levin, Volkov) (1996)
20. CDLA 9707: It's probably windy in Ovyur – Tuvan Folk Music (1995, 97)
21. ARNR 1497: Music from Tuva – Igor Keshkendey (1998)
22. Tuvinskije geroitcheskije skazanija (Rec. 1959/1982/1984) annexe to Tuvinskije geroitcheskije skazanija TyNIIJaLi, Novosibirsk (1994)

Mongolia:

23. KICC 5133 King Records: Mongolian Songs (1988) [Ganbold]
24. JVC VICG-5211 MONGOLIA: Höömii and Urtin Duu (The Folk Music Traditions 1) (1991)
25. JVC VICG-5212-2 MONGOLIA: Morin Huur (The Folk Music Traditions 2)(1992)
26. MCM 3001 : Mongolia - Living Music of the Steppes (1997) [Tserendava, Ganbold]
27. TSCD 909: Vocal & instrumental Music of Mongolia recorded by Jean Jenkins (1977) [Sundui]
28. SA 141006 Air Mail Music: Mongolia (1992) [Ensemble Mandukhai]
29. Musique & Musiciens du Monde D 8207: MONGOLIA (199.) [Sundui]
30. Musique du Monde 92591-2: Musique du Mongolie (/Musique Kazakh) (1992)
31. HUNGAROTON HCD 18013-14: Mongolian Folk Music (1990) (selected /compiled by Lajos Vargyas)
32. FM 50023 -Face Music: Duo Temuzhin : Altai-Khangain-Ayalguu (1997) [Yavgan]
33. PAN 2010 CD: TSAGAAN SAR (WHITE MOON). Traditional and popular Music from Mongolia (1992) [Erdenexüü]
34. PAN 2050 CD: Jargalant Altai. Xöömij and other vocal and instrumental music from Mongolia (1996)
35. Ocora C580051: Mongolie – Chants Kazakh et tradition épique de l'Ouest (1993)

Sampler – Central Asia/Siberia:

36. (Mongolia, Uzbekistan, Kirgizstan, Tadjikistan, Azerbaidjan, Daghestan, Kazakhstan, Turkestan, Xinjiang, Krim) YAZOO 7007 Secret Museum of Mankind – Central Asia 1925-48 (Edited bv Pat Conte)

37. (China, Mongolia, Gorno-Altai, Bourjatia, Kalymkia, Shoria, Xinjiang, Uzbekistan, Bashkordostan) ETHNIC B 6776: Musique sur les Routes de la Soie (1991)
38. (Tuva, Shoria, Kalmykia, Tadjikistan) INEDIT W260067: chants épiques et diphoniques – Asie centrale, Sibérie: Touva, Chor, Kalmouk, Tadjik vol.1 (1996)

Altai:

39. FM 50018 Face Music: Bolot & Nohon - Üch Sümer - from the golden mountains of Altai (1996)

Hakassia:

40. Hakasskij geroičeskij epos (rec. 1964)
41. Pure Nature Music: Sabjilar – Sabjilar (2000) [Kučenov,Čerkov]

Tibet:

42. RYKODISC RCD 20113: The Gyuto Monks – Freedom Chants from the Roof of the World (1989)
43. Music & Arts CD- 736: Sacred Music, Sacred Dance for Planetary Healing and World Purification - Tibetan Buddhist Monks form Drepung Loseling Monastery (1991)
44. Interra Rec. IN -5730-2: buddhist monks of maitri vihar monastery – tibetan mantras & chants (1996)
45. ELEKTRA/Nonesuch Explorer Series 7559-79198-2: Tibetan Buddhism – Tantras of Gyütöü (1973, 75)
46. Nonesuch Explorer Series 7559-72071-2: Tibetan Buddhism – The Ritual Orchestra & Chants (1976, 1995) [Khampagar Monastery]
47. elipsis arts 4050: TIBET: The Heart of Dharma (1996) [Loseling Dratsang of Drepung & Khampagar]
48. ocora (radio france) C 580016: Tibet – Traditions rituelles des Bonpos (1981,83) [Menri]
49. Celestial Harmonies 13132-2 : Sacred ceremonies vol. 3 – Ritual Music Of Tibetan Buddhism (1996) [Dip Tse Chok Ling Monastery]
50. Hannibal (Rykodisc) HNCD 1404: Chö – Choying Drolma and Steve Tibbetts (1997)

"Western" Overtone Singing:

51. Schott/Wergo SM 1812-2: Michael Vetter: OM. Eine Obertonschule (1987)

52. Fönix Musik FMF CD 1075: Christian Bollmann & Michael Reimann: EVOLUTION (1993)

53. Windpferd CD 41043: Sangit – The Circle of Healing (1992)

54. bauer Audio 8719: Bollmann - Echoes of Ladakh – Seelenkontakte (1997)

55. Schott/Wergo SM 1078-50: Michael Vetter: Overtones in Old European Cathedrals-Senanque

56. New Albions NA024: David Hykes & Djamchid Chemiran - Windhorse riders (1989)

57. Network 72025: KlangWelten Festival - Musik aus 5 Kontinenten (1990)

Afrika:

58. UMNGQOKOLO – Demonstration Tape, to accompany the paper: "Thembu Xhosa umngqokolo overtone singing ..." presented by Dr. Dave Dargie at the I.C.T.M. Conference, Berlin, Germany, June 1993 (self-distributed)

others:

59. PlayaSound PS 65189: Russian Far North – The chukchi (1997)

60. Ocora C559071: Canada – Jeux vocaux des Inuit (du Caribou, Netselilik et Iglooik) (1989)

61. wdr-World Network Nr. 31: Corsica / Sardinia : The Mystery of Polyphony (1993)

62. ellipsis arts CD 3252: Voices of forgotten worlds (30 verschiedene Völker) (1993)

63. CMX 374 1010.12: Les voix du monde (Collection du C.N.R.S. et du Musée de l'homme) (1996)

64. Overtone Singing – CD accompanying Mark van Tongeren (2002) "Overtone Singing". Fusica: Amsterdam.

65. HOSOO: Höömij Legende. indigenous production (2001)

B.2.2 Broadcasts [B] & Documentaries[F]

B1: Reise durch das sozialistische Tuva (radio broadcast, Stimme der DDR, 1988) [Kongar-ool Ondar]

F1: Le chant harmonique (1989), Hugo Zemp u. Trân Quan Hai, CNRS: Paris

F2: Dave Dargie: Xhosa Music (1993) VHS

F3: Geheimnisse des Chöömej (1996), Wolfgang Hamm, WDR

F4: Voxtours: Mongolei (1996) VOX

F5: Altai, Changai, Gobi. NDR (1998)

B2: Michael Vetter – Liebesszenen. DLR Berlin (1997)

B3: Stockhausen: Stimmungen (Radiomitschnitt, DLF 1995)

B.2.3 Field Recordings [FR] and Archive Material [AR]

FR1: (Grawunder) recording of the Tuvan national xöömej contest, 15.07.1998, Kyzyl, Tsentr Xoomeja,

FR2: (Brož) Altai field recording, summer 2000

FR3: (van Tongeren) field recordings made in the years 1993-1998

FR4: (Grawunder) Igor Köshkendey, Berlin, Nov. 2002

FR5: (Kyrgys) recording of a demonstration of styles in Tuvan throat singing held at the "Khoomei"-Symposium, July 1996, Kyzyl, Tsentr Xoomeja

AR: Archive Material (Radio archive "Radio Abakan": recordings of Hakas epic singers and čatxan player from the years 1950-80 (samples of ca. 3-4 min)

B.3 Subjects

Note that not all recordings although screened and listed above were included in the acoustic analysis. Table B.1 list all singers who were included in this study.

index	R	Singer	Abrev.	ST	index	R	Singer	Abrev.	ST
11	A	Emil Tergishev	ET	vl					
12	A	Nohon	NH	v	57	T	Alim Kountshoun	KA	v
14	A	Shinzhin	SH	v	58	T	Kuulaar Oleg	OK	a
21	H	Slava Kutshenov	SK	vl	59	T	Sevek Aldyn-ool	S2	a
22	H	Sergej Tsharkov	ST	vl	60	T	Ayas Ondar	AO	a
23	H	Juri Topoev	JT	vl	61	T	Boris Mongush	BM	a
24	H	Maxim Samuzhikov	MS	vl	62	T	Kuular Sergej	KS	a
25	H	Oleg Tshebodaev	OT	vl	63	T	Dongak Buyan	DB	a
26	H	Zhenja Ulugbashev	ZU	vl	64	T	Möngün-ool Ondar	MO	a
31	T	Andrej Mongush	AM	vl	65	T	Saryglar Aleksej	S4	a
32	T	Anton X.	AN	vl	66	T	Fedor Tau	FT	a
33	T	Stas Iril	SI	vls	67	T	Mongush Mergen	MM	a
34	T	Mosuk Radion S.	RM	vl	68	T	Mongush Sundukai	MU	a
35	T	Ondar Scholban	OS	vl	69	T	Topchun, Mihail	TM	a
36	T	Ondar Sergej	SO	vl	70	T	Marzhimal Ondar	MZ	a
37	T	Ayas Dansyrin	AD	vl	71	T	Tschasir Vasili	CV	a
38	T	Natschin Tshoodu	NT	vl	72	T	Kuular German Belekovitsh	GB	a
39	T	Zhenja Saryglar	ZS	vl	73	T	Schaktaar Scholban	SC	a
40	T	Kongal-ool Ondar	KO	vs	74	T	Dambai-ool	DO	a
41	T	Kaigal-ool Hovalyg	KX	vl	75	T	Kuular Kozak-ool	KK	a
42	T	Anatoli Kuular	AK	vl	76	T	Oyun Evgeni Datap- ool	OE	a
43	T	Ayan Schirizhik	AS	vs	77	T	Mongush B. Coldap Xonaevic	M2	a
44	T	Ondar Bady-Dorzhu	OB	vs	78	T	Mongush Andrej(2)	MA	a
45	T	Ayan-ool Sam	SA	vs	90	M	Ganbold Taravjav	TG	a
46	T	Sergej Sotpa	SS	vs	91	M	Gereltsogt	G2	a
47	T	Vadim Oorshak	VO	vs	92	M	Odsuren Badraa	BO	v
48	T	Ondar Saryglar	OO	vl	93	M	Xösöö Dangaa Xosbayar	HS	a
49	T	Sedik Mai-ool	SE	vs	94	M	Tserendavaa	T4	a
50	T	Saryglar Vadim	SV	vs	95	M	Yavgan	Y1	a
51	T	Igor Köshkendej	IK	v	96	M	Nandjid Sengedorzh	NS	a
52	T	Shanshagaj Oorshak	SC	v	97	M	Sundui	SU	a
53	T	Tshyldym-ool Andrej	TA	v	98	M	Amaryn Altanxuyag	AA	a
54	T	Oorshak Xunashtaar-ool	OX	a	99	M	Bori	BI	a
55	T	Genadi Tumat	GT	a	100	M	Tshimidorzh	CI	a
56	T	Tumat Kara-ool	TK	a	101	M	Yanjiv Tsogtbataar	YT	a

Table B.1: List of informants and used abbreviations grouped by area (R=region); ST=source Type: v = voice signal (Vx), l = laryngographic signal (Lx), s = subglottal (jugular microphone) signal (Sx); a=audio (not recorded by the author)

Bibliography

Adachi, S. and Yamada, M. (1999). An acoustical study of sound production in biphonic singing, xoomij. *J Acoust Soc Am*, 105(5):2920–32.

Agarwal, M., Scherer, R. C., and Hollien, H. (2003). The false vocal folds: shape and size in frontal view during phonation based on laminagraphic tracings. *J Voice*, 17(2):97–113.

Aksenov, A. (1967). Die Stile des tuvinischen zweistimmigen Sologesanges. In Stockmann, E., editor, *Sowjetische Volkslied- und Volksmusikforschung*, pages 293–307. Akademie Verl., Berlin.

Aksenov, A. (1973). Tuvin folk music. *Asian music*, 4:7–18.

Alku, P., Backstrom, T., and Vilkman, E. (2002). Normalized amplitude quotient for parametrization of the glottal flow. *J Acoust Soc Am*, 112(2):701–10.

Allen, E. L. and Hollien, H. (1973). A laminagraphic study of pulse (vocal fry) register phonation. *Folia Phoniatr (Basel)*, 25:241–250.

Anders, L. C. (1997). *Spektrale Analysen gestörter Stimmen*. Fischer, Jena.

Apiluck, T. (2003). A laryngoscopic study of Chong register.

Ardran, G. M. and Kemp, F. H. (1967). The mechanism of the larynx. ii. the epiglottis and closure of the larynx. *Br J Radiol*, 40(473):372–89.

Augsten, A. and Gall, V. (1997). Stimmanalyse bei gehaltenen Vokalen im Vergleich der Zeitanalyse zur Frequenz- und Formantenanalyse. *Sprache-Stimme-Gehör*, 21:111–116.

Baken, R. J. and Orlikoff, R. F. (2000). *Clinical measurement of speech and voice*. Singular Thomson Learning, San Diego, 2. edition.

Bear, T., Titze, I. R., and Yoshioka, H. (1983). Multiple simulataneous measures of vocal fold activity. In Bless, D. and Abbs, J. H., editors, *Vocal fold physiology: Contemporary research and clinical issues*, pages 229–237. College-Hill, San Diego.

Behrman, A., Dahl, L. D., Abramson, A. L., and Schutte, H. K. (2003). Anterior-posterior and medial compression of the supraglottis: signs of nonorganic dysphonia or normal postures? *J Voice*, 17(3):403–10.

Blomgren, M., Chen, Y., Ng, M. L., and Gilbert, H. R. (1998). Acoustic, aerodynamic, physiologic, and perceptual properties of modal and vocal fry registers. *J Acoust Soc Am*, 103(5 Pt 1):2649–58.

Bloothooft, G., Bringmann, E., van Cappellen, M., van Luipen, J. B., and Thomassen, K. P. (1992). Acoustics and perception of overtone singing. *J Acoust Soc Am*, 92(4 Pt 1):1827–36.

Bloothooft, G., Bringmann, E., van Cappellen, M., van Luipen, J. M., and Thomassen, K. P. (1991). A phonetic study of overtone singing. In *XIIth Conference of Phonetic Sience*, volume V, pages 14–17, Aix-en-Provence.

Boersma, P. (1993). Accurate short-term analysis of the fundamental frequency and the harmonics-to-noise ratio of a sampled sound. In *Proceedings 17*, pages 97–110, Institute of Phonetic Sciences, University of Amsterdam.

Boersma, P. and Weenink, D. (1999-2005). Praat: doing phonetics by computer (version 4.3.10) [computer program]. Retrieved `www.praat.org`.

Böhme, G. and Gross, M. (2001). *Stroboskopie und andere Verfahren zur Analyse von Stimmlippenschwingungen : Lehrbuch*. Median-Verl. von Killisch-Horn, Heidelberg.

Bollmann, C. (1999). [curriculum vitae of christian bollmann]Lebenslauf von Christian Bollmann. `http://www.lichthaus-musik.net/d_CB_Lifeline.html`, retrieved 16. Sept. 2007.

Boves, L. (1984). *The Phonetic Basis of Perceptulal Ratings of Running Speech*. Foris, Dortrecht/Cinnaminson.

Buder, E. H. (2000). Acoustic Analysis of Voice Quality: A Tabulation of Algorithms 1902-1990. In Kent, R. D. and Ball, M. J., editors, *Voice Quality Measurement*, pages 119–244. Singular, San Diego.

Butanaev, V. J. (1998). *[Ethnic culture of Xakas] Etničeskaja kul'tura xakasov*. Isdatel'stvo xakaskogo gasudarvstvennogo universiteta im. N.F. Katanova, Abakan.

Carlson, B. and Esling, J. H. (2003). Phonetics and physiology of the historical shift of uvulars to pharyngeals in Nuuchahnulth (Nootka). *JIPA*, 33:183–193.

Castrén, M. A. and Schiefner, A. (1853). *Nordische Reisen und Forschungen*. Buchdr. der Kaiserlichen Akad. der Wiss., St. Petersburg.

Charron, C. (1978). Toward transcription and analyses of inuit throat-games:micro-structure. *Ethnomusicology*, 22(2):245–259.

Chen, Y., Robb, M. P., and Gilbert, H. R. (2002). Electroglottographic evaluation of gender and vowel effects during modal and vocal fry phonation. *J Speech Lang Hear Res*, 45(5):821–9.

Chernov, B. P. and Maslov, V. T. (1987). Larynx double sound generator. In *Proceedings of the XIth Congress of Phonetic Science*, volume 6, Tallinn.

Childers, D. (1978). *Modern spectrum analysis* . IEEE Press (selected reprint series).

Childers, D. and Krishnamurthy, A. K. (1985). A critical review of electroglottography. *CRC critical reviews in biomedical engineering*, 12(2):131–161.

Colton, R. H. and Casper, J. K. (1997). *Understanding voice problems: a physiological perspective for diagnosis and treatment*. Williams & Wilkins, Baltimore, Md. [u.a.], 2. ed., [nachdr.] edition.

Colton, R. H. and Estill, J. (1981). Elements of voice quality: Perceptual, acoustic and physiologic aspects. In Lass, N. J., editor, *Speech and Language: Advances in Basic Research and Practice*, volume 5, pages 311–403. Academic Press, New York.

Comrie, B. (2001). *The Slavonic languages*. Routledge, London [u.a.], reprinted edition.

Cranen, B. (1991). Simultaneous modelling of egg, pgg, and glottal flow. In Gauffin, J., editor, *Vocal Fold Physiology: Acoustic, Perceptual, and Physiological Aspects of Voice Mechanisms*, pages 57–64. Singular, San Diego.

Cranen, B. and Boves, L. (1985). Pressure measurements during speech production using semiconductor miniature pressure transducers: impact on models for speech production. *J Acoust Soc Am*, 77(4):1543–51.

Cranen, B. and Boves, L. (1987). On subglottal formant analysis. *J Acoust Soc Am*, 81(3):734–46.

Crystal, D. (1992). *A dictionary of linguistics and phonetics*. The language library. Blackwell, Oxford [u.a.], 3. ed., repr edition.

Czermak, J. N. (1879). *Stimme und Sprache. Anatomie und Physiologie der Stimm- und Sprachwerkzeuge*. Wilhelm Engelmann, Leipzig.

Dargie, D. (1991). Umngqokolo: Xhosa overtone singing and the song non-del'ekhaya. *Journal of international library of African music*, 7(1):33–47.

Dargie, D. (1993). Thembu xhosa umngqokolo overtone singing: the use of human voice as a type of 'musical bow'. In *I.C.T.M. Conference*, Berlin.

de la Breteque, B. A. (1988). Le chant diphonique [diphonic singing]. *Rev Laryngol Otol Rhinol (Bord)*, 109(4).

Deal, R. E. and Emanuel, F. W. (1978). Some waveform and spectral features of vowel roughness. *J Speech Hear Res*, 21(2):250–64.

Deliyski, D. D. (1993). Acoustic model and evaluation of pathological voice production. In *EUROSPEECH'93*, pages 1969–1972.

Dmitriev, L. B., Cernov, B. P., and Maslov, V. T. (1992). *Tajna tuvinskovo "dueta" ili svojstvo gortani celoveka formirovatj mechanism aerodinamiceskovo svista*. samo izd., Novosibirsk.

Dmitriev, L. B., Chernov, B. P., and Maslov, V. T. (1983). Functioning of the voice mechanism in double-voice touvinian singing. *Folia Phoniatr (Basel)*, 35(5):193–7.

Edgerton, M. (2005). *The 21st-century voice: contemporary and traditional extra-normal voice*, volume 9 of *The New Instrumentation*. Scarecrow, Lanham (Maryland), Toronto, Oxford.

Edgerton, M., Bless, D., Thibeault, S., Fagerholm, M., and Story, B. (2003). The acoustic analysis of reinforced harmonics. *to appear in Journal of New Music Research*, pages 1–16.

Edmondson, J. A. (2004). The aryepiglottic sphincter & the source-filter theory: Evidence from endangered languages.

Esling, J. H. (1984). Laryngographic study of phonation type and laryngeal configuration. *JIPA*, 14:56–73.

Esling, J. H. (1996). Pharyngeal consonants and the aryepiglottic sphincter. *JIPA*, 26(2):65–88.

Esling, J. H. (1999). The IPA categories "pharyngeal" and "epiglottal": laryngoscopic observations of pharyngeal articulations and larynx height. *Lang Speech*, 42 (Pt 4):349–72.

Esling, J. H. (2002a). Laryngoscopic analysis of tibetan chanting modes and their relationship to register in sino-tibetan. In *ICSLP*, volume 2, pages 1081–184, Denver.

Esling, J. H. (2002b). The laryngeal sphincter as an articulator: Tenseness, tongue root and phonation in Yi and Bai. In *LSA Annual Meeting*, San Francisco.

Fabre, F. (1958). [Comparative study of glottograms & phonograms of the human voice.] Etude comparée des glottogrammes et de phonogrammes de la voix humaine. *Ann Otolaryngol Chir Cervicofac*, 75(10-11):767–75.

Fant, G. (1970). *Acoustic theory of speech production : with calculations based on X-ray studies of Russian articulations.* Description and analysis of contemporary standard Russian ; 2. Mouton, The Hague [u.a.], 2. printing edition.

Fant, G. (1997). Frequency domain of glottal flow: The lf-model revisited. In Kiritani, S., Hirose, H., and Fujisaki, H., editors, *Speech Production and Language*, volume 13, Speech Research. Mouton de Gruyter, Berlin, New York.

Fant, G., Ishizaka, K., Lindqvist, J., and Sundberg, J. (1972). Sub-glottal formants. *Speech Transmission Laboratory, Q. Stat. Prog. Rep.*, 1:1–11.

Firmin, H., Reilly, S., and Fourcin, A. (1997). Non-invasive monitoring of reflexive swallowing. In Smits, R., Rosen, S., and Holland, M., editors, *UCL: Speech Hearing and Language: work in progress 1997*, volume 10. Department of Phonetics and Linguistics UCL.

Fischer, P.-M. (1998). *Die Stimme des Sängers : Analyse ihrer Funktion und Leistung ; Geschichte und Methodik der Stimmbildung.* Metzler, Stuttgart [u.a.], 2., durchges. aufl edition.

Forsyth, J. (2000). *A history of the peoples of Siberia : Russia's north Asian colony, 1581 - 1990.* Cambridge Univ. Press, Cambridge [u.a.].

Fourcin, A., McGlashan, J., and Blowes, R. (2000). Measuring voice in the clinic - laryngograph speech studio analysis.

Fuks, L., Hammarberg, B., and Sundberg, J. (1998). A self-sustained vocal-ventricular phonation mode: acoustical, aerodynamic and glottographic evidences. *TMH-QPSR*, 3/1998:49–59.

Gall, V. and Berg, R. (1998). *[Glottal segmentation of voice and speech] Feinstrukturen von Stimme und Sprache.* Feinstrukturen von Stimme und Sprache : inkl. CD-ROM mit PC-Programm "Glottal segmentation of voice and speech" zur Diagnostik und Therapie von Stimm-, Sprech- und Sprachstörungen / Volker Gall; Reni Berg ; CD-ROM. Ed. Wötzel, Frankfurt am Main.

Gall, V. and Stelzig, Y. (1997). Glottale Segmentierung des Stimmsignals. *Stimme - Sprache - Gehör*, 21:117–121.

Garcia, M. P. (1855). Observations of the human voice. *Proc R Soc London*, 7(399-410).

Garcia, M. P. (1985). *École de Garcia - Traité complet de l'art du chant.* Minkoff, Genève, réimpr. de l'éd. de paris, l'auteur, 1847 edition.

Gauffin, J. (1977). Mechanisms of larynx tube constriction. *Phonetica*, 34(4):307–309.

Gerratt, B. R. and Kreiman, J. (2001). Toward a taxonomy of nonmodal phonation. *Journal of Phonetics*, 29(4):365–381.

Gibbon, D. (2000). *Handbook of multimodal and spoken dialogue systems : resources, terminology and product evaluation.* Kluwer international series in engineering and computer science ; 565. Kluwer Academic Publ., Boston, Mass. [u.a.].

Gmelin, J. G. (1751). *Johann Georg Gmelins Reise durch Sibirien von dem Jahr 1733-1743.* Sammlung neuer und merkwürdiger Reisen zu Wasser und zu Lande ; ... Vandenhoeck, Göttingen.

Gobl, C. and Chasaide, A. N. (2003). The role of voice quality in communicating emotion, mood and attitude. *Speech Commun.*, 40(1-2):189–212.

Goldmann, J. (1992). *Heilende Klänge-Die Macht der Obertöne.* Knaur, München.

Grawunder, S. (1999). *Die Erforschung eines besonderen Stimmgebrauchs – Obertongesang versus Kehlgesang.* Diploma, Martin-Luther-Universität Halle-Wittenberg.

Grawunder, S. (2003a). Comparison of voice production types of 'western' overtone singing and south siberian throat singing. In *15th ICPhS*, pages 1699–1702, Barcelona. Causal.

Grawunder, S. (2003b). Der südsibirische Kehlgesang als Gegenstand phonetischer Untersuchungen. In Krech, E.-M. and Stock, E., editors, *Gegenstandsauffassung und aktuelle Forschungen der halleschen Sprechwissenschaft*, volume 10 of *Hallesche Schriften zur Sprechwissenschaft und Phonetik*, pages 53–91. Peter Lang, Frankfurt am Main.

Greisbach, R. (2001). *Experimentelle Testmethodik in Phonetik und Phonologie : Untersuchungen zu segmentalen Grenzphänomenen im Deutschen.* Lang, Frankfurt am Main [u.a.].

Gundermann, H. (1994). *Phänomen Stimme.* Reinhardt, München [u.a.].

Hacki, T. (1996). Electroglottographic quasi-open quotient and amplitude in crescendo phonation. *J Voice*, 10(4):342–7.

Hanson, H. M. (1997). Glottal characteristics of female speakers: acoustic correlates. *J Acoust Soc Am*, 101(1):466–81.

Hanson, H. M. and Chuang, E. S. (1999). Glottal characteristics of male speakers: acoustic correlates and comparison with female data. *J Acoust Soc Am*, 106(2):1064–77.

Hartmann, W. M. (1997). *Signals, sound, and sensation.* AIP Press, Woodbury.

Hasumi, H. (1980). Understanding mongolian music. In Emmert, R. and Minegishi, Y., editors, *Musical Voices of Asia*, pages 234–238. Heibonsha Publishers, Tokyo.

Henke, W. L. (1974). Signals from external accelerometer during phonation: Attributes and their internal physical correlates. *Quarterly progress report MIT*, 114:224–231.

Henrich, N., d'Alessandro, C., Doval, B., and Castellengo, M. (2004). On the use of the derivative of electroglottographic signals for characterization of nonpathological phonation. *J Acoust Soc Am*, 115(3):1321–32.

Henton, C. and Bladon, A. (1988). Creak as sociophonetic marker. In Hyman, L. M. and Li, C. N., editors, *Language, Speech and Mind: Studies in the honour of Victoria A. Fromkin.* Routledge, London, New York.

Hertegard, S. and Gauffin, J. (1995). Glottal area and vibratory patterns studied with simultaneous stroboscopy, flow glottography, and electroglottography. *Journal of Speech, Language and Hearing Research*, 38(1):85–100.

Hirano, M. and Bless, D. (1993). *Videostroboscopic examination of the larynx.* Whurr Singular Pub. Group, San Diego.

Hirose, H. (1997). Investigating the physiology of laryngeal structures. In Hardcastle, W. J. and Laver, J., editors, *The Handbook of Phonetic Sciences*, Blackwell Handbooks in Linguistics. Blackwell, Oxford, Cambridge.

Hoffman-Ruddy, B., Lehman, J., Crandell, C., Ingram, D., and Sapienza, C. (2001). Laryngostroboscopic, acoustic, and environmental characteristics of high-risk vocal performers. *J Voice*, 15(4):543–52.

Hollien, H. (1974). On vocal registers. *Journal of Phonetics*, 2:125–143.

Hollien, H. and Michel, J. F. (1968). Vocal fry as a phonational register. *J Speech Hear Res*, 11(3):600–4.

Ishiki, N. (1964). Regulatory mechanisms of vocal intensity variation. *J Speech Hear Res*, 7(1):17–29.

Ishizaka, K., Matsudaira, M., and Kaneko, T. (1976). Input acoustic-impedance measurement of the subglottal system. *J Acoust Soc Am*, 60(1):190–7.

Johanson, L. (1998). *The Turkic languages.* Routledge language family descriptions. Routledge, London [u.a.].

KAY-ELEMETRICS-CORP. (1993). Operations manual: Multi-dimensional voice program (MDVP) model 4305.

Keating, P. (1980). Patterns of fundamental frequency and vocal registers. In *Infant Communication: Cry and Early Speech*, pages 209–233. College-Hill Press: Houston, Texas.

Keller, E. (2004). The analysis of voice quality in speech processing. In *Lecture notes in computer science.* Springer, Berlin.

Kent, R. D. and Ball, M. J. (2000). *Voice quality measurement.* Singular Pub. Group, San Diego.

Kent, R. D. and Read, C. (1992). *The Acoustic Analysis of Speech.* Singular, San Diego, London.

Klasmeyer, G. (1999). *Akustische Korrelate des stimmlich emotionalen Ausdrucks in der Lautsprache [Acoustical correlates of emotional vocal expressions in speech]*, volume 67 of *Forum Phoneticum.* Hector, Frankfurt/Main.

Klatt, D. H. and Klatt, L. C. (1990). Analysis, synthesis, and perception of voice quality variations among female and male talkers. *J Acoust Soc Am*, 87(2):820–57.

Klingholz, F. (1992). Obertonsingen[overtone singing]. *Sprache-Stimme-Gehör*, 16:168–170.

Klingholz, F. (1993). Overtone singing: productive mechanisms and acoustic data. *J Voice*, 7(2):118–22.

Kob, M. (2002). *Physical Modeling of the Singing Voice*. Dissertation, RWTH.

Kob, M., Neuschaefer-Rube, C., and Saus, W. (2001). Untersuchungen der akustischen eigenschaften des obertongesanges [investigations of acoustical properties of overtone singing].

Kotby, M. N., Kirchner, J. A., Kahane, J. C., Basiouny, S. E., and el Samaa, M. (1991). Histo-anatomical structure of the human laryngeal ventricle. *Acta Otolaryngol*, 111(2):396–402.

Koufman, J. A., Radomski, T. A., Joharji, G. M., Russell, G. B., and Pillsbury, D. C. (1996). Laryngeal biomechanics of the singing voice. *Otolaryngol Head Neck Surg*, 115(6):527–37.

Kreiman, J. and Gerratt, B. R. (1998). Validity of rating scale measures of voice quality. *J Acoust Soc Am*, 104(3 Pt 1):1598–608.

Kreiman, J. and Gerratt, B. R. (2005). Perception of aperiodicity in pathological voice. *J Acoust Soc Am*, 117(4):2201–2211.

Kruse, E. (1981). Der Mechanismus der Taschenfaltenstimme [The mechanism of the ventricular fold voice. a critical alternative response to the concepts of Rethi]. *Folia Phoniatr (Basel)*, 33(5):294–313.

Kruse, E. (1991). Funktionale Stimmtherapie - Therapeutisch-konzeptionelle Konsequenz der laryngealen Doppelventilfunktion. [Functional Voice Therapy - Therapeutic-conceptual Consequences of the Laryngeal Double Valve Function]. *Sprache-Stimme-Gehör*, 15:127–134.

Kruse, E., Kleinsasser, O., and Schönhärl, E. (1975). Muskelfasern in den Taschenfalten des menschlichen Kehlkopfs. [Muscle fibers in the false folds of the human larynx]. *Arch Ohr Nas Kehlk Heilk*, 210:248–250.

Kruskal, W. and Wallis, W. (1952). Use of ranks in one-criterion analysis of variance. *Journal of the American Statistical Association*, 47:583–621.

Kyrgys, Z. K. (1992). Hoomej-pamjatnik samobytnoj kultury tuvinskogo i drugix narodov Asii. *Melodii «Choomeja»Kyzyl 1994*, pages 13–16.

Kyrgys, Z. K. (2002). *Tuvinskoe gorlovoe penie - etnomuzikovečeskoe issledovanie[Tuvan Throat Singing - ethnomusicological studies]*. Nauka, Novosibirsk.

Ladefoged, P. (1975). *A Course in Phonetics*. Harcourt Brace Jovanovich, N.Y., Chicago, San Francisco.

Ladefoged, P. (2003). *Phonetic data analysis : an introduction to fieldwork and instrumental techniques*. Blackwell, Malden, Mass. [u.a.], 1. publ edition.

Ladefoged, P. and Maddieson, I. (1996). *The sounds of the world's languages*. Phonological theory. Blackwell, Oxford [u.a.], 1. publ edition.

Lass, N. J. (1974). *Experimental phonetics*. MSS Information Corp, New York.

Lass, N. J. (1996). *Principles of experimental phonetics*. Mosby, St. Louis [u.a.].

Laufer, A. and Condax, I. (1979). The epiglottis as an articulator. *JIPA*, 9:50–56.

Laufer, A. and Condax, I. (1981). The function of the epiglottis in speech. *Language and Speech*, 24(1):39–61.

Laurion, C. (1996). *[Music with Overtones] Musik mit Obertönen*. Diploma, Hochschule Hildesheim.

Laver, J. (1980). *The phonetic description of voice quality*. Cambridge studies in linguistics ; 31. Cambridge Univ. Press, Cambridge [u.a.].

Laver, J. (1999). Phonetic evaluation of voice quality. In Kent, R. D. and Ball, M. J., editors, *Voice Quality Measurement*, pages 37–48. Singular, San Diego.

Laver, J. (2002). *Principles of phonetics*. Cambridge textbooks in linguistics. Cambridge Univ. Press, Cambridge [u.a.], repr edition.

Levin, T. C. and Edgerton, M. E. (1999). The throat singers of tuva. *Sci Am*, 281(3):80–7.

Levin, T. C. and Süzükei, V. (2006). *Where Rivers and Mountains Sing: Sound, Music, and Nomadism in Tuva and Beyond*. Indiana University Press.

Lindestad, P. A., Blixt, V., Pahlberg-Olsson, J., and Hammarberg, B. (2004). Ventricular fold vibration in voice production: a high-speed imaging study with kymographic, acoustic and perceptual analyses of a voice patient and a vocally healthy subject. *Logoped Phoniatr Vocol*, 29(4):162–70.

Lindestad, P. A., Sødersten, M., Merker, B., and Granqvist, S. (2001). Voice source characteristics in mongolian "throat singing" studied with high-speed imaging technique, acoustic spectra, and inverse filtering. *J Voice*, 15(1):78–85.

Lomax, A. (1968). *Folk Song Style and Culture.* American Association for the Advancement of Science. Publication ; 88. American Association for the Advancement of Science, Washington.

Ludlow, C. L., Coulter, D., and Gentges, F. (1983). The diferential sensitivity of frequency perturbation to laryngeal neoplasms and neuropathologies. In Bless, D. M. and Abbs, J. H., editors, *Vocal fold physiology: contemporary research & clinical issues*, pages 381–392. College Hill, San Diego.

Mann, H. and Whitney, D. (1947). On a test of whether one of two random variables is stochastically larger than the other. *Annals of Mathematical Statistics*, 18(1):50–60.

Marasek, K. (1997). *Electroglottographic description of voice quality.* Dissertation, Inst. für Maschinelle Sprachverarbeitung.

Maslov, V. T. and Černov, B. P. (1980). [the secret of the "solo-duet"] tajna "sol'nogo dueta". *Sovjetskaja Etnografija*, pages 157–159.

Massey, F. (1951). The Kolmogorov-Smirnov test for goodness of fit. *Journal of the American Statistical Association*, 46(253):68–78.

Matern, G., Neuschaefer-Rube, C., Saus, W., and Kob, M. (2001). Ansatzrohrgestaltung beim obertonsingen. In Gross, M., editor, *Aktuelle phoniatrisch-pädaudiologische Aspekte 2000/2001*, volume 8, pages 16–19. Median, Frankfurt.

McLaren, J. (1936). *A concise Xhosa-English Dictionary.* Longmans, Green and Co., London, New York, Toronto.

Michaelis, D. (1999). Das göttinger heiserkeits-diagramm - entwicklung und prüfung eines akustischen verfahrens zur objektiven stimmgütebeurteilung pathologischer stimmen.

Miller, J. E. and Mathews, J. (1963). Investigation of the glottal waveshape by automatic inverse filtering. *J Acoust Soc Am*, 67:1876.

Miller, R. L. (1959). On the nature of the vocal cord wave. *J Acoust Soc Am*, 31:667–677.

Misun, V. and Prikryl, K. (2002). The source voice generation on the basis of the "compressed air bubble" principle. In *ICVPB 2004 - INTERNATIONAL CONFERENCE ON VOICE PHYSIOLOGY AND BIOMECHANICS*, Marseille.

Misun, V. and Prikryl, K. (2003). The modeling of the vocal folds function. In *AQL 2003*, Hamburg.

Ní Chasaide, A. and Gobl, C. (1997). Voice source variation. In Hardcastle, W. J. and Laver, J., editors, *The Handbook of Phonetic Sciences*, pages 427–461. Blackwell, Oxford.

Nadoleczny, M. (1923). *Über den Kunstgesang - Atem- und Kehlkopfbewegungen*, volume 1. Springer, Berlin.

Nagakawa, S. (1980). A study of urtiin duu - its melismatic elements and musical form. In Emmert, R. and Minegishi, Y., editors, *Musical voices of Asia*, pages 149–161. Heibonsha Publishers, Tokyo.

Nasri, S., Jasleen, J., Gerratt, B. R., Sercarz, J. A., Wenokur, R., and Berke, G. S. (1996). Ventricular dysphonia: a case of false vocal fold mucosal traveling wave. *Am J Otolaryngol*, 17(6):427–31.

Nattiez, J.-J. (1999). Inuit throat-games and siberian throat singing: A comparative, historical, and semiological approach. *Ethnomusicology*, 43(3):399–418.

Nawka, T., Anders, L. C., Cebulla, M., and Zurakowski, D. (1997). The speaker's formant in male voices. *J Voice*, 11(4):422–8.

Nettle, B. (2005). *The Study of Ethnomusicology: Thirty-one Issues and Concepts*. University of Illinois Press, Urbana and Chicago, 2nd edition.

Neumann, K., Gall, V., Schutte, H., and Miller, D. (2001). Subglottale druckverläufe - vergleich intratrachealer druckmessungen und simultaner externer kontaktmikrofonregistrierungen. In Gross, Manfred; Kruse, E., editor, *Aktuelle phoniatrische-pädaudiologische Aspekte 2000/2001*, volume 8, pages 19–23. Median-Verlag, Heidelberg.

Neumann, K., Gall, V., Schutte, H. K., and Miller, D. G. (2003). A new method to record subglottal pressure waves: potential applications. *J Voice*, 17(2):140–59.

Neuschaefer-Rube, C., Saus, W., Matern, G., Kob, M., and Klajman, S. (2001). Sonographische und endoskopische untersuchungen beim obertonsingen. In Geissner, H., editor, *Stimmkulturen - 3. Stuttgarter Stimmtage 2000*, pages 219–222. Röhrig Universitätsverlag, St. Ingbert.

Omori, K. (1997). Acoustic characteristics of rough voice:subharmonics. *J o Voice*, 11(1):40–47.

Orlikoff, R. F., Baken, R. J., and Kraus, D. H. (1997). Acoustic and physiologic characteristics of inspiratory phonation. *J Acoust Soc Am*, 102(3):1838–45.

Painter, C. (1991). The laryngeal vestibule, voice quality and paralinguistic markers. *Eur Arch Otorhinolaryngol*, 248(8):452–8.

Panconcelli-Calzia, G. (1953). *Die Taschenbandstimme: Dysphonia plicarum ventricularium*. Akademie-Verl., Berlin.

Pegg, C. (1992). Mongolian conceptualizations of overtone singing (xöömij). *British Journal of Ethnomusicology*, 1(1):31–54.

Pegg, C. (2001). *Mongolian music, dance, & oral narrative : performing diverse identities*. University of Washington Press, Seattle [u.a.].

Pegg, C. (2003). Overtone singing. In Sadie, S., editor, *The New Grove Dictionary of Music and Musicians*, volume 20, pages 821–824. Oxford University Press, London, Washington.

Pereira Jotz, G., Cervantes, O., Abrahao, M., Parente Settanni, F. A., and Carrara de Angelis, E. (2002). Noise-to-harmonics ratio as an acoustic measure of voice disorders in boys. *J Voice*, 16(1):28–31.

Press, W., Teukolsky, S., Vetterling, W., and Flannery, B. (1992). *Numerical Recipes in C: The Art of Scientific Computing (2d ed.; Cambridge*. Cambridge Univ. Press.

Ptok, M. (1993a). [pseudoglottis after laryngeal trauma with bilateral recurrent laryngeal nerve paralysis]. *Hno*, 41(1):41–6.

Ptok, M., Ptok, A., Bootz, F., and Arold, R. (1993). [comparative studies of various phonation substitution mechanisms] vergleichende untersuchungen verschiedener phonationsersatzmechanism. *Stimme - Sprache - Gehör*, 17(2):164–168.

Pützer, M. (2001). [multiparametric description of voice quality for normal male and female voices]. *Folia Phoniatr Logop*, 53(2):73–84.

Rabinov, C. R., Kreiman, J., Gerratt, B. R., and Bielamowicz, S. (1995). Comparing reliability of perceptual ratings of roughness and acoustic measure of jitter. *J Speech Hear Res*, 38(1):26–32.

Ranke, O. F. and Lullies, H. (1953). *Gehör. Stimme. Sprache.* Lehrbuch der Physiologie in zusammenhängenden Einzeldarstellungen. Springer-Verl., Berlin [u.a.]. Otto F. Ranke.

Reidenbach, M. M. (1998a). Aryepiglottic fold: normal topography and clinical implications. *Clin Anat*, 11(4):223–35.

Reidenbach, M. M. (1998b). The muscular tissue of the vestibular folds of the larynx. *Eur Arch Otorhinolaryngol*, 255(7):365–7.

Reidenbach, M. M. (1998c). Subglottic region: normal topography and possible clinical implications. *Clin Anat*, 11(1):9–21.

Rethi, A. (1952). [role of the stylopharyngeal muscular system in defective phonation due to ventricular bands and in dysphonia spastica]. *Folia Phoniatr (Basel)*, 4(4):201–16.

Rohmert, W. (1991). *Grundzüge des funktionalen Stimmtrainings : ein Leser-Service der Zeitschrift für Arbeitswissenschaft.* Dokumentation Arbeitswissenschaft ; 12. Schmidt, Köln, 6., unaltered ed. edition.

Rothenberg, M. (1979). Some relations between glottal air flow and vocal fold contact area. *Proceedings of the Conference on the Assessment of Vocal Pathology, ASHA Reports, No. 11*, pages 88–96.

Rothenberg, M. (1992). A multichannel electroglottograph. *J Voice*, 6(1):36–43.

Sadie, S., editor (2001). *The New Grove Dictionary of Music and Musicians.* Grove, London, New York.

Sakakibara, K.-I., Fuks, L., Imagawa, H., and Tayama, N. (2004a). Growl voice in ethnic and pop styles. In *International Symposium on Musical Acoustics (ISMA2004)*, Nara.

Sakakibara, K.-I., Imagawa, H., Niimi, S., and Osaka, N. (2002a). Synthesis of the laryngeal source of throat singing using a 2x2-mass model. In *ICMC*, pages 5–8.

Sakakibara, K.-I., Imagawa, H., Niimi, S., and Osaka, N. (2003). The laryngeal flow model for pressed-type singing voices. In *Stockholm Music Acoustics Conference (SMAC)*, Stockholm, Sweden.

Sakakibara, K.-I., Kimura, M., Imagawa, H., Niimi, S., and Tayama, N. (2004b). Physiological study of the supraglottal structure.

Sakakibara, K.-I., Konishi, T., Murano, E. Z., Imagawa, H., Kumada, M., Kondo, K., and Niimi, S. (2002b). Observation of laryngeal movements for throat singing - vibrations of two pairs of folds in the human larynx. In *Acoustical Society of America 144th Meeting - First Pan-American/Iberian Meeting on Acoustics*, Lay Language Papers, Cancun.

Sakakibara, K.-I., Konishi, T., Murano, E. Z., Imagawa, H., Kumada, M., Kondo, K., and Niimi, S. (2002c). Observation of the laryngeal movements for throat singing. *J Acoust Soc Am*, 112(5):2264.

Sanders, I. and Mu, L. (1998). Anatomy of the human internal superior laryngeal nerve. *Anat Rec*, 252(4):646–56.

Sanders, I., Wu, B. L., Mu, L., Li, Y., and Biller, H. F. (1993). The innervation of the human larynx. *Arch Otolaryngol Head Neck Surg*, 119(9):934–9.

Saus, W. (2004). *Oberton singen - Das Geheimnis einer magischen Stimmkunst.* Traumzeit-Verlag, Schönau, Odenwald.

Schiel, R., Olthoff, A., and Kruse, E. (2003). Anatomische untersuchungen zur taschenfaltenmuskulatur. In Pädaudiologie, D. G. f. P. u., editor, *20. Wissenschaftl. Jahrestagung der DGPP*, Rostock. Düsseldorf, Köln: German Medical Science.

Schutte, H. K. (1980). *The efficiency of voice production.* Kemper/Groningen, Groningen.

Schutte, H. K. and Miller, D. G. (1988). [resonance spectrum of the singing voice relative to supra- and sub-glottal pressure changes; consequences for the theory of voice production]. *Folia Phoniatr (Basel)*, 40(2):65–73.

Seidner, W. and Wendler, J. (1997). *Die Sängerstimme : phoniatrische Grundlagen der Gesangsausbildung.* Henschel, Berlin, 3., erw. aufl edition.

Shapiro, S. S. and Wilk, M. B. (1965). An analysis of variance test for normality (complete samples). *Biometrika.*

Shearer, W. M. (1997). Experimental design and statistics in speech sciences. In Hardcastle, W. J. and Laver, J., editors, *The Handbook of Phonetic Sciences.* Blackwell, Oxford, Cambridge.

Smith, H. and Stevens, K. N. (1967). Unique vocal abilities of certain tibetan lamas. *Am Anthropol*, 69(2):209–212.

Smith, H., Stevens, K. N., and Tomlinson, R. S. (1967). On an unusual mode of chanting by certain tibetan lamas. *J Acoust Soc Am*, 41(5):1262–1264.

Smith, S. (1981). Research on the principle of electroglottography. *Folia Phoniatr (Basel)*, 33(2):105–14.

Stager, S. V., Bielamowicz, S. A., Regnell, J. R., Gupta, A., and Barkmeier, J. M. (2000). Supraglottic activity: evidence of vocal hyperfunction or laryngeal articulation? *J Speech Lang Hear Res*, 43(1):229–38.

Stelzig, Y. (1996). *[Soundwave cascading of pathologically disordered voice signals and its pathophysiological background] Schallwellenkaskadierung von krankhaft veränderten Stimmsignalen und deren pathophysiologische Hintergründe.* Md, Johann Wolfgang Goethe University.

Stelzig, Y., Hochhaus, W., Gall, V., and Henneberg, A. (1999). [laryngeal manifestations in patients with parkinson disease]. *Laryngorhinootologie*, 78(10):544–51.

Stevens, K. N. (1977). Physics of laryngeal behaviour and larynx modes. *Phonetica*, 34:264–279.

Stevens, K. N. (1989). On the quantal nature of speech. *J Phonetics*, 17(2-45).

Stevens, K. N. (2000). *Acoustic phonetics.* Current studies in linguistics ; 30. MIT Press, Cambridge, Mass. [u.a.], 1. paperback ed edition.

Stevens, K. N. and Hanson, H. M. (1995). Classification of glottal vibration from acoustic measurements. In Fujimura, O. and Hirano, M., editors, *Vocal Fold Physiology: Voice Quality Control.* Singular, San Diego.

Stone, R. E., J., Cleveland, T. F., Sundberg, P. J., and Prokop, J. (2003). Aerodynamic and acoustical measures of speech, operatic, and broadway vocal styles in a professional female singer. *J Voice*, 17(3):283–97.

Strahlenberg, P. J. v. (1730). *Das nord- und östliche Theil von Europa und Asia : in so weit solches das gantze rußische Reich mit Siberien und der grossen Tartarey in sich begreiffet ; in einer historisch-geographischen Beschreibung der alten und neuern Zeiten, und vielen andern unbekannten Nachrichten vorgestellet, nebst einer noch niemahls ans Licht gegeben tabula polyglotta von zwey und dreyßigerley Arten tartarischer Völcker Sprachen und einem kalmuckischen Vocabulario ... bey Gelegenheit der schwedischen Kriegs-Gefangenschaft in Russland aus eigener sorgfältigen Erkundigung auf denen verstatteten weiten Reisen zusammen gebracht und ausgefertiget.* In Verlegung des Autoris, Stockholm.

Sundberg, J. (1983). Chest wall vibrations in singers. *J Speech Hear Res*, 26(3):329–40.

Sundui, M. M. (2000). [some musical specialties of styles and dissimilitudes of tuvan hööömej] nekotoryje muzykal'nyje osobennosti stilej i raznovidnostej tuvinskogo xoomeja. unpublished manuscript.

Süzükei, V. Y. (1993). *[Burdon-overtone foundations of Tuvan traditional instrumental music]*. Tuvinskij naučno-issledovatel'skij institut yazyka, literatura i istorii republikanskij tsentr traditsionnoj kultury, Kyzyl.

Svec, J. G., Schutte, H. K., and Miller, D. G. (1996). A subharmonic vibratory pattern in normal vocal folds. *J Speech Hear Res*, 39(1):135–43.

Takahashi, H. and Koike, Y. (1976). Some perceptual dimensions and acoustical correlates of pathologic voices. *Acta Otolaryngol Suppl*, 338:1–24.

Tatarintsev, B. I. (1998). *Poblems of the origin of Tuvan throat-singing.* MNZ «XOOMEJ», Kyzyl.

Titze, I. R. (1980). Comments on the myoelastic - aerodynamic theory of phonation. *J Speech Hear Res*, 23(3):495–510.

Titze, I. R. (1992). Voice quality ii. *The NATS Journal. September/October.*

Titze, I. R. (1994a). *Principles of voice production*. Prentice Hall, Englewood Cliffs, NJ.

Titze, I. R. (1994b). Workshop on acoustic voice analysis - summary statement.

Titze, I. R. (2001). Acoustic interpretation of resonant voice. *J Voice*, 15(4):519–28.

Titze, I. R. and Story, B. H. (1997). Acoustic interactions of the voice source with the lower vocal tract. *J Acoust Soc Am*, 101(4):2234–43.

Traill, A. (1986). The laryngeal sphincter as a phonatory mechanism in !xóõ bushman. In Singer, R. and Lundy, J. K., editors, *Variation, Culture and Evolution in African Populations - Papers in honour of Dr Hertha de Villiers*, pages 123–131. Witwatersrand UP, Johannesburg.

Trân, Q. H. (1991). New experiments about the overtone singing style. *Bulletin d' Audiophonologie. Ann. Sc. Univ. Franche-Comté*, Vol. VII(N°5&6):607–618.

Trân, Q. H. and Guillou, D. (1980). Original research and acoustical analysis in connection with the Xöömij style of biphonic singing. *Musical Voices of Asia, Individual research reports: Mongolia*, pages 162–173.

Tsai, C.-G. (2003). Overtone singing - perception, physical modeling of sygyt, kargyraa and sub-cortical structures.

van Buuren, L. (1983). Observations on phonation. *JIPA*, 13(1):13–23.

van den Berg, J. (1958). Myoelastic-aerodynamic theory of voice production. *Journal of Speech and Hearing Research*, 1(3):227–244.

van den Berg, J. (1960). An electrical analogue of the trachea, lungs and tissues. *Acta Physiol. Pharmacol. Neerlandica*, 9(1-24).

van Tongeren, M. (1994). *Xöömej in Tuva - New Developments, New Dimensions.* Ma, Universiteit van Amsterdam.

van Tongeren, M. (2002). *Overtone Singing - physics and metaphysics of harmonics in east and west*, volume 1 of *The Harmonic Series*. fusica, Amsterdam.

Vary, P., Heute, U., and Hess, W. (1998). *Digitale Sprachsignalverarbeitung*. Informationstechnik. Teubner, Stuttgart.

Vieira, M. N., McInnes, F. R., and Jack, M. A. (1997). Comparative assessment of electroglottographic and acoustic measures of jitter in pathological voices. *J Speech Lang Hear Res*, 40(1):170–82.

Vieira, M. N., McInnes, F. R., and Jack, M. A. (2002). On the influence of laryngeal pathologies on acoustic and electroglottographic jitter measures. *J Acoust Soc Am*, 111(2):1045–55.

Walcott, R. (1974). The chöömij of Mongolia - A Spectral Analyses of Overtone Singing. *Selected Reports in Ethnomusicology*, II(1):55–60.

Waldeyer, A. and Mayet, A. (1986). *Anatomie des Menschen, Band 2*. Berlin: deGruyter, 15th edition.

Williams, P. L., Warwick, R., and Gray, H. (1989). *Gray's anatomy*. Livingstone, Edinburgh [u.a.], 37. ed edition.

Wulff, B. (2001). Bericht über die erste eurasische Kultur-Konferenz "Bridge" 9.-11. März 2001 in Ulan-Baator.

Yanagisawa, E., Estill, J., Kmucha, S. T., and Leder, S. B. (1989). The contribution of aryepiglottic constriction to "ringing" voice quality - a videolaryngoscopic study with acoustic analysis. *J Voice*, 3(4):342–350.

Zemp, H. and Trân, Q. H. (1991). Recherches expérimentales sur le chant diphonique. *Cahiers de musiques traditionelles*, 4:27–68.

Abstract

This study focuses on phonation types which result, in addition to the normal activity of the vocal folds, from various combinations of phonation activities involving the aryepiglottic sphincter (AES), the ventricular folds (VTF) and sometimes even the aryepiglottic folds (AEF). Such extraordinary phonatory outcomes occur in the context of South-Siberian throat singing (ThS), which is the theme of this study. The voice production types serve – in the sense of source-filter theory – as source, which is subject to various ways of formant shaping, formant merging, formant adjustment, and formant reinforcement, all of which function to enhance individual harmonics. These harmonics serve as carriers of musical phrases and thus are used to create tunes and melodies.

Two main types are proposed for voice production in South-Siberian throat singing: a voice production by means of the vocal folds featuring a constriction of the AES (Phonation Mode 1), and a voice production with involvement of the ventricular folds (Phonation Mode 2). The VTF involvement appears as a double cyclic period, whith the vocal folds vibrating twice as fast as the ventricular folds; every second cycle consists of a (near-)synchronous closure of VF and VTF. An additional proposed mechanism for phonation mode 2 is the involvement of the AEF. Accordingly, the specific anatomical mechanisms of the constriction of VTF and AEF are discussed and the basic voice production types assumed for ThS are described in terms of their physical configurations (anatomical settings). Furthermore a simple schematic model for the articulation types in throat singing is suggested. This model is based upon observations in the field as well upon previous studies (incl. X-ray, ultrasound and endoscopy) and an additional small-scale video-endoscopic investigation of one subject (the author).

One of the basic questions throughout this study is whether the phenomenon of throat singing shows fairly clear regional variants in different parts of southern Central Siberia or whether the variation is chiefly a matter of individual styles with no link to geography.

In search of a non-invasive but meaningful research technique a 3-channel parallel recording of the acoustic (Vx), the electroglottographic (Lx) and a so-called "chest-resonance" (Sx) signal was adopted. Using this technique data from 25 singers was collected during fieldwork in Southern Siberia. For analysis 25 VxLx-samples of 15 singers and 10 VxSx-samples of 10 singers were included in a core corpus. 44 Vx-samples (of 44 singers) were added in order to represent areal sub-varieties (Gorno-Altai, Hakassia, Tuva, Mongolia). The acoustic analysis of the Vx-signal and the Lx-signal focusses on the desciption of wavefrom shapes as well as perturbation measures (F0, Jitter, Shimmer, HNR), formant measures (F, B, A, H), energy band measures and spectral component analysis. The analysis of

Lx-signal also addresses, besides perturbation measures, various EGG-quotients (closing quotient, open quotient, quasi-open quotient, speed quotient and contact index).

Analysis of the differences between groupings based on geographical area, phonation mode and articulation type was carried out, and relations between acoustic and electrophysiological characteristics were described.

Although the findings from the acoustic and electrophysiological analyses suggest group-specific areal differences in the parameters investigated, the variation across individual singers' productions can in part be fairly large. In many cases also a strong influence of the particular articulation type (overtone articulation type) must be considered, although unfortunately the corpus is too small to properly assess such influence.

Other findings regard the ultra-structure of the signals (Vx, Lx, Sx). Here for phonation mode 1 (AES-VF) the impression of a tensed (sometimes pressed) voice seems to be justified. However, for phonation mode 2 there was only one singer for whom the involvement of a AEF-VF phonation type seemed reasonably secure. The majority of the singers investigated uses the VTF-VF phonation type of doublec-cycle ventricular fold - vocal fold oscillation. The synchronous analysis of Vx, Lx and inverse filtered Vx signal may help to explain the function of VTF-VF voice. Here it is assumed that the vocal tract is excited during the closure phase of the 'pure' vocal fold cycle.

Regarding the formant (harmonic) reinforcement a linear coupling of multiple resonators is suggested as a model, where the size of the epilaryngeal space formed by the AES may be of particular relevance.

Zusammenfassung

Die Arbeit widmet sich im Kern solchen Phonationsarten, die neben der Aktivität der Stimmlippen (SL) auf Basis des aryepiglottischen Sphinkters (AES) sowohl mit zusätzlichem Einsatz der Taschenfalten sowie z.T. der aryepiglottischen Falten (AEF) entstehen. Diese außergewöhnlichen phonatorischen Möglichkeiten treten zusammen im für die Untersuchung ausgewählten musikalischen Kontext als Stimmen des südsibirischen Kehlgesangs (sKG) auf. Diese Stimmproduktionsarten dienen hierbei – im Sinne der Quelle-Filter-Theorie – als Quelle für verschiedene Wege der Formantschärfung, -bündelung und -anpassung, die wiederum der Hervorhebung einzelner Teiltonbereiche dienen, um mit Hilfe der auf diese Weise verstärkten Obertöne einen Träger musikalischer Phrasen bzw. Melodien zu erzeugen. Anhand bereits vorliegender Studien sowie einer zusätzlichen endoskopischen Untersuchung an einer VP (dem Autor) werden die als grundlegend angenommenen Stimmproduktionsvarianten im KG in ihrer atomisch-physiologischen Konfiguration beschrieben.

Grundsätzlich werden 2 Hauptformen der Stimmproduktion im sKG vorgeschlagen: eine Stimmproduktion der Stimmlippen mit starker Verengung des AES (Phonationsmodus 1) und eine Stimmproduktion mit Beteiligung der Taschenfalten (TF/VTF)(Phonationsmodus 2). Diese TF-Beteiligung zeigt sich zumeist als doppelzyklische Periode, bei der jeder zweite Zyklus mit einem zeitgleichen Schließen von SL und TF verbunden ist. Eine zweite Stimmproduktionsform für Modus 2 wird in einer ähnlichen Beteiligung der AEF vermutet. Auf Grundlage vorliegender histo-anatomischer Befunde wird eine funktionale Beschreibung der AES-SL-Phonation und der hier beschriebenen (nicht-pathologischen) Taschenfaltenstimme vorgeschlagen. Hinsichtlich der Obertonartikulationstechnik bzw. den stilistisch umschrieben Varianten der Formantartikulation ist ein einfaches Modell von 3 Artikulationstypen vorgeschlagen worden. Dieses Modell basiert sowohl auf den Beobachtungen im Feld als auch auf denen an bereits bestehenden röntgenologischen u.ä. Untersuchungen.

Hauptsächlich wurde für die weitere Analyse 1. die Hypothese einer arealen Specifik auf Basis phonatorischer Parameter (und artikulatorischer Faktoren) und 2. die Hypthese einer für Phonationsmodus 2 differenzierten Charakteristik von VTF-SL-Phonation versus AEF-SL-Phonation geprüft.

Unter Auswahl einer nichtinvasiven aber aussagekräftigen und für die Feldforschung geeigneten Methode, wurden an 25 Kehlsängern synchrone 3-Kanal-Aufnahmen des Mikrophon-, EGG- und Brustresonanz-Signals (Vx, Lx und Sx) vor Ort in Südsibirien erstellt. Hievon konnten für das Kernkorpus 25 VxLx-Proben von 15 Sängern und 10 VxSx-Proben von 10 Sängern sowie eine VxLxSx-Probe für die Analyse verwendet werden. Um das Korpus auch hinsichtlich der regionalen Varietäten (Gorno-Altai, Hakassia, Tuva, Mongolei) zu komplettieren, wurden für die akustische Analyse des Stimmsignals weitere 44 Aufnahmen ergänzt (insges. 44 Sänger). Die akustische Analyse von Mikrophonsignal (Vx) und Brustresonanz-Signal (Sx) konzentrierte sich auf die Beschreibung der angetroffenen Wellenformen sowie die Perturbationsanalyse (F0, Jitter, Shimmer, HNR), Formantstrukturanalyse (F, B, A, H), Energiebandanalyse und Analyse einzelner Spektralkomponenten. Die Signalanalyse des EGG (Lx) widmet sich neben der Perturbation den EGG-Quotienten (Schließ-, Offen-, Quasi-Offen-, Versatzquotient and Kontaktindex). Schließlich wurden die Unterschiede zwischen den Gruppierungen analysiert, die sich aufgrund von Phonationsmodus, regionaler Herkunft (Stil) und des Artikulationstyps (Obertonartikulationsstrategie) ergeben. Dabei werden die Beziehung der akustischer und elektrophysiologischer Eigenschaften der Stimmproduktionstypen zu den gebildeten Gruppen aber auch zwischen den einzelnen Messwerten untersucht.

Die Befunde aus den akustischen und elektroglottographischen Analysen lassen zwar auf regionalgruppenspezifische Unterschiede schließen, doch ist die Streuung der Ausprägung der individuellen Sänger teilweise so stark, dass keine eindeutigen Tendenzen zu beschreiben sind. Vielfach muss auch ein starker Einfluss der jeweiligen Artikulationsstrategie (Obertonartikulationstyp) angenommen werden.

Andere Befunde betreffen die Ultrastruktur der gewonnen Signale (Vx, Lx und Sx). So ist für Phonationsmodus 1 (AES-VF) der Eindruck einer gespannten (in einigen Fällen auch gepressten) Stimme gerechtfertigt. Im Phonationsmodus 2 konnte auf Basis des vorliegenden Materials nur für einen Sänger die Verwendung eines AEF-VF Phonationstyps nicht ausgeschlossen werden. Die Mehrheit der untersuchten Sänger verwenden vermutlich den Phonationstyp TF-VF mit einer doppelzyklischen Taschenfalten-Stimmlippen-Oszillation. Die synchrone Analyse von Vx, Lx und invers gefiltertem Vx Signal kann dabei helfen, die Funktionsweise der 'TF-Stimme' aufzuklären. Dabei muss angenommen werden, dass nur die Schlussphase des 'reinen' SL-Zyklus als Moment der Anregung des Vokaltrakts (VT) dient. Hinsichtlich der Formantverstärkung kann modellhaft eine aneinandergereihte Kopplung von 'kleineren' Resonatoren angenommen werden. Diese werden durch mehrfache Konstriktion des VT an verschiedenen Stellen erreicht. Dabei könnte das Maß des durch den AES gebildeten epilaryngealen Raums von Bedeutung sein.

